the CSIRO
total wellbeing diet
Complete
Recipe Collection

Introduction by Professor Manny Noakes

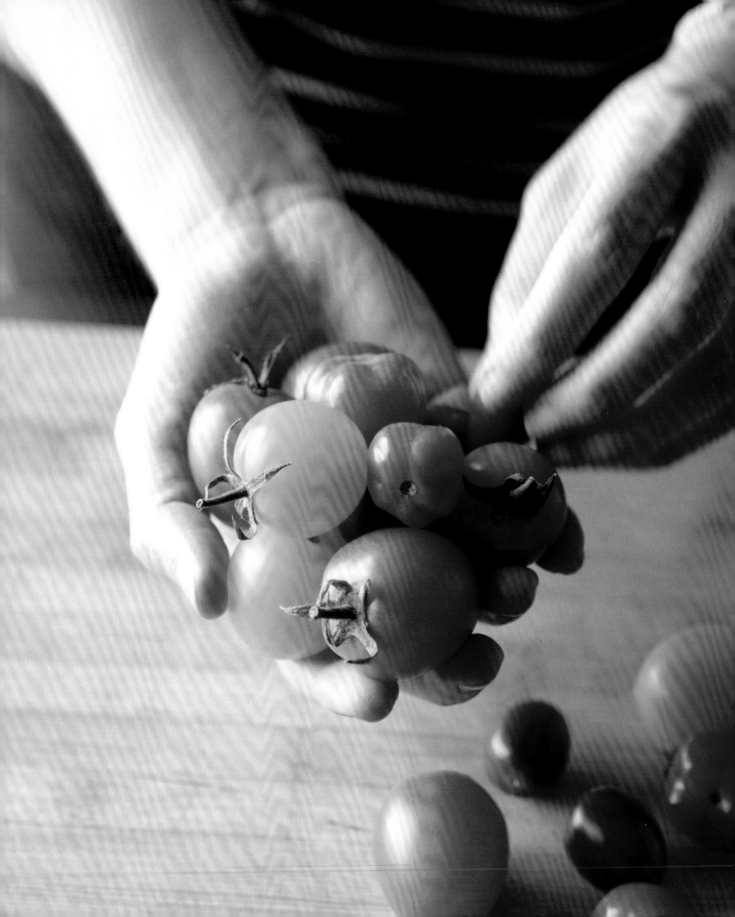

contents

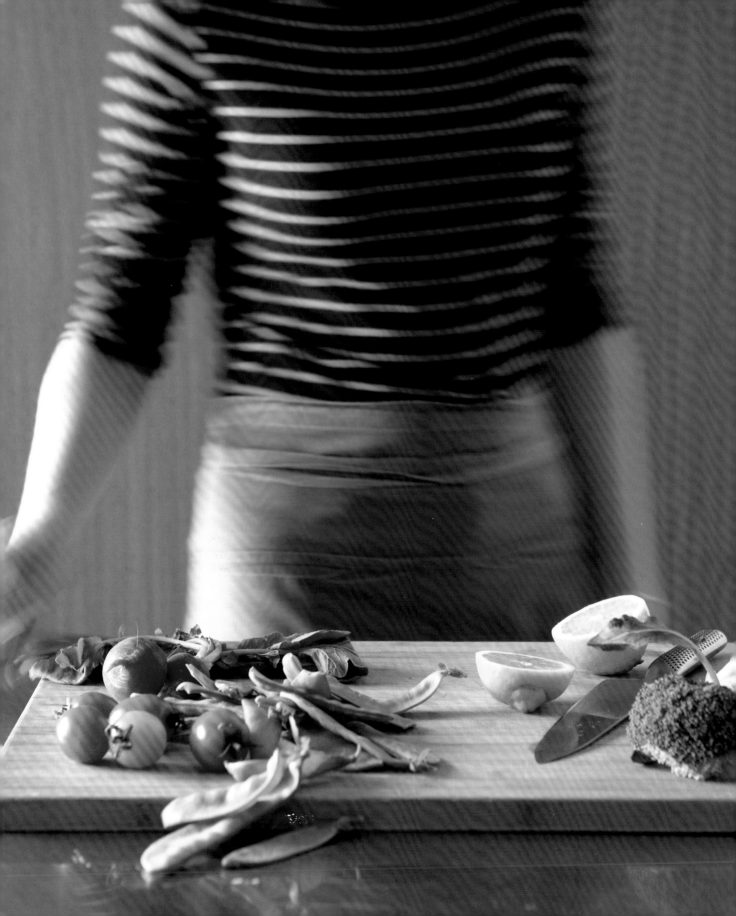

introduction

Cooking nourishing, delicious food provides immense rewards – not least the pleasure it brings to others, and the health and wellbeing benefits we see and feel.

The CSIRO Total Wellbeing Diet Complete Recipe Collection brings together the best recipes from our first four books, with TWD favourites as well as wonderfully easy recipes that take precious little time to prepare. All these recipes are based on the same principles of the TWD, which has been so successful for many thousands of Australians who have wanted to eat better and watch their waistlines. Every year, more and more international research confirms that a diet higher in protein has many benefits – from helping to control hunger to reducing the amount of muscle and bone loss that can occur when dieting, as well as providing a rich concentration of nutrients when kilojoules are being counted. A very large international study has shown that a higher protein diet that is combined with low glycaemic index (GI) carbohydrates is best for the maintenance of weight loss.

As a result, we have placed a little more emphasis on choosing low GI breads and cereals in the food group section of this edition. The combination of higher protein foods with low GI carbohydrate foods seems to be particularly beneficial in preventing regain of weight after weight loss.

One of our current areas of interest is how we can use technology to help people lose and maintain weight. We have experimented with online versions of the Total Wellbeing Diet where over 5000 people lost a combined total of over 3000 kilograms. The internet can be a powerful way of connecting the TWD community and providing ongoing support for those who have completed the eight-week plan. Our aim has been to produce a comprehensive and informative website in order to reach as many people as possible, regardless of location.

We are very excited to have now launched an online version of Total Wellbeing Diet now available at **www.totalwellbeingdiet.com**. In doing so, CSIRO have teamed with the GI Foundation, bringing the combined benefits of low GI foods to a higher protein eating plan. I encourage you to go to the website to learn more about TWD online.

If you have previously experienced success with the TWD, we hope this ultimate collection of recipes will be your go-to guide to TWD and keep you motivated to continue. If this is your first encounter with TWD, we hope you will find the eating plan simple and the recipes fresh and fantastic!

Professor Manny Noakes

the CSIRO **Total Wellbeing Diet basic plan**

your daily food allowance

LEAN PROTEIN FOODS

– 2 units a day for dinner

1 unit is equal to 100 g raw weight of protein food, including red meat, chicken or fish. Eat red meat, such as beef, lamb, pork and kangaroo, three times a week for dinner. Eat fish at least twice a week for dinner.

– Up to 1 unit a day for lunch

Eat up to 100 g of any lean protein food (tinned or fresh seafood, chicken, turkey, red meat or 2 eggs) each day for lunch. Eat red meat, such as beef, lamb, pork and kangaroo, once a week for lunch. We recommend limiting processed meats such as ham.

LOW GI HIGH FIBRE BREADS AND CEREALS

– 3 units a day

1 unit is equal to:
- 1 slice low GI bread, such as Burgen, rye or sourdough (40 g)
- 2 Ryvita
- 150 g sweet potato
- 1 medium low GI potato, such as Carisma (150 g)
- 4 tablespoons cooked basmati rice
- ½ cup (about 50 g) cooked pasta or quinoa
- 4 tablespoons baked beans, or cooked lentils, kidney beans or other legumes
- 40 g low GI cereal, such as rolled oats or All Bran

DAIRY

– 3 units a day

1 unit is equal to:
- 250 ml reduced-fat milk
- 200 g diet yoghurt
- 150 g reduced-fat custard
- 25 g cheddar or other full fat cheese

FRUIT

– 2 units a day

1 unit is equal to 150 g fresh or tinned unsweetened fruit, juice or 30 g dried fruit.

VEGETABLES

– At least 2½ units a day from free list

1 unit is equal to 1 cup cooked vegetables. See free list (right) for vegetables you can eat. We recommend at least ½ unit salad and 2 cups raw or cooked vegetables each day.

HEALTHY FATS AND OILS

– 3 units added oils or fats a day

1 unit is equal to:
- 1 teaspoon trans-fat-free margarine
- 2 teaspoons light margarine
- 1 teaspoon oil
- 20 g avocado
- 7 g nuts or seeds

INDULGENCE FOODS

– Up to 1 units a day

This depends on the level of plan best for you (see *The CSIRO Total Wellbeing Diet* books 1 and 2). As a general rule, 1 unit is equal to 450 kilojoules, such as 15 ml wine or 20 g chocolate.

THE FREE LIST: ANYTIME FOODS

The vegetables below contain minimal kilojoules, so eat them freely with your meals.

Artichokes, asparagus, bamboo shoots, bean sprouts, beetroot, bok choy, broccoli, broccolini, brussels sprouts, cabbage, capsicum, carrots, cauliflower, celeriac, celery, chilli, chives, choko, choy sum, corn, cucumber, eggplant, fennel, fresh and dried herbs, green beans, kohlrabi, leeks, lettuce, marrow, mushrooms, onion, parsnip, peas, pumpkin, radish, rhubarb, rocket, silverbeet, snowpeas, spinach, swedes, tomato, turnip, zucchini.

MISCELLANEOUS FOODS

These foods are also very low in kilojoules and can be used as desired.

Soda and mineral water, diet soft drinks, condiments such as salt-reduced soy, fish and tomato sauce, Worcestershire sauce, low kilojoule sweeteners, coffee, tea, herbal teas, vegemite, vinegar, lemons, mustard, horseradish, curry powder, oil-free salad dressings, diet jelly, verjuice, unprocessed bran, parsley and fresh and dried herbs, salt-reduced stock.

> **NOTE:** It is acceptable to use small amounts (1–2 level teaspoons per person) of cornflour, custard powder or sugar to thicken or sweeten dishes. 1 level teaspoon has 40–60 kilojoules. This is low enough not to worry about if you use only occasionally. Always use salt sparingly.

READING THE RECIPES IN THIS BOOK

The nutritional units contained in each recipe are displayed above the recipe.

FOR MORE INFORMATION

Please refer to *The CSIRO Total Wellbeing Diet* books 1 and 2 for more extensive diet and lifestyle information.

sample daily meal plan

A suggested way to distribute your food group units over the day is as follows:

BREAKFAST
1 unit HIGH FIBRE LOW GI BREAD/CEREAL
1 unit DAIRY
1 unit FRUIT

LUNCH
2 units HIGH FIBRE LOW GI BREAD/CEREAL
Up to 1 unit PROTEIN FOOD
½ unit FREE VEGETABLES
1 unit HEALTHY FATS/OILS

DINNER
2 units PROTEIN FOODS
At least 2 units FREE VEGETABLES
2 units HEALTHY FATS/OILS
1 unit DAIRY

SNACKS
1 unit DAIRY
1 unit FRUIT

EXAMPLE MEAL PLAN

BREAKFAST
40 g oats
1 cup (250 ml) reduced-fat milk
1 banana
Coffee/tea

LUNCH
Sandwich with 2 slices Burgen bread, 50 g tuna, salad, 2 teaspoons light margarine

DINNER
Veal scaloppine with caponata (recipe page 401)
Side salad with reduced-fat dressing
1 carton vanilla diet yogurt and stewed rhubarb

SNACKS
Cappuccino on reduced-fat milk
Fresh peach

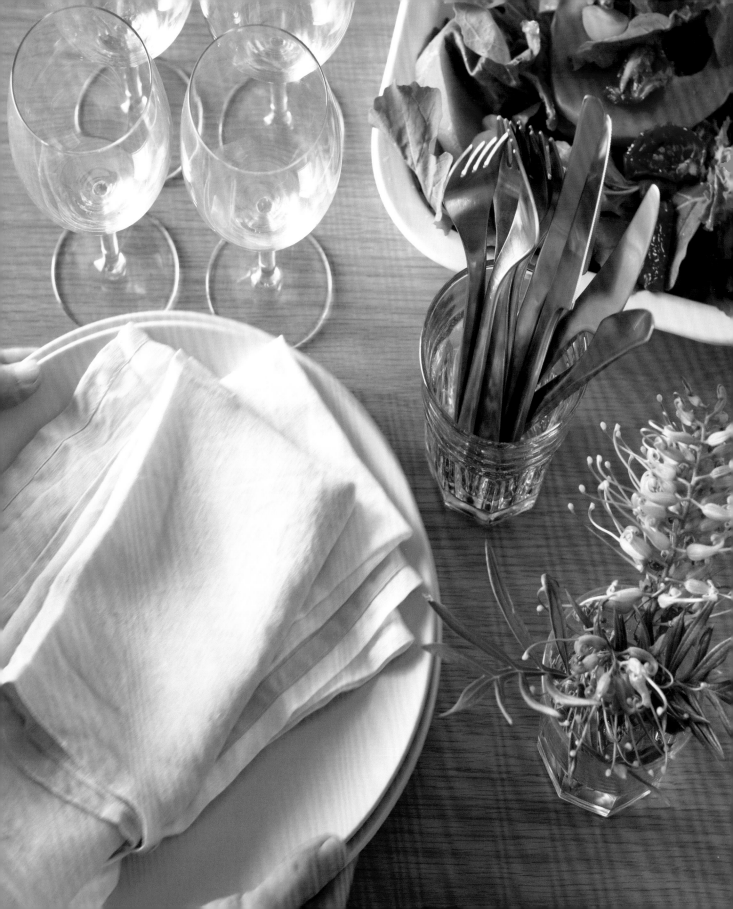

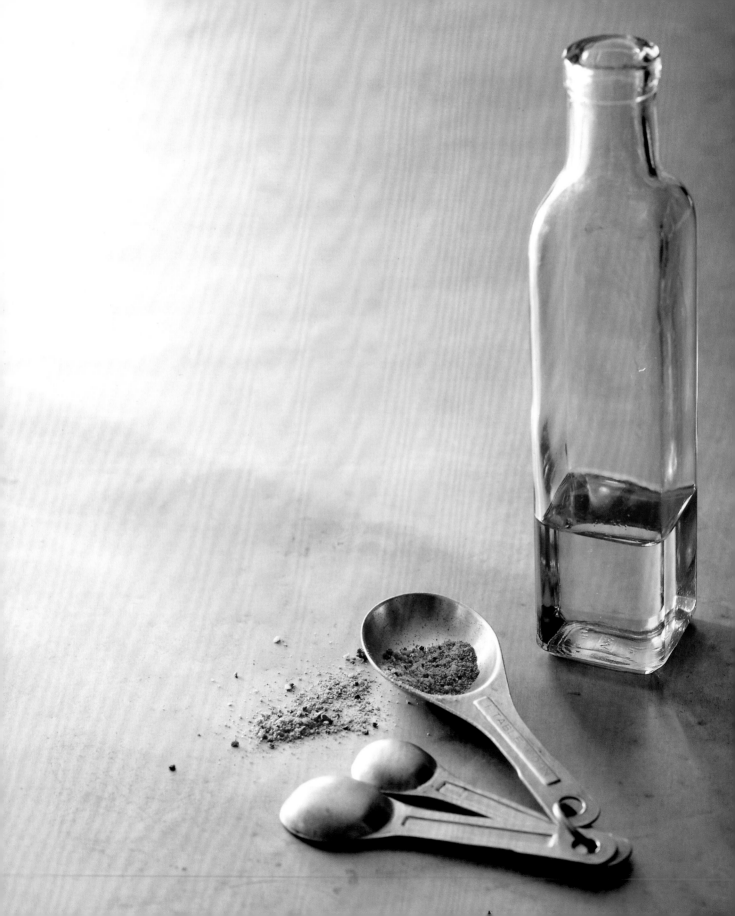

stocking your kitchen

IN THE FRIDGE OR FREEZER

- Cheeses, such as bocconcini, gruyere, pecorino, reduced-fat cheddar, reduced-fat feta, reduced-fat parmesan and reduced-fat ricotta
- Eggs
- Filo pastry
- Fresh fruit and vegetables, particularly those in season
- Fresh herbs (or grow your own)
- Frozen fruit, such as mixed berries and raspberries
- Frozen vegetables, such as broad beans, corn kernels and peas
- Lean meat and poultry
- Light margarine
- Reduced-fat custard
- Reduced-fat cottage cheese
- Reduced-fat cream cheese
- Reduced-fat milk
- Reduced-fat sour cream
- Reduced-fat vanilla, natural or Greek-style yoghurt
- Seafood, such as prawns, smoked salmon, white fish fillets and mussels
- Tofu

CONDIMENTS

- Chilli paste
- Curry paste, such as laksa, red or green curry paste
- Fish sauce
- Hoisin sauce
- Horseradish cream
- Lemon juice
- Lime juice
- Mirin
- Mustard: Dijon, hot English and/ or seeded
- Olive tapenade
- Oyster sauce
- Pesto
- Reduced-fat hummus
- Reduced-fat mayonnaise
- Reduced-fat tartare sauce
- Salt-reduced soy sauce
- Salt-reduced tomato salsa
- Sweet chilli sauce
- Tabasco sauce
- Teriyaki sauce
- Tomato ketchup
- Vegemite
- Wasabi
- White miso
- Worcestershire sauce

IN THE PANTRY

- Baking powder
- Breadcrumbs
- Breads, such as flour tortillas, mountain bread and wholemeal flatbreads
- Capers
- Chinese Shaohsing rice wine
- Cornflour
- Crispbread
- Curry powder
- Dried fruit, such as apples, apricots, cranberries and sultanas
- Dried herbs and ground spices
- Dried pasta, such as lasagna sheets, penne and spaghetti; try wholegrain varities
- Dried yeast
- Dry sherry
- Flour, such as white and wholemeal plain flours
- Grains, such as couscous, pearl barley and polenta
- Honey
- Noodles, such as egg or rice noodles
- Nuts, such as flaked and slivered almonds, pine nuts and walnuts
- Oils, such as extra virgin olive oil, olive oil spray, sesame oil and vegetable oil
- Olives
- Peppercorns
- Powdered gelatine
- Reduced-fat coconut-flavoured evaporated milk or reduced-fat coconut milk
- Rice, preferably basmati and brown
- Rolled oats
- Salt-reduced beef, chicken and vegetable stock
- Salt-reduced tomato passata
- Seeds, such as caraway, poppy, sesame and sunflower seeds
- Semi- or sun-dried tomatoes
- Spices, such as caraway seeds, chilli powder, cinnamon, cloves, cumin seeds, curry powder, dried chilli flakes, dried oregano, fennel seeds, ground allspice, ground coriander, ground cumin, ground turmeric, Moroccan spice mix, mustard seeds, nutmeg, smoked paprika, star anise and sweet paprika
- Sugar or powdered sweetner
- Tahini
- Tinned anchovy fillets
- Tinned or dried beans, chickpeas, lentils and other legumes
- Tinned salmon and tuna
- Tinned unsweetened fruit
- Tinned vegetables, such as artichokes, baby beetroot, bamboo shoots, corn kernels and tomatoes
- Tomato paste (puree)
- Vanilla bean paste or extract
- Vegetable staples, such as onion, garlic, sweet potato and pumpkin
- Verjuice
- Vinegars, such as balsamic, cider, white, rice, white-wine and red wine vinegar

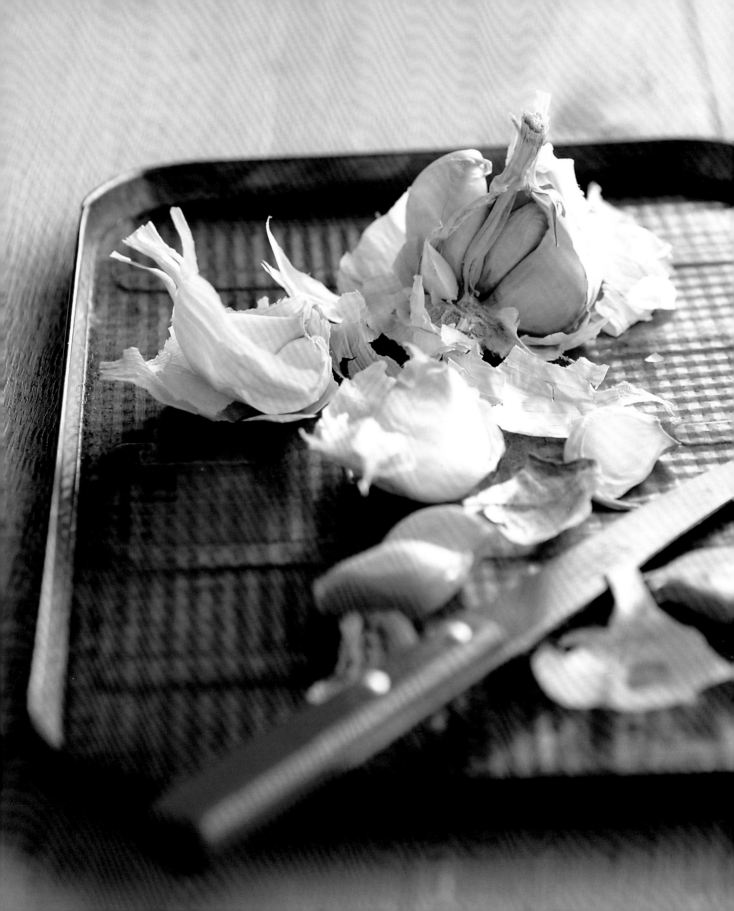

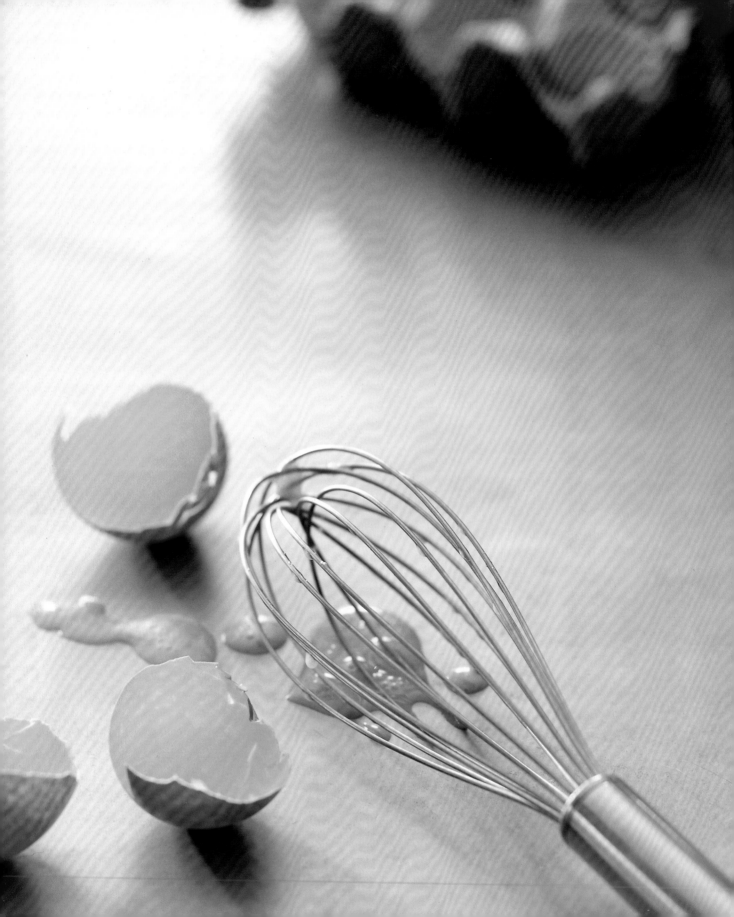

breakfast

Mixed berry smoothie

SERVES 4   **PREP** 5 mins

This fresh, fruity smoothie is a great option for busy mornings when you don't have time for a sit-down breakfast.

2 cups (500 ml) reduced-fat milk
400 g reduced-fat vanilla yoghurt
2 cups (300 g) frozen mixed berries
2 tablespoons unprocessed bran

1   Process all the ingredients in a blender until smooth. Pour into four glasses and serve.

Banana smoothie

SERVES 4   **PREP** 5 mins

1 teaspoon Equal
4 bananas
3 cups reduced-fat milk
200 g reduced-fat vanilla yoghurt
2 teaspoons ground cinnamon

1   Place all ingredients in a blender and process until smooth. Divide between 4 glasses and sprinkle with a little extra cinnamon.

VARIATIONS

Try smoothies made with other fruits, such as mango or apple, for an alternative refreshing snack.

Mango and berry frappe

SERVES 4   **PREP** 5 mins

150 g frozen berries
150 g fresh mango
300 ml orange juice
1 tablespoon mint
ice

1   Place all ingredients in a blender and process until smooth. Divide between 4 glasses.

Fresh fruit salad

SERVES 4   **PREP** 10 mins

2 mangoes
8 strawberries
2 passionfruit
2 kiwifruit

1   Slice fresh fruit, toss and serve. Easy!

Dried fruit compote

SERVES 4   PREP 10 mins, plus overnight soaking

120 g dried apricots
100 g prunes, pitted
20 g sultanas
1 tablespoon honey
1 cinnamon stick
400 g reduced-fat vanilla yoghurt
1 tablespoon finely grated
    orange zest (optional)

**Put this compote together the night before and bring
something special to your morning. It also makes a great
addition to a weekend brunch with friends, or a fabulous
dessert with 1½ tablespoons brandy or Grand Marnier
added to the marinade.**

1 Combine the apricots, prunes, sultanas, honey and cinnamon stick
   in a large bowl and pour over just enough boiling water to cover.
   Stir and refrigerate overnight.

2 Combine the yoghurt and zest (if using) and serve with the fruit.
   The fruit can be served warm or cold.

Muesli

SERVES 8   PREP 10 mins   COOK 20 mins

4 cups (360 g) rolled oats
100 g slivered almonds
60 g sunflower seeds
100 g dried apricots, chopped
80 g dried cranberries (craisins)
60 g dried apple, chopped

Muesli is a really good way to fuel up in the morning and this homemade version will keep you going until lunch time.

1   Preheat the oven to 180°C and line a baking tray with baking paper.

2   Spread the oats and almonds on the tray and bake for 15–20 minutes, tossing occasionally until toasted and lightly golden. Cool, then mix with sunflower seeds, apricots, cranberries and apple. Store in an airtight container.

TIP You can vary this muesli by incorporating different dried fruit, such as figs, prunes or pears, and nuts, such as hazelnuts, pecans or macadamias.

Bircher muesli with bran

SERVES 8 (makes 4 cups)   **PREP** 15 mins + soaking and refrigerating time

1 cup (90 g) rolled oats
1 cup (110 g) untoasted muesli
1 cup (60 g) unprocessed wheatbran
2 cups (500 ml) hot water
2 tablespoons lemon juice
¼ cup (40 g) almonds
200 g reduced-fat flavoured yoghurt
1 large green apple, grated
150 g seasonal fruit (berries, peaches,
    nectarines, bananas) per serve
2 tablespoons honey

1   Place the oats, muesli and bran in a large ceramic dish and pour water and lemon juice over. Allow to soak for 30 minutes. Add almonds, yoghurt and apple and stir to combine thoroughly. Cover and refrigerate overnight.

2   Serve with fruit and a drizzle of honey, plus extra yoghurt from your dairy allowance, if desired.

TIP Bircher muesli keeps for – and actually improves over – about four days. Make this recipe on Sunday night and enjoy a nutritious and easy breakfast well into the week.

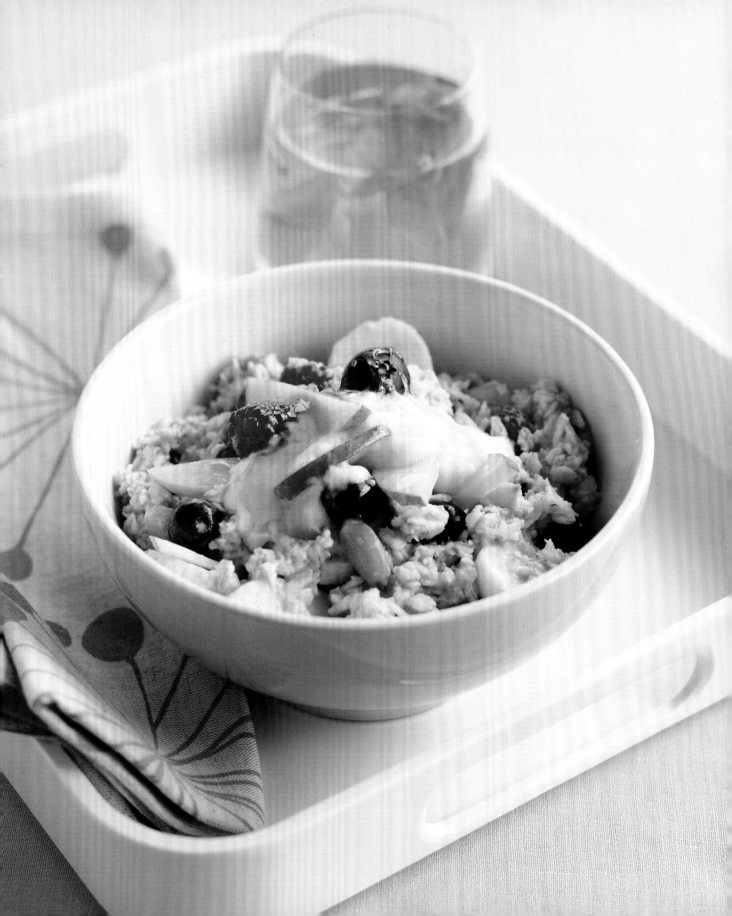

Cinnamon and sultana porridge

SERVES 4   **PREP** 5 mins   **COOK** 5 mins

2 cups (180 g) rolled oats
2 cups (500 ml) reduced-fat milk
1 teaspoon ground cinnamon
120 g sultanas or chopped
   dried apricots
1 tablespoon honey (optional)

Warm yourself up on a cool morning with this breakfast favourite. The cinnamon and dried fruit add a flavour burst to every mouthful.

1 Place all the ingredients in a saucepan with 2 cups (500 ml) water and bring to the boil. Reduce the heat and simmer for 3–4 minutes or until cooked. Alternatively, follow the microwave instructions on the packet of oats.

TIP The milk can be replaced with additional water, if desired.

Ricotta hotcakes

SERVES 4   PREP 10 mins   COOK 15 mins

250 g reduced-fat ricotta
¾ cup (185 ml) reduced-fat milk
2 egg yolks
½ cup (80 g) wholemeal plain flour
½ cup (75 g) plain flour
2 teaspoons baking powder
2 tablespoons sugar or
    powdered sweetener
2 egg whites
olive oil spray

These light and fluffy hotcakes may be served with a variety of toppings. They are sure to be popular with kids and adults alike.

1   Combine the ricotta, milk and egg yolks in a large bowl and mix until smooth. Sift the flours, baking powder and sugar or sweetener (tipping the bran back in) into the ricotta mixture and stir until smooth.

2   Whisk the egg whites to form soft peaks. Gently fold half the egg white into the ricotta mixture, then fold in the remaining egg white.

3   Heat a non-stick frying pan over medium heat and spray with olive oil. For each hotcake, spoon about 3 tablespoons of the mixture into the pan and spread to form a 10 cm round. Cook until bubbles appear on the surface, then turn and cook the other side until golden. Remove and keep warm while you make the remaining hotcakes. Serve with your choice of toppings (see left).

TIP Drizzle with a teaspoon of maple syrup or honey. Top with mixed berries and reduced-fat yoghurt. Spoon over stewed fruit of your choice, such as apple, apricot, pear, or stewed rhubarb and strawberry.

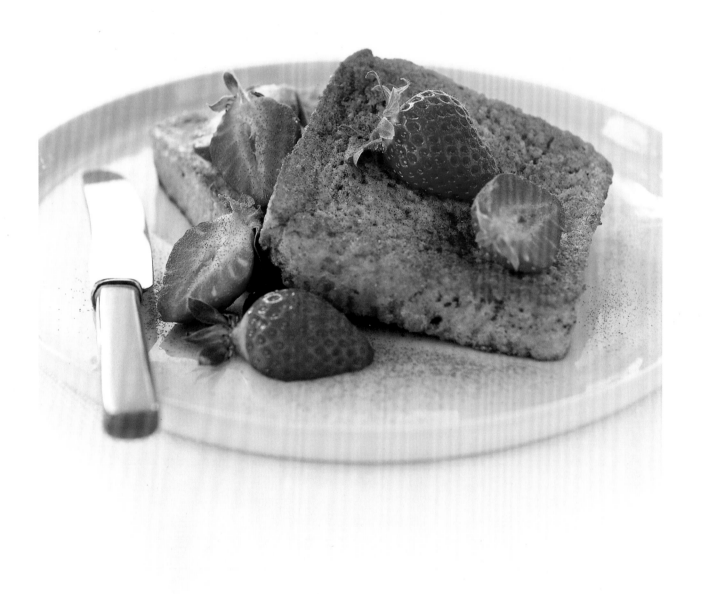

French toast

SERVES 4   PREP 10 mins   COOK 5 mins

4 eggs
¹/₃ cup reduced-fat milk
1 teaspoon ground cinnamon
4 slices wholegrain bread
olive oil spray
fresh strawberries

1 In a shallow bowl, lightly beat eggs with milk and cinnamon.
   Add 1 slice of bread to bowl and soak thoroughly in egg mixture.

2 Meanwhile, spray a non-stick frying pan with oil and heat over medium
   heat. Add soaked bread to pan and cook each side for 30 seconds, or
   until lightly browned. Repeat with remaining bread and egg mixture.

3 Serve sprinkled with a little extra ground cinnamon and with fresh
   strawberries from your daily fruit allowance.

Scrambled eggs

SERVES 4   PREP 5 mins   COOK 5 mins

8 eggs
200 ml reduced-fat milk
¼ cup chopped flat-leaf (Italian)
    parsley

1   In a small bowl, lightly whisk eggs and milk together and lightly season.

2   Heat a non-stick frying pan over medium heat. Pour in egg mixture and cook, repeatedly dragging the cooked egg to the centre and tilting the pan to allow uncooked egg to run to the sides, until all the egg is cooked.

3   Sprinkle with parsley and serve immediately.

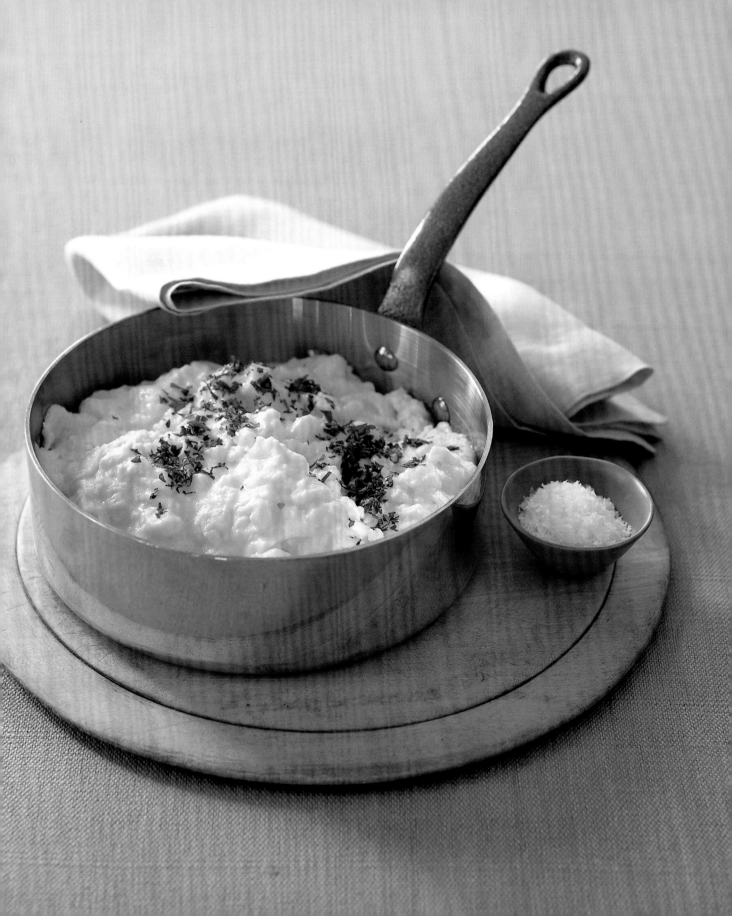

1 SERVE =
1 unit protein
½ unit dairy
¼ unit vegetables

Warm mushroom salad on toast

SERVES 4 **PREP** 10 mins **COOK** 10 mins

The nutty flavours of this dish are great for those who enjoy a savoury start to the morning.

2 teaspoons extra virgin olive oil
350 g mixed mushrooms (such as Swiss
   brown, oyster and field), sliced
1 clove garlic, crushed
2 spring onions, finely chopped
1 tablespoon red wine vinegar
15 g pine nuts, toasted and chopped
50 g rocket
4 slices wholegrain bread
100 g reduced-fat ricotta

1 Heat the olive oil in a large frying pan over high heat. Add the mushrooms and cook, stirring, for 5 minutes or until they are coloured. Add the garlic and spring onion and stir for 1 minute. Remove from the heat and stir in the vinegar and a pinch of pepper. Combine the mushrooms with pine nuts and rocket.

2 Meanwhile, toast the bread. Spread with the ricotta and top with the mushroom mixture.

Tomato and cheese mini frittatas

SERVES 4 **PREP** 10 mins **COOK** 20 mins

These frittatas offer a lovely savoury start to your day, and also make a great light lunch or afternoon snack.

olive oil spray
8 eggs
2 tomatoes, diced
2 tablespoons chopped flat-leaf
   (Italian) parsley
100 g grated reduced-fat cheddar

1 Preheat the oven to 180°C. Spray eight ½ cup (125 ml) muffin holes with olive oil.

2 In a large bowl, whisk the eggs until well combined. Mix through the tomato, parsley, half the cheddar and a pinch of pepper.

3 Divide the mixture among the muffin holes and top with the remaining cheddar. Bake for 20 minutes or until puffed and golden.

1 SERVE =
½ unit protein
1 unit vegetables
1 unit fats

Mexican eggs

SERVES 4   PREP 10 mins   COOK 25 mins

1 tablespoon extra virgin olive oil
1 onion, finely chopped
3 cloves garlic, crushed
½–1 teaspoon chilli flakes
1 teaspoon ground cumin
2 × 400 g tins chopped tomatoes
½ cup chopped flat-leaf (Italian)
   parsley or coriander (cilantro),
   plus extra to serve
4 eggs

For those days when you need a bit of a kickstart to get you going, these Mexican eggs are a feisty option.

1   Heat the olive oil in a large frying pan over medium heat. Add the onion and cook, stirring, for 5 minutes or until softened. Stir in the garlic, chilli and cumin and cook for 1 minute or until fragrant. Add the tomato and simmer for 10 minutes or until the mixture thickens. Season to taste, then stir in the parsley or coriander.

2   Make four hollows in the tomato mixture, then break an egg into each hollow. Cover and simmer gently for 5–10 minutes or until the eggs are cooked to your liking. Serve topped with extra parsley or coriander.

TIP These are great served on wholegrain toast. Make the sauce the night before for a quick breakfast the next day. If you like, add some finely sliced capsicum with the tomatoes for extra flavour.

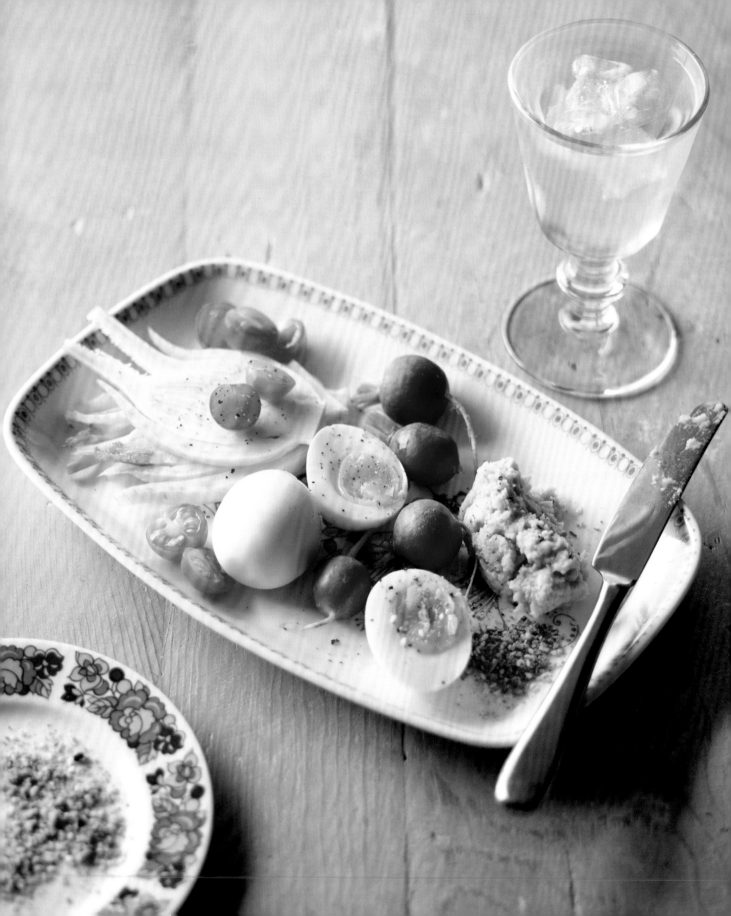

1 SERVE =
1 unit protein
1 unit bread
1½ units vegetables
½ unit fats

Boiled eggs with dukkah, hummus and crudites

SERVES 4   PREP 20 mins   COOK 8 mins

8 eggs
1 bulb fennel, trimmed and sliced
16 radishes
400 g cherry tomatoes, halved
2 tablespoons dukkah

HUMMUS
1 clove garlic, crushed
1 × 400 g tin chickpeas, drained
¼ cup (60 ml) salt-reduced chicken
    or vegetable stock

Dukkah is a mixture of crushed spices and nuts that is commonly used for dipping. It is available in packets from larger supermarkets and specialty food stores. Use whatever vegetables you have to hand here – raw carrot, zucchini, celeriac or steamed broccoli, cauliflower or brussels sprouts.

1   To make the hummus, place all the ingredients in a food processor and combine to a coarse paste. Season to taste with salt and pepper.

2   Meanwhile, place the eggs in a small saucepan of cold water, then bring to simmering point. Simmer for 2 minutes, then drain well and run under cold water. Peel the eggs and cut in half.

3   Divide the eggs, vegetables, dukkah and hummus among plates, then serve.

> **TIP** If you have a spare dairy unit, you might like to add a few cubes of reduced-fat feta to each plate.

Tuna, artichoke and white-bean omelettes

SERVES 4   PREP 10 mins   COOK 10 mins

8 eggs
olive oil spray
12 tinned artichoke hearts,
    drained and quartered
1 × 425 g tin tuna in spring water,
    drained and coarsely flaked
2 spring onions, trimmed and
    thinly sliced (optional)
1¹/₃ cups (265 g) tinned cannellini
    beans, drained
large handful watercress sprigs
1½ tablespoons balsamic vinegar

Tuna and cannellini beans are a classic Italian combination. Using them to top an omelette makes for a more satisfying meal.

1   Place the eggs and 2½ tablespoons cold water in a large bowl, then whisk to combine well and season with salt and pepper.

2   Heat a small non-stick frying pan over medium heat and, once hot, spray with olive oil. Add a quarter of the egg mixture, swirling to coat the pan, then cook for 2–3 minutes or until the omelette is just set, pushing the edges in towards the middle of the pan as they cook. Invert the omelette onto a plate, then slip it back into the pan to cook the other side for about 30 seconds. Remove the omelette to a warm plate while you cook the remaining mixture: you'll have enough for four omelettes.

3   Place the artichoke, tuna, spring onion (if using), beans, cress and balsamic vinegar in a large bowl and gently toss to combine.

4   Serve one omelette per person topped with the tuna salad.

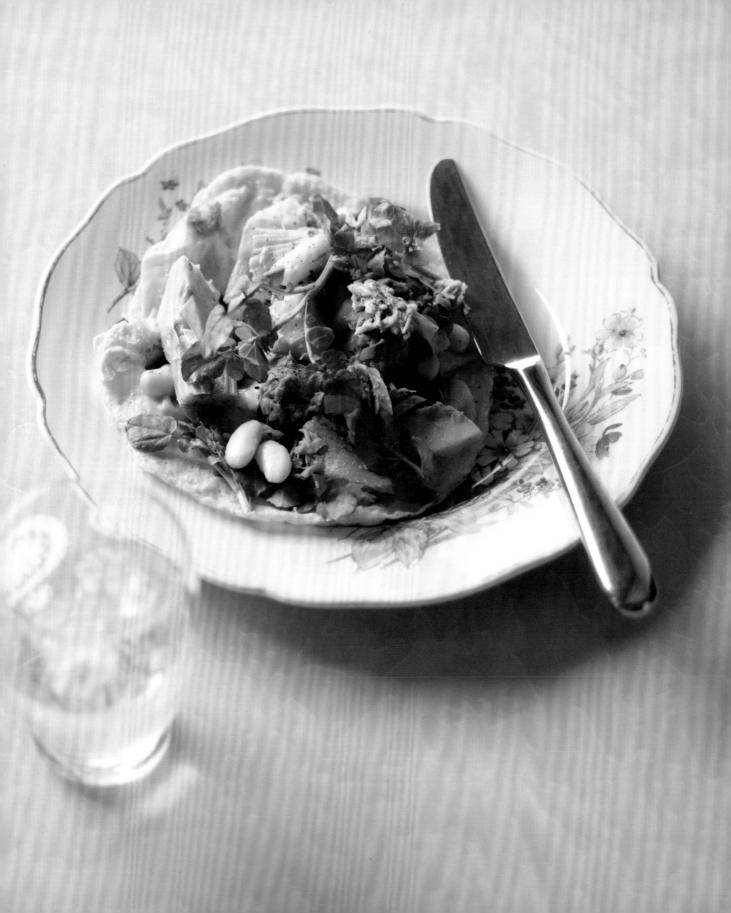

1 SERVE =
2 units bread
2 units dairy
1 unit vegetables

Grilled vegetable and lemon-cream bruschetta

SERVES 4   PREP 10 mins   COOK 10 mins

olive oil spray
1 eggplant (aubergine),
    trimmed and sliced
2 red capsicums (peppers), trimmed,
    seeded and cut into wide strips
8 slices wholegrain bread
2½ teaspoons finely grated
    lemon zest
2 cups (400 g) reduced-fat
    cottage cheese
12 tinned artichoke hearts,
    drained and quartered
flat-leaf (Italian) parsley leaves,
    to garnish (optional)

Spread each slice of bread lightly with pesto for a burst of flavour if you have a fat unit to spare. You can also flavour the cottage cheese – add chopped herbs (basil, oregano or chives) or some finely grated orange zest.

1 Heat a chargrill plate or large, heavy-based frying pan over medium heat. Spray the eggplant and capsicum with olive oil and, working in batches, cook for about 3 minutes on each side or until lightly charred and cooked through.

2 Meanwhile, preheat the grill to medium and toast the bread lightly on both sides.

3 Place the lemon zest and cottage cheese in a bowl, then season to taste and stir to combine well.

4 Place the toast on a board, then divide the eggplant and capsicum between the toast slices. Top with the artichokes and cottage cheese mixture, scatter with parsley (if using), then serve.

Bran muffins

MAKES 24   **PREP** 20 mins + standing time   **COOK** 20 mins

½ cup (125 ml) canola oil
½ cup (175 g) honey
1 cup (240 g) (about 2 carrots)
   grated carrot
2 bananas, mashed
2 apples, unpeeled and grated
3 eggs, lightly beaten
2 cups (500 ml) reduced-fat milk
1½ cups (90 g) unprocessed
   wheatbran
1½ cups (180 g) oat bran
2 cups (320 g) plain wholemeal flour
1 tablespoon baking powder
1 teaspoon ground cinnamon
1 cup (115 g) pecans or walnuts,
   finely chopped
½ cup (75 g) raisins

1 Preheat oven to 190°C. Lightly grease two 12-cup muffin tins.

2 In a large bowl, mix oil, honey, carrot, bananas, apples, eggs and milk. Stir through the two kinds of bran and let sit for 10 minutes.

3 In a separate bowl, combine flour, baking powder and cinnamon. Fold dry ingredients, along with pecans and raisins, through bran mixture until just mixed. Fill muffin cups two-thirds full with mixture and bake for 20 minutes, or until muffins are firm to the touch. Turn muffins out onto a wire rack to cool.

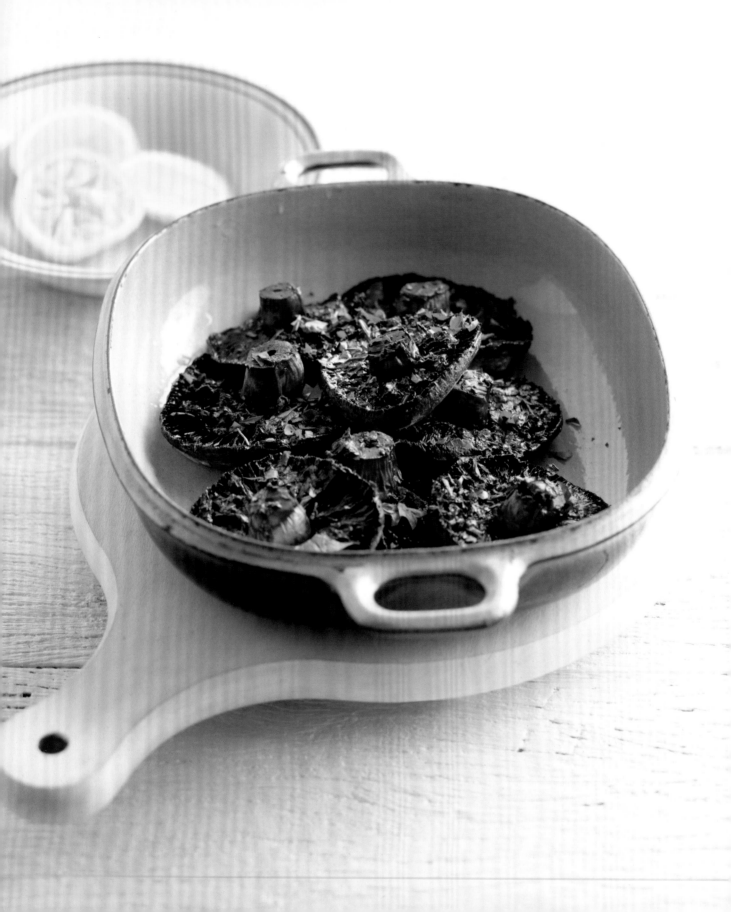

Balsamic-baked field mushrooms

SERVES 4   PREP 10 mins   COOK 10 mins

olive oil spray
12 field mushrooms, peeled
2 tablespoons balsamic vinegar
small handful basil leaves, torn
lemon slices (optional), to serve

If you are after a hearty side dish, perhaps to serve alongside grilled steak or lamb, then look no further. Peeling mushrooms is a good idea when cooking them in small amounts of oil, as the skins tend not to soften and are better removed.

1 Preheat the oven to 180°C.

2 Place the mushrooms in a baking dish and spray with olive oil, then bake for 15–20 minutes or until deep golden and tender.

3 Drizzle the mushrooms with balsamic vinegar and scatter with basil leaves. Season to taste with salt and pepper, then serve with lemon slices to squeeze over (if using).

TIP Experiment with different herbs here – use parsley, oregano or sage if you prefer.

1 SERVE =
½ unit protein
2 units bread
½ unit vegetables
1 unit fats

Mushroom, leek and asparagus tartlets

MAKES 6   PREP 15 mins   COOK 55 mins

12 slices wholegrain bread,
   crusts removed
1½ tablespoons olive oil
1 leek, white part only, finely
   sliced and washed
150 g Swiss brown mushrooms,
   quartered
250 g asparagus spears, cut
   into 2 cm pieces
freshly ground black pepper
25 g grated parmesan
6 eggs
½ cup (125 ml) reduced-fat milk

1 Preheat oven to 180°C. Lightly grease a 6-cup non-stick 'Texan' (or large) muffin tin.

2 Place two slices of bread on top of one another and, using a rolling pin, roll slices to a thickness of approximately 5 mm. Repeat with remaining slices. Place bread in each muffin cup, pushing down firmly to mould the bread to the tin. Bake for 5–10 minutes, or until golden. Set aside and reduce oven to 160°C.

3 In a heavy-based frying pan, heat oil over medium heat. Add leek and cook for 5 minutes, or until soft. Add mushrooms and cook for a further 5 minutes. Add asparagus, season with pepper then transfer to a bowl to cool.

4 In a separate bowl, whisk together parmesan, eggs and milk. Add the vegetables and stir to combine. Spoon the mixture into the bread cases and bake for 35 minutes, or until firm to the touch. Serve warm or cool, with a salad.

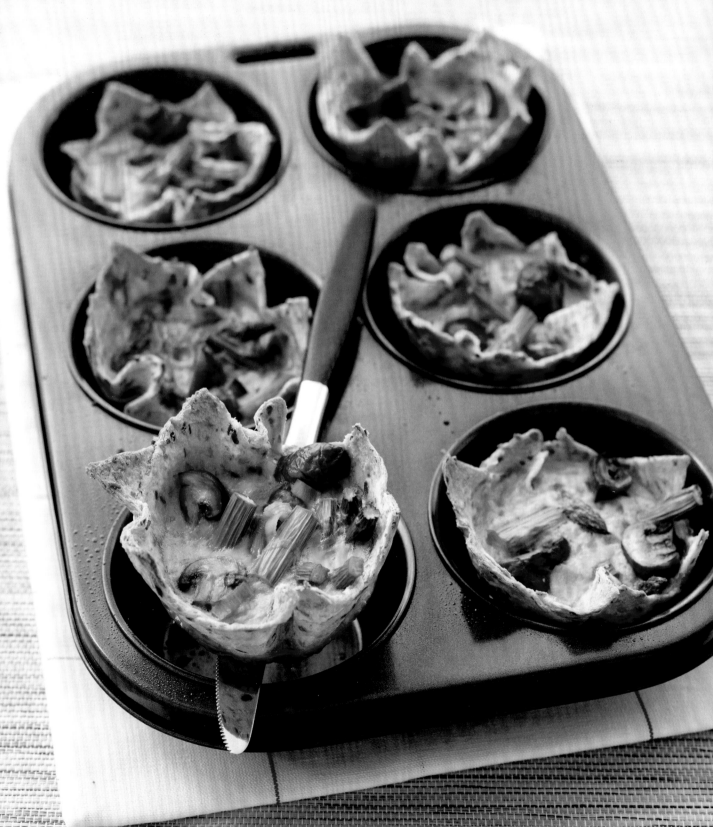

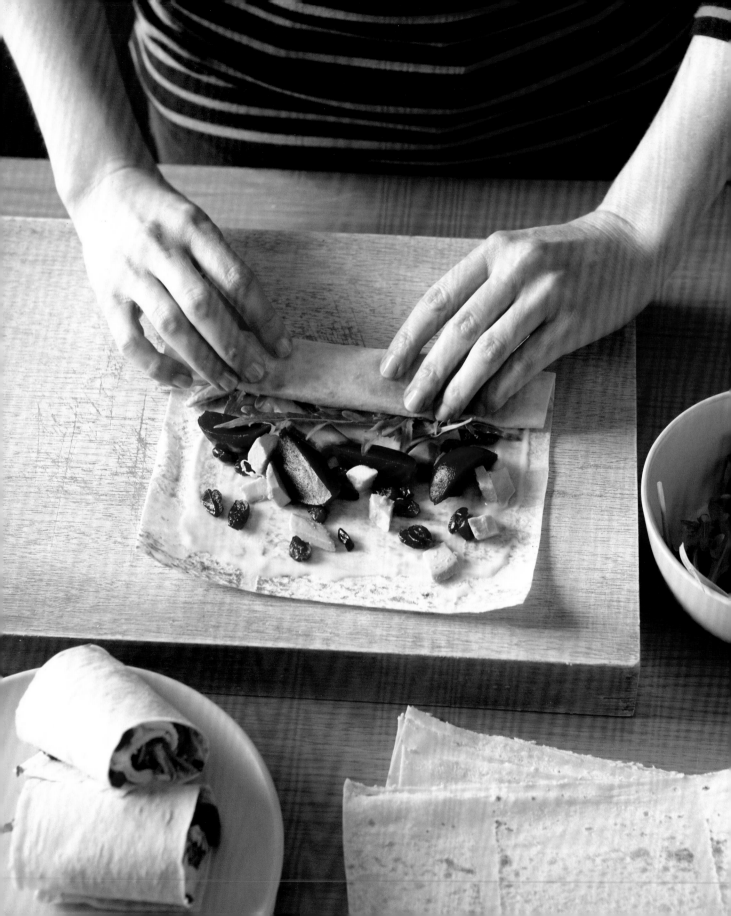

lunch and light meals

1 SERVE =
1½ units protein
½ unit dairy
½ unit vegetables*
* or 1½ units with serving suggestion

Smoked salmon and asparagus frittata

SERVES 4   PREP 15 mins   COOK 30 mins

12 spears asparagus (preferably
    thin stemmed), trimmed
8 eggs
3 tablespoons chopped dill
200 g smoked salmon,
    cut into strips
50 g grated parmesan

A slice of this lovely frittata makes a great packed lunch, or serve it with baby salad leaves as a starter at your next dinner party.

1 Preheat the oven to 150°C. Line a 20 cm square cake tin with baking paper.

2 Bring a large saucepan of water to the boil, add the asparagus and cook until just tender. Drain and rinse under cold water, then cut into 1 cm lengths.

3 Whisk together the eggs and dill in a bowl. Season, then stir in the asparagus and smoked salmon. Pour into the prepared tin and sprinkle with grated parmesan. Bake for 25 minutes or until just set. Remove from the oven and allow to cool. Cut into pieces and serve with a green salad.

TIP Try replacing the smoked salmon with smoked trout, or well-drained tinned salmon or tuna could be used for a budget option. Once opened, smoked salmon can be kept in the fridge for up to a week as long as it is tightly wrapped in plastic film. Or freeze it for up to 3 months.

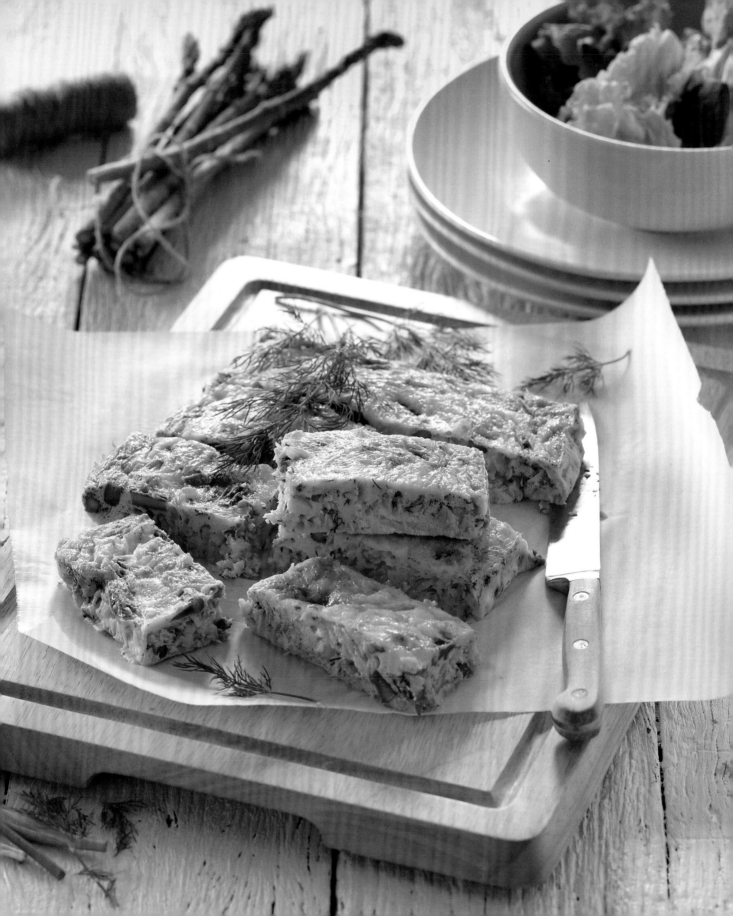

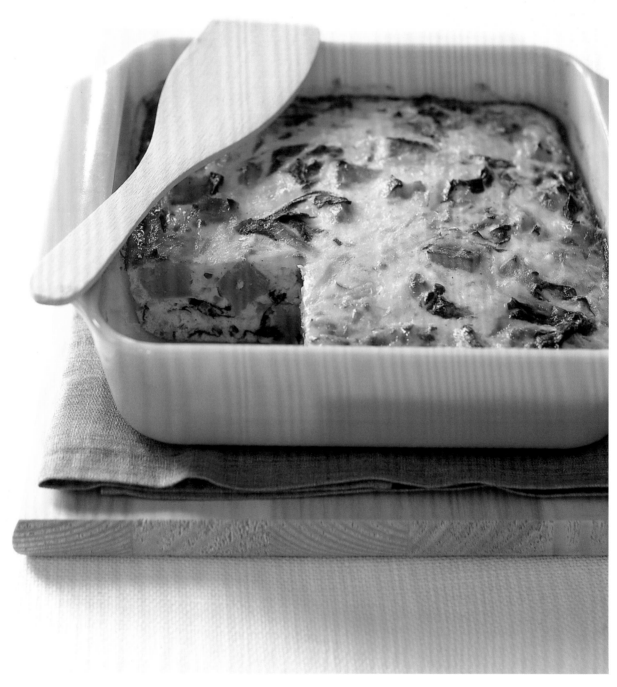

1 SERVE =
1 unit protein
1 unit dairy
2 units vegetables
1 unit fats

Pumpkin and spinach frittata

SERVES 4   **PREP** 15 mins   **COOK** 50 mins

400 g pumpkin, peeled and
   cut into 3 cm cubes
1 tablespoon olive oil
1 teaspoon soy sauce
2 leeks, finely sliced and washed
2 cloves garlic, crushed
300 g baby spinach leaves
freshly ground black pepper
8 eggs
400 g reduced-fat natural yoghurt
50 g matured cheese, grated

1 Preheat oven to 170°C. Grease a small baking dish with a little oil.

2 Place pumpkin in a bowl with 1 teaspoon oil and soy sauce and toss to coat. Tip pumpkin onto a baking tray and roast for 25 minutes.

3 Heat remaining oil in a frying pan over medium heat. Add leek and cook for 5 minutes, or until soft. Add garlic and spinach leaves and cook until spinach has wilted. Tip mixture onto work surface and chop roughly. Season to taste with pepper.

4 Whisk eggs, yoghurt and cheese together lightly in a large bowl. Add pumpkin and spinach mixture and gently stir to combine. Pour mixture into prepared dish and bake in oven for 20 minutes, or until set. Serve with a salad.

1 SERVE =
1 unit protein
1 unit bread
1 unit dairy
1½ units vegetables

Corn and cheddar frittata with tomato and bean salad

SERVES 4   PREP 30 mins   COOK 15 mins

2 cups (320 g) corn kernels
   (tinned or frozen)
8 eggs
100 g cheddar, grated
olive oil spray
1 teaspoon cumin seeds
400 g cherry tomatoes, halved
1 × 400 g tin kidney beans,
   rinsed and drained
½ small red (Spanish) onion,
   finely chopped
handful coriander (cilantro) leaves
   or flat-leaf (Italian) parsley leaves,
   chopped (optional)
1½ tablespoons lemon juice
1 tablespoon extra virgin olive oil
dried chilli flakes (optional)

Instead of corn, you could substitute any vegetables you like here – leftover cooked pumpkin or parsnip cut into small pieces, a combination of peas and broccoli, or zucchini (if using zucchini, grate it and cook in a large non-stick frying pan, stirring often, for 4–5 minutes, to allow the excess liquid to evaporate).

1   Cook the corn kernels in a saucepan of boiling water for 5–6 minutes or until tender, then drain well.

2   Whisk the eggs in a large bowl, stir in the grated cheddar and corn, then season with salt and pepper.

3   Heat a heavy-based 16 cm frying pan over medium–high heat and, once hot, spray the base and sides lightly with olive oil. Pour in the egg mixture and cook for 5–7 minutes or until browned on the underside and just set in the centre, using a spatula to push the sides of the mixture into the centre of the pan as the mixture cooks around the edge. Slide the frittata onto a dinner plate, then carefully place the frying pan over the frittata and invert so that the underside is now uppermost.

4   Return the pan to the heat and cook for 2 minutes or until firm. Remove the pan from the heat and set aside for 10–15 minutes to firm and cool slightly, then turn out and cut into four.

5   For the salad, place a small, heavy-based frying pan over low–medium heat. Add the cumin seeds to the pan then cook, shaking the pan often, for about 3 minutes or until the seeds are fragrant and lightly toasted. Remove from the heat, leave to cool slightly then tip into a bowl and add the tomato, kidney beans, onion and coriander or parsley (if using). Drizzle over the lemon juice and olive oil, then season and scatter with chilli flakes (if using).

6   Serve a wedge of fritatta with some salad to the side.

2-egg omelette

SERVES 1   PREP 10 mins   **COOK** 5 mins

2 eggs
1 tablespoon cold water
2 teaspoons olive oil
100 g shaved lean ham
¼ zucchini (courgette), finely sliced
2 teaspoons finely chopped flat-leaf
   (Italian) parsley
1 spring onion (scallion), finely sliced

1 Lightly beat eggs with water in a small bowl.

2 Heat oil in a non-stick frying pan over high heat. Pour in eggs and tilt pan so eggs cover base. Cook for 2 minutes, or until mixture just begins to set.

3 Place ham and zucchini in an even layer on top of egg mixture. Continue to cook until omelette has set. Sprinkle over parsley and spring onion and lightly season. Fold omelette in half and serve immediately.

VARIATIONS

Omelettes make a wonderful base for almost any ingredient. Experiment with roasted pumpkin, leek and thyme; red onion, capsicum (pepper) and basil; smoked salmon, chives and spinach; or stick with the more traditional tomato and bacon.

Corn fritters with smoked salmon and spinach

SERVES 4 (makes 8 fritters) **PREP** 15 mins **COOK** 15 mins

1 cup (160 g) wholemeal
  self-raising flour or 8 slices
  wholegrain bread, made
  into breadcrumbs
2 eggs
1 cup (250 ml) buttermilk
1 × 125 g tin corn, or 2 cooked
  corn cobs, kernels removed
4 spring onions (scallions),
  finely sliced
¼ cup roughly chopped
  flat-leaf (Italian) parsley
½ red capsicum (pepper),
  seeded and finely diced
1 tablespoon lemon juice
½ cup (140 g) reduced-fat
  natural yoghurt
¼ cup roughly chopped
  coriander (cilantro) leaves
1 tablespoon olive oil
300 g smoked salmon
100 g baby spinach

1 In a large bowl, sift flour and make a well in the centre. In a separate
   bowl, mix eggs and buttermilk. Pour egg mixture into flour and stir to
   make a smooth batter. Add corn, spring onions, parsley and capsicum
   and fold through.

2 In a small bowl, mix lemon juice, yoghurt and coriander, and set aside.

3 Heat oil in a large non-stick frying pan over medium heat. Drop
   $^1/_3$-cupfuls of mixture into the pan and cook for 3 minutes, or until
   golden. Turn and cook for a further 3 minutes, or until mixture is firm
   and set.

4 Serve 2 fritters per person, topped with a quarter of the smoked
   salmon and spinach, and drizzled with a little yoghurt dressing.

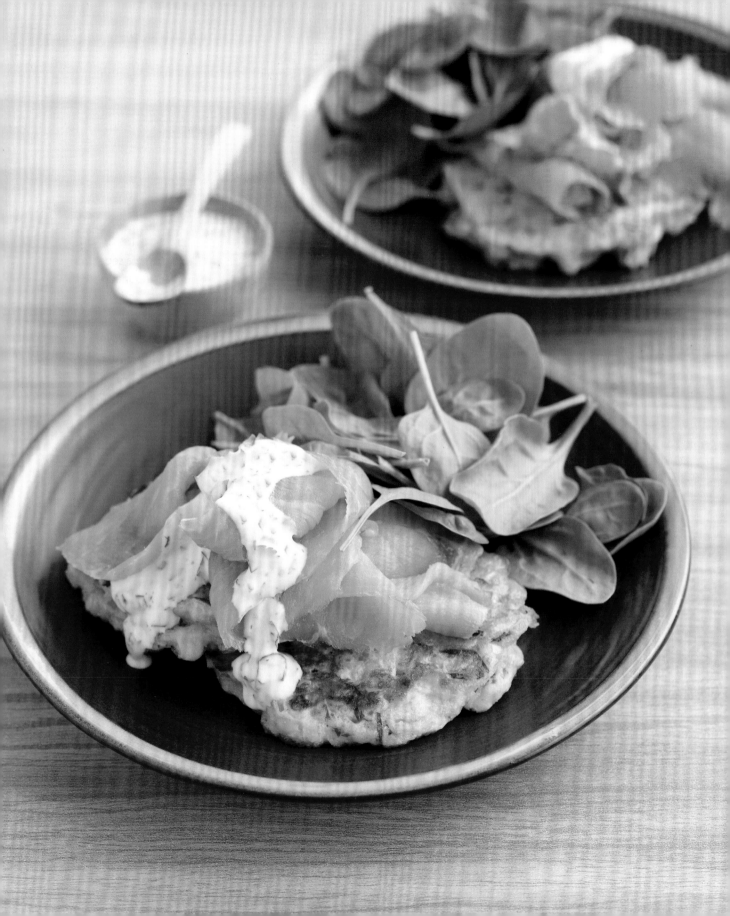

1 SERVE =
1 unit protein
2 units bread
1½ units vegetables
2 units fats

Barbecued lamb and vegetable wrap with pesto

SERVES 4   PREP 10 mins + resting time   COOK 15 mins

400 g lamb rump steaks
2 zucchini (courgettes),
    thinly sliced lengthways
2 red capsicums (peppers),
    seeded and sliced
1 red (Spanish) onion, sliced
    into thick rings
2 teaspoons picked thyme leaves
1 tablespoon olive oil
4 large wholemeal Lebanese
    flatbreads
⅓ cup (90 g) pesto
2 cups rocket (arugula)

1   Preheat a grill plate or barbecue grill to high. Cook lamb steaks for 4 minutes each side, or until done to your liking. Remove to a plate, cover with foil and set aside to rest for 5 minutes.

2   Place zucchini, capsicums, onion and thyme in a bowl. Add olive oil and toss to coat. Transfer mixture to grill plate and cook, turning occasionally, for 2–5 minutes, or until charred and soft. Set aside.

3   Slice lamb across the grain into thin strips. To serve, spread each flatbread with a quarter of the pesto. Top with a quarter each of the chargrilled vegetables, lamb and rocket. Fold up the bottom of the wrap, then cross the sides over each other. Repeat with remaining wraps and serve immediately.

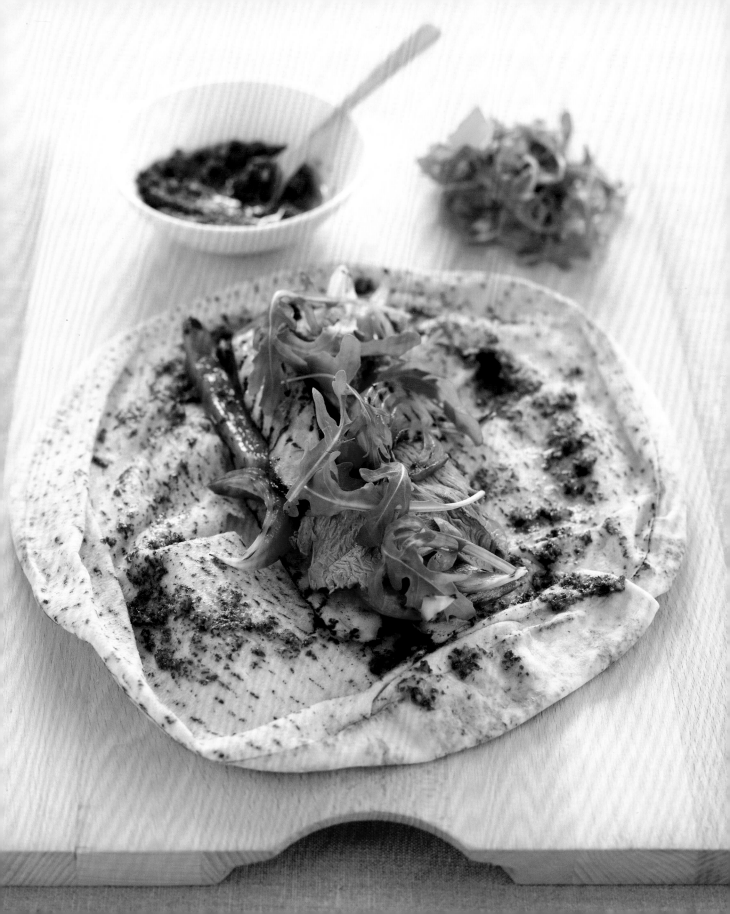

1 SERVE =
1 unit protein
1 unit vegetables*
1½ units fats
* or 2 units with serving suggestion

Chinese mushroom omelette

SERVES 4   PREP 15 mins   COOK 15 mins

8 eggs, lightly beaten
3 spring onions, finely sliced
1 tablespoon vegetable oil
coriander (cilantro) leaves,
    to serve
2 spring onions, finely sliced,
    extra, to serve

FILLING
2 teaspoons vegetable oil
1 × 1 cm piece ginger, grated
1 clove garlic, crushed
400 g mixed mushrooms
1 cup (80 g) bean sprouts

SAUCE
2 teaspoons rice vinegar
1 tablespoon oyster sauce
¼ teaspoon sesame oil

This scrumptious dish looks and tastes a treat. It's simple and quick to whip up at short notice.

1   To prepare the sauce, combine all the ingredients in a small bowl and set aside.

2   To prepare the filling, heat the oil in a wok or large frying pan over high heat. Add the ginger, garlic and mushrooms and stir-fry for 3–4 minutes or until the mushrooms are just cooked. Remove the mixture to a plate and wipe the wok clean.

3   Combine the eggs and spring onion in a large bowl. Reheat the wok or frying pan over medium–high heat and add 1 teaspoon of the oil. When the oil is hot, add a quarter of the egg mix and swirl it around the wok.

4   When the base of the omelette is cooked and the top is still slightly soft, spread a quarter of the mushroom mix over half the omelette. Top with a quarter of the bean sprouts and fold the other half of the omelette over the top. Remove from the wok and keep warm while you make the remaining three omelettes.

5   Drizzle the sauce over the omelettes and garnish with the coriander leaves and extra spring onion. Serve with a green salad.

TIP Try using a mix of shiitake, oyster, enoki and/or button mushrooms for this recipe.

Turkey, beetroot and cranberry wrap

SERVES 4 PREP 10 mins

4 pieces mountain bread
4 tablespoons reduced-fat
 mayonnaise
²/₃ cup (100 g) dried cranberries
1 ripe avocado (250 g), halved,
 seeded and chopped
400 g cooked sliced turkey
1 × 440 g tin baby beetroot,
 drained and quartered
2 large handfuls rocket

Turkey and cranberries are just made for each other. These tasty wraps can be prepared up to 4 hours in advance and kept in the fridge until lunchtime.

1 Spread one side of each piece of mountain bread with mayonnaise.

2 Divide the cranberries, avocado, turkey, beetroot and rocket among the wraps, then roll up firmly.

3 Serve immediately, or wrap in plastic wrap and refrigerate until ready to serve.

> **TIP** You can use cooked chicken instead of turkey if you prefer.

1 SERVE =
1 unit protein
2 units bread
1½ units vegetables
1 unit fats

Chicken tortillas with roasted corn salsa

SERVES 4   PREP 20 mins   COOK 10 mins

¹/₃ cup (80 ml) reduced-fat sour cream
4 large wholemeal tortillas
1 iceberg lettuce, shredded
2 tomatoes, diced
400 g cooked skinless chicken breast,
    finely sliced

CORN SALSA
2 corn cobs
1 tablespoon olive oil
¹/₃ cup roughly chopped coriander
    (cilantro)
¼ cup roughly chopped mint
½ small red (Spanish) onion,
    finely diced
juice of 1 lime

1   To make corn salsa, preheat grill plate or barbecue grill to high. Lightly brush corn with half the oil, then grill, turning occasionally, for 10 minutes, or until lightly browned all over. Remove from the grill and allow to cool. Cut kernels from cobs and transfer kernels to a small bowl. Add remaining oil plus coriander, mint, onion and lime juice, and toss to combine.

2   To serve, spread 1 tablespoon of sour cream down the centre of each tortilla. Top sour cream with a small handful of lettuce, some chopped tomato and a quarter of the sliced chicken, leaving a little room at the top and bottom of the tortilla. Spoon a quarter of the corn salsa on top. Fold up bottom of tortilla, then wrap each side over the tortilla. You should have a neat, tight wrap. Repeat with the remaining tortillas and serve immediately.

1 SERVE =
1 unit protein
1 unit bread
½ unit dairy
½ unit vegetables
3 units fats

Salmon and broccoli tart

SERVES 4   PREP 15 mins   COOK 1 hour 20 mins

**1 quantity olive oil pastry
   (see page 54)**
1 tablespoon olive oil
**1 leek, white part only, finely
   sliced and washed**
1 clove garlic, crushed
**200 g tinned salmon, drained
   and flaked**
1 cup broccoli, cut into small florets
50 g grated reduced-fat cheddar
4 eggs
½ cup (125 ml) reduced-fat milk
**½ cup (140 g) reduced-fat natural
   yoghurt**
1 tablespoon chopped dill

1   Preheat oven to 200°C. Lightly grease a 20 cm fluted flan tin.

2   Roll out pastry and use it to line the flan tin. Cover base of pastry case
    with baking paper, then cover paper with dried beans or rice to stop
    the pastry base from puffing up during cooking. Bake for 15 minutes.
    Remove beans and paper and bake for a further 10 minutes. Remove
    from oven and reduce temperature to 160°C.

3   Heat oil in a large frying pan over high heat. Add leek and cook for
    5 minutes, or until soft. Add garlic and cook for a further 2 minutes.
    Remove pan from heat and set aside.

4   Cover tart base with salmon, broccoli and cheese. In a small bowl,
    mix eggs, milk, yoghurt and dill. Add leek and garlic, season lightly
    and pour over tart filling.

5   Bake for approximately 45 minutes, or until lightly browned and puffy
    in the centre. Serve with a green salad.

1 SERVE =
1 unit protein
2 units bread
½ unit vegetables
3 units fats

Open steak sandwich

SERVES 4   PREP 10 mins + resting time   COOK 10 mins

4 × 100 g rump steaks
1 tablespoon olive oil
100 g rocket (arugula) leaves
2 ripe tomatoes, sliced
1 small avocado, sliced
4 thick slices wholegrain sourdough
    bread, lightly toasted
1 red (Spanish) onion, thinly sliced
1 teaspoon balsamic vinegar

1 Heat a large non-stick frying pan over high heat. Coat steaks with oil and cook for 3 minutes each side, or until done to your liking. You may need to do this in batches – if you crowd the pan, the steaks will stew rather than sear. Place steaks in a warm place, or cover with foil, and set aside for 5 minutes to rest.

2 Meanwhile, layer rocket, tomato and avocado on the toast.

3 Thickly slice each piece of beef and place on a sandwich. Top with onion and drizzle with the remaining oil and balsamic vinegar.

4 Serve with salad.

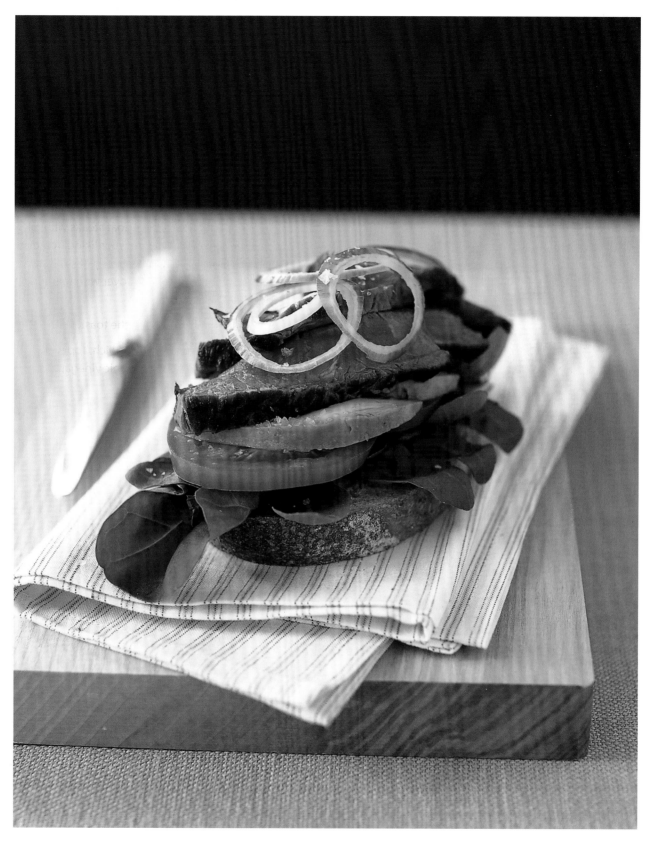

Steak and mushroom pie

SERVES 4   PREP 15 mins + cooling time   COOK 1 hour 15 mins

1 tablespoon olive oil
400 g rump steak, cut into cubes
1 onion, chopped
2 cloves garlic, crushed
350 g large flat mushrooms, sliced
2 teaspoons dried mixed herbs
1 × 400 g tin diced tomatoes
1 cup (250 ml) salt-reduced beef stock
1 tablespoon cornflour (cornstarch)
   mixed with 2 tablespoons
   cold water
1 quantity olive oil pastry
   (see below)
reduced-fat milk, for brushing

1 Heat oil in a large saucepan over medium heat. Add beef in batches
   and cook for 5 minutes, or until browned. Return all meat to pan, add
   onion and garlic and cook for 3 minutes, or until onion is soft.
   Add mushrooms, dried herbs, tomatoes and stock and bring to
   a boil. Reduce heat and simmer, covered, for 30 minutes. Pour in
   cornflour mixture and simmer, uncovered, for a further 10 minutes,
   or until thick. Spoon pie filling into a 2 litre ovenproof pie dish and
   set aside to cool slightly.

2 Preheat oven to 200°C.

3 Roll out pastry to 5 mm thickness and the size of the pie dish. Brush
   rim of pie dish with a little milk, then drape pastry over, pressing the
   edges firmly onto the rim of the dish. Brush pastry with a little more
   milk and bake for 20 minutes. Serve with steamed green vegetables
   or a crisp green salad.

OLIVE OIL PASTRY

Place 100 g wholemeal plain flour and a pinch of salt in a bowl. Add
2 tablespoons olive oil and rub into flour, using your fingers, until mixture
resembles breadcrumbs. Sprinkle in 50 ml cold water, a little at a time,
and mix together. Knead briefly, then set aside, covered with a clean tea
towel, for 1 hour. Use as specified in recipe.

Zucchini and mint pie

SERVES 4   PREP 15 mins + cooling time   COOK 45 mins

1 tablespoon olive oil
1 onion, finely chopped
5 zucchini (courgettes), finely sliced
8 eggs
400 g reduced-fat natural yoghurt
½ cup roughly chopped mint
4 spring onions (scallions), finely sliced
25 g coarsely grated parmesan
25 g feta

1 Preheat oven to 170°C. Lightly grease a 20 cm
   ovenproof flan dish.

2 Heat oil in a large non-stick frying pan over medium
   heat. Add onion and saute for 5 minutes, or until soft.
   Add zucchini and cook for 2 minutes. Transfer to
   a bowl to cool.

3 In a separate bowl, whisk eggs and yoghurt. Add
   remaining ingredients and zucchini mix, season
   lightly and stir to combine. Spoon mixture into
   prepared dish and bake for 35 minutes, or until
   golden and firm to the touch. Cut into slices and
   serve warm or cold with a crisp salad.

Chicken and leek pie

SERVES 4   PREP 15 mins   COOK 1 hour

1 tablespoon olive oil
400 g skinless chicken thigh fillets,
   trimmed of fat, cut into 4 cm pieces
2 sticks celery, sliced
2 leeks, white part only,
   sliced and washed
1 cup (250 ml) chicken stock
1 tablespoon cornflour (cornstarch)
   mixed with ½ cup (125 ml) white wine
1 tablespoon chopped tarragon
1 tablespoon chopped flat-leaf (Italian) parsley
½ cup (60 g) frozen peas
1 quantity olive oil pastry (see page 54)
reduced-fat milk, for brushing

1 Heat oil in a large heavy-based saucepan over
   medium heat. Add chicken in batches and cook for
   5 minutes, or until browned. Return all chicken pieces
   to pan, add celery and leek and cook for 5 minutes, or
   until leek is soft. Pour in chicken stock and cornflour
   mixture and bring to a boil. Reduce heat, cover and
   simmer for 20 minutes. Stir in herbs and peas and
   season lightly. Spoon chicken filling into a 2 litre
   ovenproof pie dish and set aside to cool slightly.

2 Preheat oven to 200°C.

3 Roll out pastry to 5 mm thickness and the size of
   the pie dish. Brush rim of dish with a little milk, then
   drape pastry over, pressing edges firmly onto the rim
   of the dish. Brush pastry lid with a little more milk and
   bake for 20 minutes. Serve with your favourite green
   vegetables.

Minute steak sandwiches with pesto and grilled vegetables

SERVES 4   **PREP** 10 mins   **COOK** 5 mins

2 small zucchini (courgettes), trimmed
   and sliced on the diagonal
1 large red capsicum (pepper),
   trimmed, seeded and
   cut into thick slices
olive oil spray
4 × 100 g lean beef or veal minute
   steaks, trimmed of fat
4 slices wholegrain bread
2 tablespoons pesto
2 tomatoes (optional), thinly sliced
handful watercress sprigs

These super-quick sandwiches are a satisfying lunch. If you have a spare dairy unit, you might like to add 25 g shaved parmesan to each sandwich.

1   Heat a chargrill plate or heavy-based frying pan over medium–high heat. Spray the zucchini and capsicum with olive oil. Cook the zucchini for 3–4 minutes, turning once, or until lightly charred and tender, then set aside. Cook the capsicum for 4–5 minutes, turning once, or until lightly charred and tender, then set aside. Cook the steak for 1 minute on each side or until cooked through but still a little pink in the middle.

2   Lay out the bread slices on a board and spread with pesto. Divide the zucchini and tomato (if using) among the slices, then cut the steaks into two or three pieces and place on top. Add the capsicum and watercress, season to taste with salt and pepper, then serve.

> **TIP** Substitute the pesto with horseradish, mustard or tapenade, if you prefer. For a change from red meat, chargrill some thinly sliced chicken breast instead.

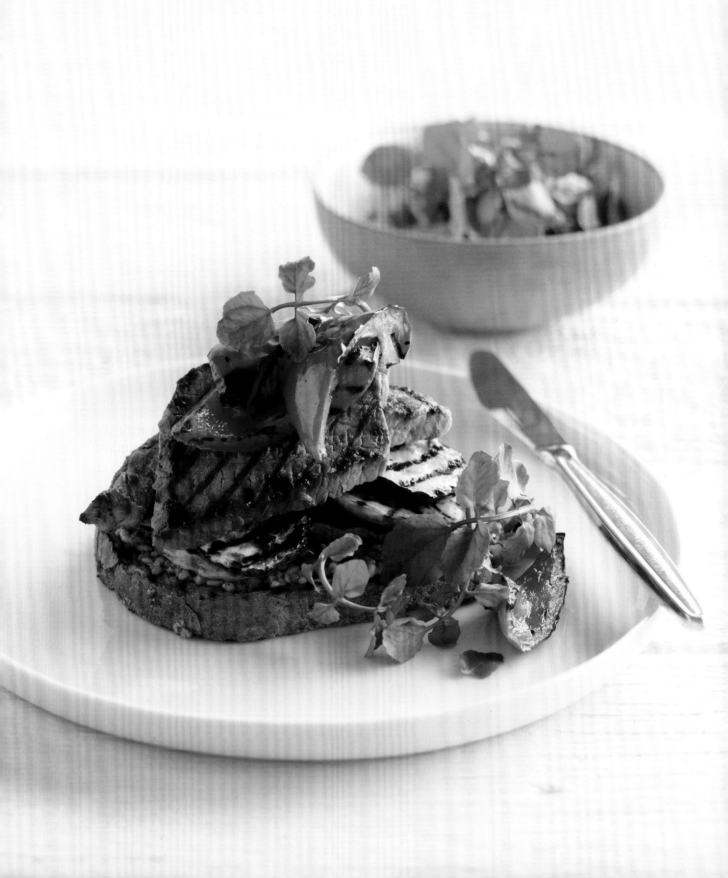

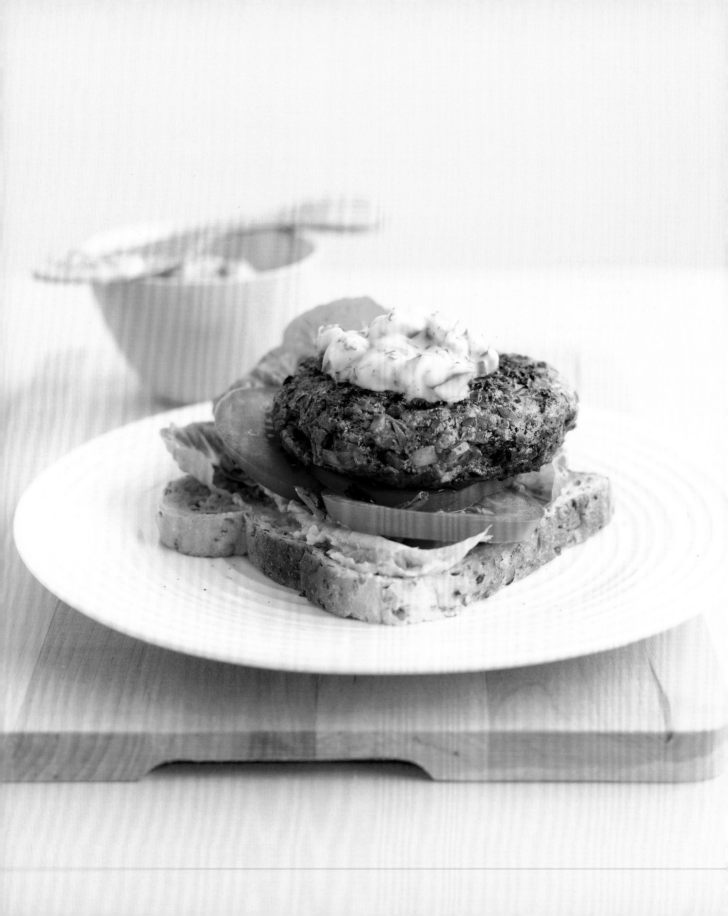

Spicy lamb burger with tzatziki

SERVES 4   PREP 20 mins   COOK 16 mins

2 tablespoons reduced-fat Hummus
   (see page 530)
4 slices wholegrain bread,
   lightly toasted
2 baby cos lettuces, outer leaves
   discarded, leaves separated
2 ripe tomatoes, sliced

BURGER PATTIES
400 g lean minced (ground) lamb
1 red (Spanish) onion, finely diced
1 small red chilli, seeded and
   finely chopped
½ cup roughly chopped
   coriander (cilantro)
1 clove garlic, crushed
2 teaspoons freshly grated ginger

TZATZIKI
½ cup (140 g) reduced-fat
   natural yoghurt
1 Lebanese cucumber, seeded
   and finely diced
1/3 cup roughly chopped mint

1   In a large bowl, mix all patty ingredients thoroughly. Form mixture
    into 4 patties.

2   Preheat a grill plate or barbecue grill to high. Add patties and cook
    for 8 minutes each side, or until cooked through. Meanwhile, in
    a small bowl, mix yoghurt, cucumber and mint.

3   To serve, spread a quarter of the hummus on each slice of bread.
    Layer with cos leaves, tomato and a burger patty, and top with
    a dollop of tatziki.

TIP A versatile lunch or dinner meal, burgers freeze extremely well.
Make double the recipe and freeze for later use.

1 SERVE =
1 unit protein
½ unit vegetables*
* or 1½ units with serving suggestion

Chicken cakes

SERVES 4   PREP 15 mins   COOK 25 mins

olive oil spray
400 g lean minced chicken
½ small onion, chopped
2 cloves garlic, crushed
¼ red capsicum (pepper), diced
1 small zucchini (courgette), diced
1 tablespoon soy sauce
1 egg
2 tablespoons roughly chopped
   coriander (cilantro)
sweet chilli sauce, to serve (optional)

Kids love these chicken cakes and they're delicious hot or cold. Wrap any leftovers in plastic film and pack them into a lunchbox for a tasty treat the next day.

1   Preheat the oven to 180°C. Spray eight ½ cup (125 ml) muffin holes with olive oil.

2   Place all the ingredients (except the chilli sauce) in a food processor and process until smooth. Spoon into the prepared muffin holes.

3   Bake for 20–25 minutes or until golden and firm. Serve two per person with mixed baby salad leaves and sweet chilli sauce, if liked.

TIP These cakes also work well with minced pork or turkey.

Lemon tuna patties

SERVES 4 (makes 8 patties)   PREP 20 mins   COOK 10 mins

300 g tinned tuna, drained
1 small red (Spanish) onion,
   finely chopped
2 tablespoons chopped
   coriander (cilantro)
2 teaspoons finely grated lemon zest
2 eggs, separated
2 tablespoons wholemeal plain flour
2 tablespoons vegetable oil

1 Place tuna, onion, coriander and lemon zest in a bowl and mix lightly with a fork. Add egg yolks (reserving whites for later) and continue to mix. Season lightly. Sift flour into mixture, and gently fold through.

2 Place the egg whites in a clean bowl and whisk until soft peaks form. Spoon the whites into the tuna mixture and gently fold through. With slightly wet hands, form the mixture into 8 patties.

3 Heat oil in a large non-stick frying pan over medium heat. Add patties and cook for 5 minutes each side, or until golden brown. Drain on paper towels. Serve tuna patties with a mixed-leaf salad tossed with an oil-free dressing.

TIP The patties are fantastic lunchbox options, and keep well in the fridge for several days. Take them to work for lunch, and eat them cold or warm, with a side salad or vegetables (see pages 465–520).

1 SERVE =
1 unit protein
¼ unit vegetables*
2 units fats
* or 1¼ units with serving suggestion

Thai fishcakes with lime and chilli sauce

SERVES 4   **PREP** 20 mins   **COOK** 10 mins

400 g white fish fillets, skin
   and bones removed
1–2 tablespoons red curry paste
1 egg white
1 tablespoon chopped coriander
   (cilantro)
2 teaspoons fish sauce
1 red chilli, chopped (optional)
2 spring onions, thinly sliced
50 g green beans, thinly sliced
1 tablespoon vegetable oil
lime wedges, to serve

LIME AND CHILLI SAUCE
¹/₃ cup (80 ml) light soy sauce
1½ tablespoons lime juice
2 teaspoons grated ginger
1 small red chilli, seeded and
   finely chopped
1 tablespoon finely chopped
   coriander (cilantro)

Everybody's favourite, these spicy fishcakes make an impressive weekend lunch to share with family or friends.

1   To make the lime and chilli sauce, combine all the ingredients in a bowl.

2   Place the fish fillets, curry paste, egg white, chopped coriander, fish sauce and chilli (if using) in a food processor and process until smooth. Place in a bowl with the spring onion and beans and mix well. Form the mixture into 12 patties.

3   Heat the oil in a non-stick frying pan over medium heat. Cook the patties for 3–4 minutes on each side until golden. Serve with the sauce and a salad, with lime wedges to the side.

TIP   If you're running short of time, use a shop-bought sweet chilli sauce instead of making your own. These can be made into bite-sized balls and served as finger food with the sauce as a dipping sauce. The cooking time will be reduced to 2–3 minutes.

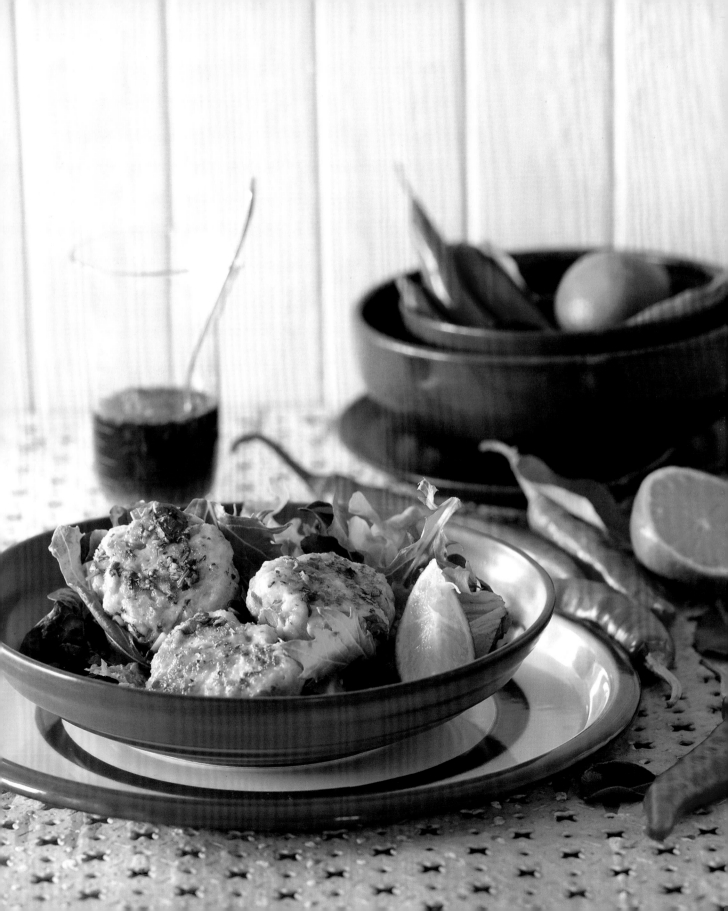

1 SERVE =
1 unit protein
1 unit bread
1 unit vegetables
3 units fats

Salmon fishcakes with red capsicum and basil salad

SERVES 4 (makes 8 patties)   PREP 30 mins + refrigerating time   COOK 30 mins

400 g tinned salmon, drained
6 spring onions (scallions),
    finely sliced
400 g desiree potatoes, peeled,
    boiled and mashed
finely grated zest of 1 lemon
¼ cup roughly chopped mint
¼ cup roughly chopped flat-leaf
    (Italian) parsley
¼ cup (35 g) plain flour
2 tablespoons vegetable oil

RED CAPSICUM & BASIL SALAD
2 roasted red capsicums
    (peppers), sliced
½ cup basil leaves
12 cherry tomatoes, halved
1 clove garlic, crushed
2 teaspoons red wine vinegar
1 tablespoon olive oil
1 tablespoon salted baby capers,
    rinsed well

1   Combine salmon, spring onions, mashed potato, lemon zest, mint
    and parsley in a bowl, and roll into 8 balls. Transfer to a plate, cover
    with plastic wrap and refrigerate for at least 1 hour.

2   Preheat oven to 180°C. Sprinkle flour onto a board. Roll fish balls in
    flour and flatten gently. Heat half the oil in a large non-stick frying
    pan over medium heat. Cook 4 fishcakes for 5 minutes each side, or
    until golden brown. Transfer to a baking tray. Repeat with 4 remaining
    cakes. Bake cakes for 8 minutes, or until heated through.

3   Meanwhile, mix all salad ingredients in a bowl. Divide fishcakes
    among four plates and serve with the salad.

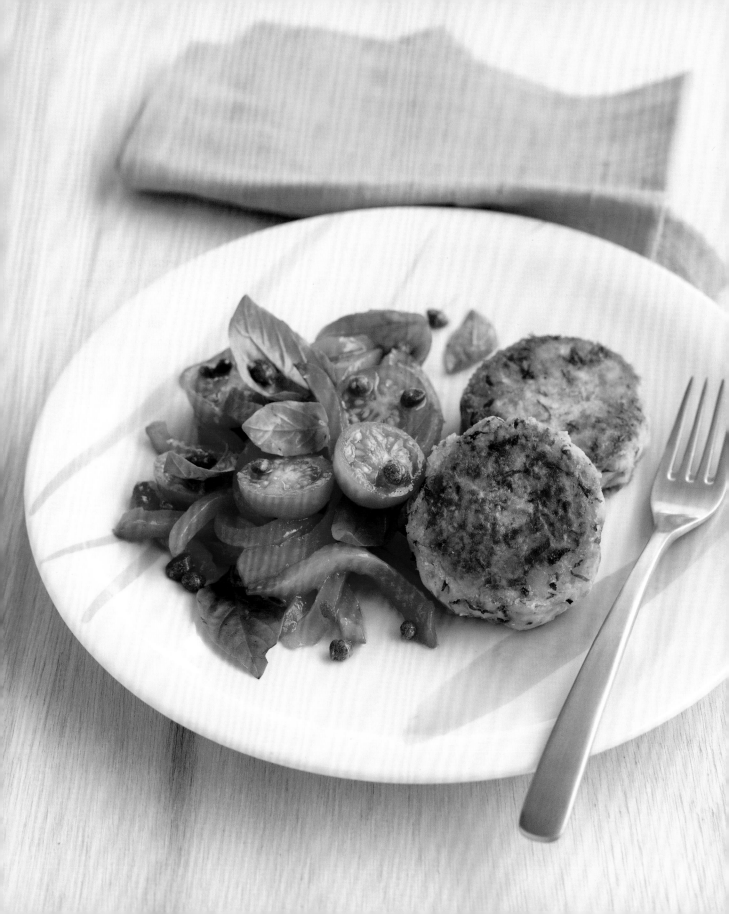

Homemade pizza dough

SERVES 4   PREP 25 mins + standing time   COOK 20 mins

1½ teaspoons dried yeast
½ teaspoon sugar
1½ cups (240 g) wholemeal plain flour
½ cup (75 g) plain flour
olive oil spray

There's no need to be daunted by the idea of making your own pizza dough. The recipe below is clear and straightforward, and the delectable results will make you so pleased you took the time.

1 Combine the yeast and sugar with 1 cup (250 ml) warm water in a small bowl. Set aside for 10 minutes or until frothy.

2 Place the flours in a large bowl, add the yeast mixture and mix with clean hands to form a dough. Turn out onto a floured surface and knead for several minutes until the dough is smooth and elastic and springs back when pressed.

3 Spray a large, clean bowl with olive oil and add the dough. Cover with a clean tea towel and set aside for 45–60 minutes or until the dough has doubled in size.

4 Preheat the oven to 220°C. Dust a large baking tray or two pizza trays with flour.

5 Turn out the dough onto a lightly floured surface and punch it down. Roll out to a 40 cm × 30 cm rectangle, or divide the dough in half and roll to make two 25 cm round pizza bases. Transfer the dough to the prepared tray or trays and add your choice of toppings (see facing page). Bake for 15–20 minutes or until the base is crisp and cooked through.

TIP If you don't have time to make the pizza base, you can use wholemeal pita or mountain bread instead.

SPINACH AND RICOTTA

Spread ²/₃ cup (170 g) salt-reduced tomato passata or pasta sauce over the pizza base, then sprinkle evenly with 2 large handfuls baby spinach leaves, 200 g reduced-fat ricotta and 100 g pitted black olives. Bake according to the pizza dough recipe instructions.

> **TIP** You can add smoked salmon and/or semi-dried tomatoes to this pizza, if liked. Sprinkle your cooked pizza with fresh herbs or rocket and perhaps drizzle with a little balsamic vinegar.

MARGHERITA

Spread ²/₃ cup (170 g) salt-reduced tomato passata or pasta sauce over the pizza base, then top with 200 g grated or sliced reduced-fat mozzarella. Bake according to the pizza dough recipe instructions. Sprinkle with a handful of basil leaves and serve.

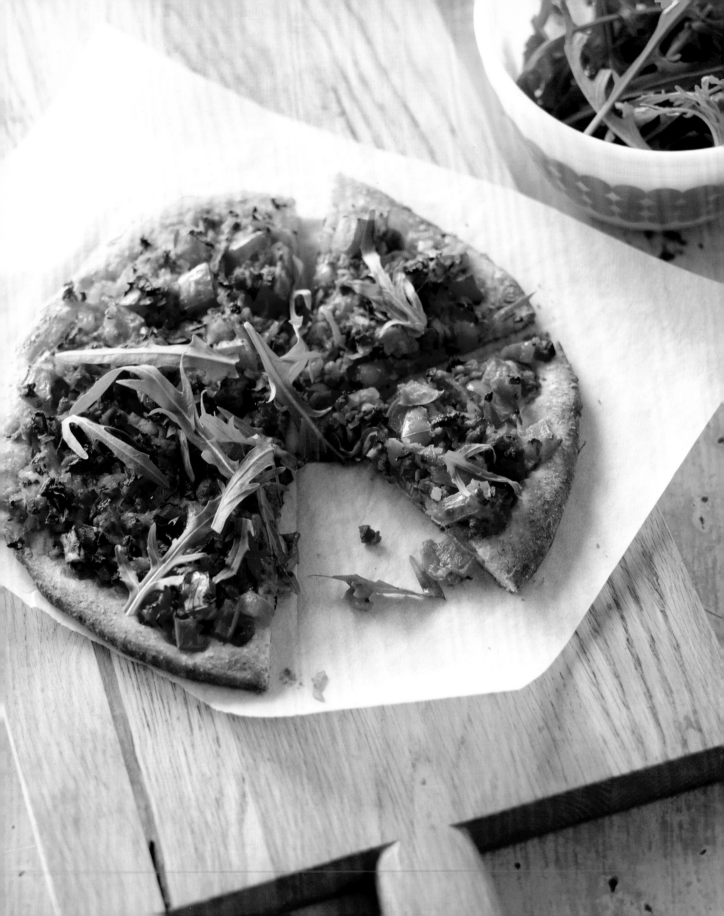

1 SERVE =
1 unit protein
2 units bread
1 unit vegetables
1 unit fats

Spiced lamb and carrot pizzas

SERVES 4   PREP 30 mins + dough rising time   COOK 30 mins

2 teaspoons olive oil
1 onion, finely chopped
1½ teaspoons cumin seeds
    or ground cumin
400 g lean minced lamb
2 carrots, grated
1 tablespoon tomato paste (puree)
2½ teaspoons dried mint or oregano
4 roma (plum) tomatoes (about
    300 g), seeded and finely chopped
large handful rocket, to serve
1 quantity Homemade Pizza Dough
    (see page 66)

The Middle Eastern-inspired combination of flavours here make this one a real standout. When making the pizza dough, use 280 g wholemeal flour instead of white and wholemeal flour. Use small pita breads for the pizza bases if you don't have time to make your own dough.

1 Heat the oil in a saucepan over medium heat. Add the onion and cook, stirring, for 5 minutes or until soft. Add the cumin and lamb and cook, stirring to break up the mince, for another 2 minutes or until fragrant. Add the carrot, tomato paste and dried mint or oregano, then bring the mixture to simmering point. Cook over medium heat for 4–5 minutes or until any excess liquid has evaporated, then season to taste with salt and pepper. Remove from the heat and stir in the tomato.

2 Preheat the oven to 220°C.

3 Using your fist, deflate the dough, then turn it out onto a lightly floured work surface. Divide the mixture into quarters. Working with one piece at a time, roll each piece out to form a 20 cm round. Line two baking trays with baking paper, then place two rounds on each tray. Divide the lamb mixture among the rounds, spreading it to cover each, leaving a 1 cm border around the edge.

4 Bake for 15 minutes or until the base is golden and crisp. Sprinkle over some of the rocket leaves, then cut into wedges and serve immediately with the remaining rocket alongside.

TIP Once cooked, these can be frozen for up to 1 month. Thaw in the fridge, then bake for 8–10 minutes at 180°C.

Chicken, tomato and zucchini pizza

SERVES 4 PREP 15 mins COOK 10 mins

4 small wholemeal pita breads

$^1/_3$ cup (95 g) tomato paste

2 teaspoons dried Greek oregano

2 ripe tomatoes, thinly sliced

2 zucchini (courgettes), thinly
sliced lengthways

400 g cooked skinless chicken
breast, sliced

100 g feta or mozzarella

1$^1/_3$ cups rocket (arugula)

1 tablespoon olive oil

1 Preheat oven to 200°C.

2 Spread pita breads with tomato paste and sprinkle with oregano. Divide tomato and zucchini between pitas, add a layer of sliced chicken and crumble feta or mozzarella over the top. Bake for 10 minutes.

3 Serve topped with rocket leaves and a drizzle of olive oil and with a salad alongside.

TIP Pizzas are a delicious way to use up leftovers. Keep a packet of pita breads in the freezer for emergency meals, and use any toppings you like.

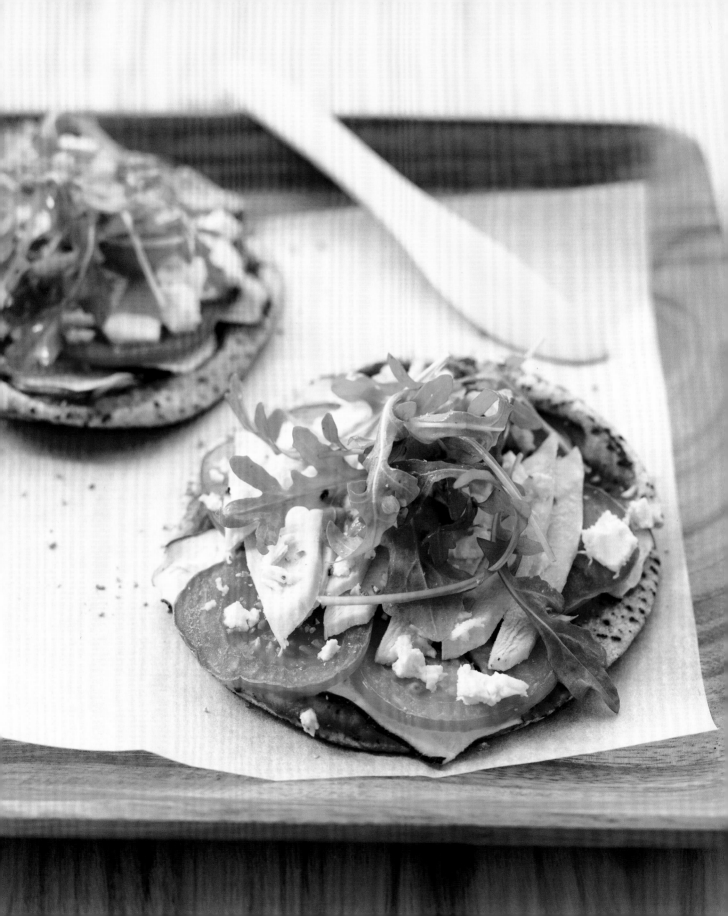

Bruschetta

SERVES 4 PREP 5 mins COOK 5 mins

**8 slices good-quality crusty bread
1 clove garlic**

This recipe for bruschetta is simple to prepare, and with three flavoursome topping options it is bound to appeal to a variety of tastes.

1 Toast the bread in a toaster, under the grill or on a chargrill. Cut the garlic clove in half, then rub the cut side over the toast while it is still warm.

2 Add your choice of topping (see below) and eat straight away. Or, if you are packing the toast for a lunchbox, allow it to cool before wrapping. Seal the topping in an airtight container and add it when you are ready to eat.

TOMATO AND BASIL
Combine 6 diced tomatoes, 1 tablespoon balsamic vinegar, 1 tablespoon extra virgin olive oil and some shredded basil and season with salt and pepper. Spoon onto the bread and top with 100 g sliced bocconcini (optional). Garnish with small basil leaves, if liked.

ARTICHOKE AND ROCKET
Combine 8 marinated artichokes, drained well and sliced, 1 crushed clove garlic, 1 teaspoon capers, rinsed and drained, 8 olives, pitted and chopped, 1 tablespoon chopped flat-leaf (Italian) parsley, 1 tablespoon lemon juice and 40 g rocket leaves. Spoon onto the bread.

TUNA AND OLIVE
Drain a 425 g tin tuna in spring water and break the tuna into large flakes. Place in a bowl with 3 tablespoons reduced-fat mayonnaise, 8 large black olives, pitted and chopped, 1 diced tomato, 2 teaspoons lemon juice, 1 tablespoon roughly torn flat-leaf (Italian) parsley and a dash of Tabasco sauce (optional). Gently combine the ingredients so as not to break up the tuna too much, then season to taste. Spoon onto the bread and top with lettuce or rocket leaves.

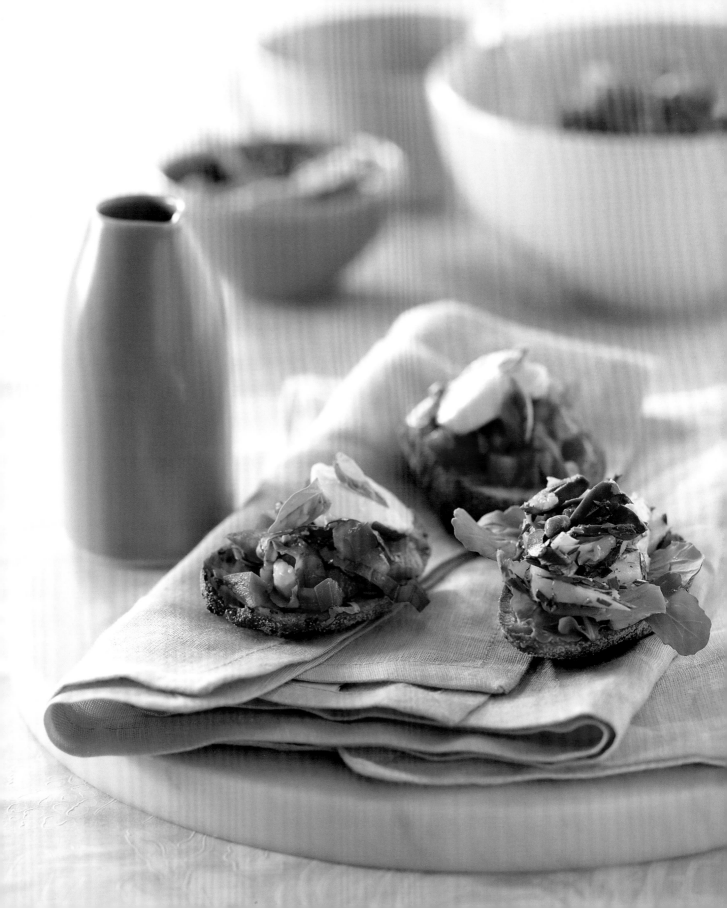

Pinwheel sandwiches

SERVES 4   PREP 15 mins

4 slices wholemeal mountain bread

These attractive sandwiches make a nice change from the traditional version. We've suggested a few fillings below, but try experimenting with your own combinations.

1   Spread your choice of filling (see below) over the bread and roll up tightly. Cut into 2 cm thick slices and serve.

1 SERVE =
½ unit protein
1 unit dairy
½ unit vegetables

SALMON AND RICOTTA

Combine 200 g reduced-fat ricotta, 2 teaspoons horseradish cream, 2 teaspoons lemon juice and 2 tablespoons finely chopped dill or mint in a bowl. Spread over 4 slices mountain bread, top with 200 g smoked salmon and 2 handfuls of baby rocket leaves, and roll up tightly.

1 SERVE =
½ unit protein
1 unit dairy

HAM AND CHEESE

Spread 2 tablespoons Dijon mustard over 4 slices mountain bread and top with 200 g thinly sliced reduced-fat ham and 200 g grated reduced-fat cheddar. Roll up tightly.

1 SERVE =
½ unit protein
(if using hummus or bean dip)
1 unit vegetables

CHARGRILLED VEGETABLE

Spread 1 cup (250 g) grilled eggplant dip (see page 531), hummus (see page 530) or other vegetable dip over 4 slices mountain bread. Top with 4 slices chargrilled eggplant (aubergine), roughly torn, 8 slices chargrilled zucchini (courgette), 1 chargrilled capsicum (pepper), cut into strips, and a scattering of flat-leaf (Italian) parsley. Roll up tightly.

Cucumber bites

SERVES 4   PREP 15 mins

**2 Lebanese (small) cucumbers, cut
into 5 mm thick slices**

**These refreshing nibblies take just minutes to prepare, and the
choice of toppings is limited only by your imagination (and
what you have in the pantry). Below are a few suggestions to
get you started.**

1   Spread your choice of topping (see below) over the cucumber rounds
and serve.

1 SERVE =
¼ unit protein

PRAWN AND WATERCRESS
Combine 200 g chopped cooked prawns, 1–2 tablespoons reduced-fat
mayonnaise, 1 teaspoon lemon juice and a splash of Tabasco sauce in
a bowl. Place at spoonful of the prawn mixture on each cucumber round
and top with a watercress or parsley leaf. Serve with lemon wedges.

1 SERVE =
¼ unit protein
¼ unit dairy

SMOKED SALMON AND RICOTTA
Combine 50 g reduced-fat ricotta and ½ teaspoon grated horseradish
in a bowl. Spread over the cucumber rounds and top with 100 g smoked
salmon, torn into pieces. Garnish with snipped chives.

1 SERVE =
¼ unit protein

OLIVE AND EGG
Spread 2 tablespoons olive tapenade over the cucumber rounds and top
with a slice of hard-boiled egg (you will need 2 hard-boiled eggs for this).
Finish with a grinding of black pepper.

Marinated chicken rice paper rolls

SERVES 4 (makes 8 rolls)   **PREP** 25 mins + marinating and cooling time
COOK 15 mins

400 g skinless chicken breast fillets
8 sheets rice paper
1 cup (80 g) bean sprouts
16 mint leaves
¼ cup loosely packed coriander
   (cilantro) leaves
½ red capsicum (pepper),
   seeded and sliced
1 carrot, cut into sticks

MARINADE
2 tablespoons char siu sauce
   (Chinese barbecue sauce)
1 teaspoon Chinese five-spice powder
2 teaspoons freshly grated ginger
1 teaspoon rice wine vinegar

1 Preheat oven to 180°C.

2 Mix marinade ingredients together in a bowl. Add chicken and toss to coat thoroughly. Cover bowl and allow the chicken to marinate for 10–15 minutes.

3 Transfer chicken to a baking dish and cook for 15 minutes, or until cooked through. Remove from the oven and allow to cool. Slice chicken into long strips and set aside.

4 Fill a large, shallow bowl with cold water. One by one, soak sheets of rice paper in cold water for 2 minutes, then drain and lay on a clean cloth. Divide chicken and remaining ingredients equally among the centres of the rice paper sheets. Tuck in both sides and roll up securely.

5 Serve with a sweet-chilli dipping sauce and a mixed-leaf salad.

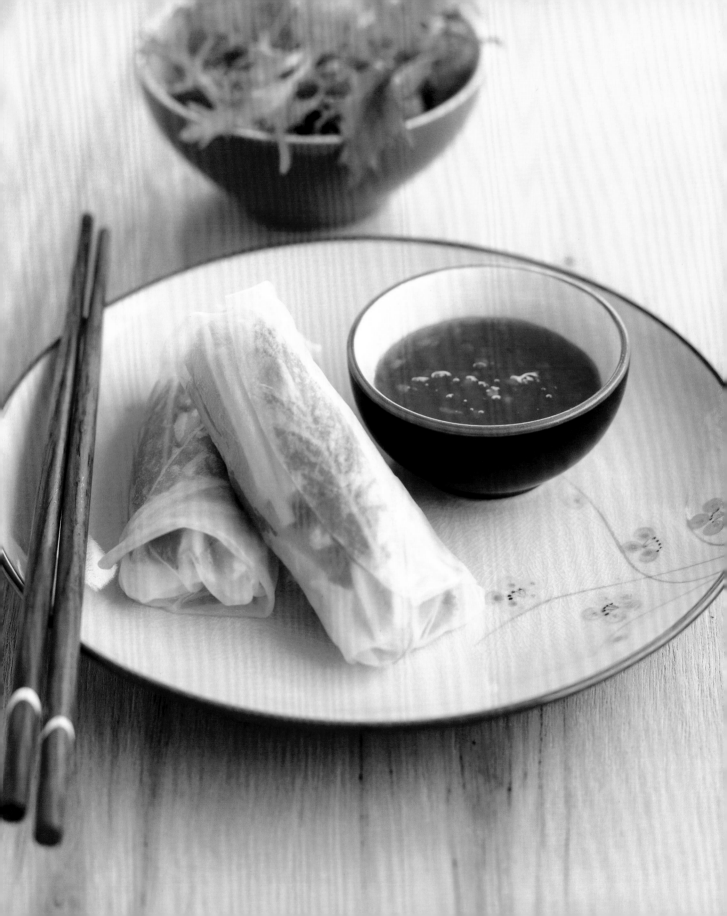

Layered sushi

SERVES 4   PREP 15 mins   COOK 20 mins

1¹/₃ cups (265 g) short-grain rice
¹/₃ cup (80 ml) rice vinegar
3 teaspoons sugar
4 sheets nori
light soy sauce, to serve
wasabi, to serve

Even if you aren't a fan of raw fish, this sushi recipe is still worth trying. There is plenty of scope for designing healthy fillings to suit individual tastes.

1   Steam the rice according to the packet instructions and spread out on a tray while still hot. Combine the vinegar and sugar and pour over the rice, stirring to mix through. Set aside to cool.

2   Lay two sheets of nori on a tray and top each with a quarter of the rice mixture. Layer your choice of filling (see left) over the rice, then top with the remaining rice and another sheet of nori. Press firmly to flatten, then cut into squares with a serrated knife. Cover with plastic wrap and store in the fridge until ready to eat. Serve with soy sauce and wasabi.

TIP Any combination of grated carrot, sliced cucumber, strips of capsicum (pepper), raw or smoked salmon, raw, cooked or tinned tuna, and pickled ginger would make an excellent filling.

1 SERVE =
½ unit dairy
2 units vegetables
1 unit fats

1 SERVE =
1 unit protein
¼ unit vegetables

Stuffed capsicums

SERVES 4   PREP 15 mins + cooling time   COOK 25 mins

1 tablespoon olive oil
1 small onion, finely chopped
2 cloves garlic, crushed
2 large tomatoes, chopped
12 button mushrooms, sliced
150 g baby spinach leaves
1 egg, lightly beaten
1 tablespoon water
4 yellow capsicums (peppers),
   halved lengthways and seeded
40 g grated parmesan
2 tablespoons shredded basil

1 Preheat oven to 180°C.

2 Heat oil in a medium-sized non-stick frying pan over
   high heat. Add onion, garlic, tomato, mushrooms
   and spinach leaves and cook for 5 minutes, or until
   vegetables are soft.

3 Transfer to a bowl and allow to cool slightly. Add
   egg and water, lightly season and stir to combine.
   Spoon mixture into capsicum shells and sprinkle
   tops with parmesan and basil. Place on a baking
   tray and bake for 15–20 minutes, or until capsicum
   is soft and cheese is brown. Serve with salad.

Spicy meatballs with chilli tomato sauce

SERVES 4   PREP 10 mins   COOK 25 mins

**A simplified version of the popular classic dish,
the meatballs are baked in the oven then added
to a homemade sauce to serve.**

400 g lean minced beef or chicken
1 small onion, grated
1 clove garlic, crushed
1 teaspoon ground coriander
1 teaspoon ground cumin
¼ teaspoon ground cinnamon
½ teaspoon chilli powder (or to taste)
1 tablespoon chopped coriander (cilantro)

CHILLI TOMATO SAUCE
1 × 400 g tin chopped tomatoes
1 tablespoon brown sugar
1 tablespoon white wine vinegar
2 small red chillies, seeded and finely chopped

1 Preheat the oven to 180°C and line a baking tray
   with baking paper.

2 Place the beef or chicken, onion, garlic, ground
   spices, chilli powder and chopped coriander in
   a food processor and process until well combined.
   Roll tablespoons of the meat mixture into balls and
   place on the prepared baking tray. Bake for about
   20–25 minutes or until cooked through, turning
   from time to time.

3 Meanwhile, combine the chilli tomato sauce
   ingredients in a saucepan. Bring to the boil, then
   reduce the heat and simmer for 15 minutes or
   until thickened. Season to taste and serve with
   the meatballs.

Stuffed baked tomatoes with bocconcini salad

SERVES 4   PREP 30 mins + draining time   COOK 30 mins

8 firm, ripe tomatoes
¹/₃ cup (65 g) long-grain rice
1 tablespoon olive oil
1 onion, finely chopped
2 cloves garlic, crushed
100 g baby spinach leaves, chopped
8 sun-dried tomatoes, drained of oil
   and chopped
small handful basil leaves
200 g bocconcini, torn into
   small pieces
2–3 tablespoons balsamic vinegar

The summery flavours of the rice filling also work well with red capsicums; just replace the tomato flesh with chopped olives.

1   Using a large sharp knife, slice a lid off each tomato, about 1 cm from the top; reserve the tomato lids. Hollow out the tomatoes with a spoon, placing the seeds and membrane into a sieve placed over a bowl to collect the juices. Leave to drain for 30 minutes, then pour the juice into a jug and top it up with water to make 1 cup (250 ml). Coarsely chop the tomato flesh in the sieve and set aside.

2   Preheat the oven to 180°C.

3   Place the rice and the 1 cup (250 ml) tomato liquid in a small saucepan, then cover and bring to simmering point. Reduce the heat to low and cook for 10 minutes or until the liquid has been absorbed. Meanwhile, heat half the oil in another saucepan, then add the onion and garlic and cook, stirring, for 5 minutes or until softened. Add the spinach and reserved tomato flesh, cover and cook for 2 minutes or until the spinach just starts to wilt. Remove the pan from the heat, add the rice and sun-dried tomatoes and stir to mix well. Season to taste with salt and pepper, then divide the mixture among the tomato shells. Place the stuffed tomatoes in a roasting tin or baking dish and top with the tomato lids. Bake for 20 minutes or until heated through.

4   Place the basil leaves and bocconcini in a bowl, drizzle with the remaining oil and the vinegar and toss to combine. Divide the salad and stuffed tomatoes among plates and serve.

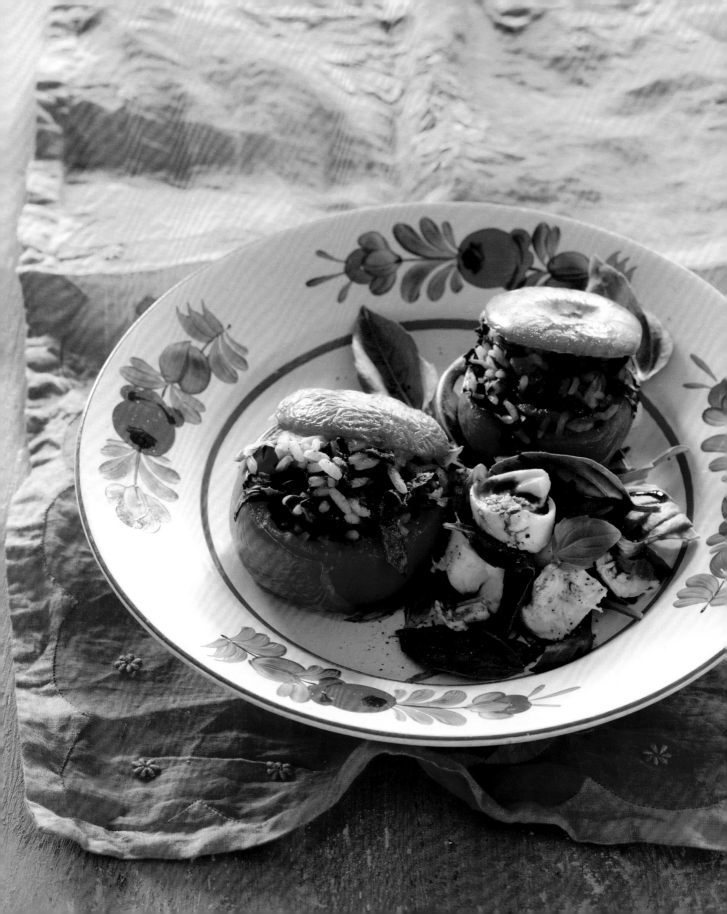

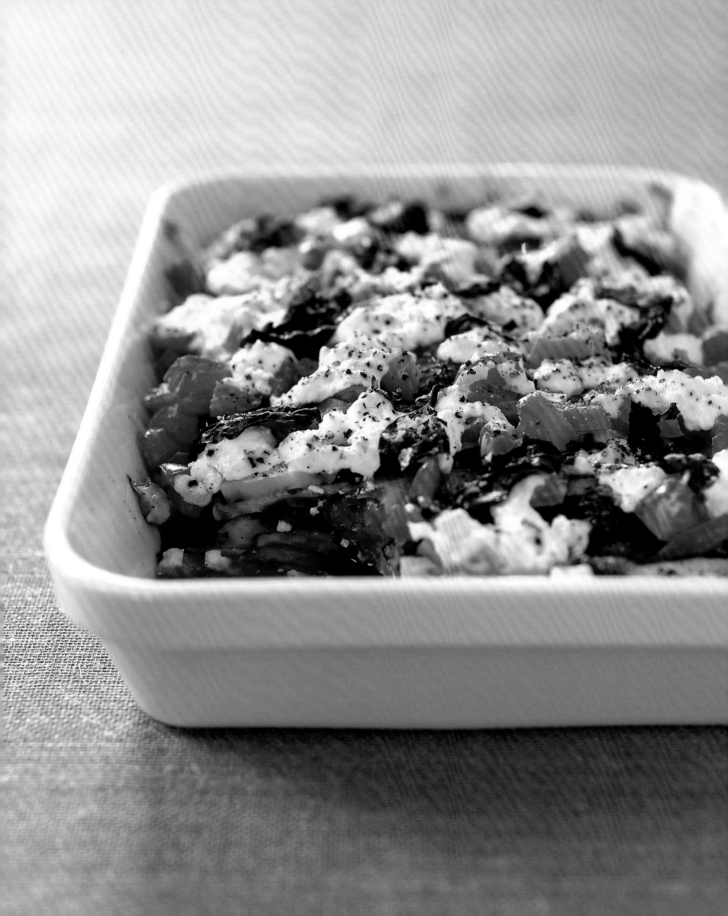

1 SERVE =
1 unit dairy
2 units vegetables
1 unit fats

Baked Mediterranean vegetables with ricotta

SERVES 4   PREP 20 mins + cooling time   COOK 1 hour

1 red capsicum (pepper),
   halved and seeded
1 yellow capsicum (pepper),
   halved and seeded
4 zucchini (courgette), finely
   sliced lengthways
1 eggplant (aubergine), finely sliced
1 tablespoon olive oil
1 clove garlic, crushed
2 red (Spanish) onions, finely sliced
4 Roma (plum) tomatoes, diced
½ cup torn basil
200 g reduced-fat ricotta

1   Heat oven to 180°C.

2   Place capsicums, skin-side up, in a baking dish and drizzle with a little olive oil. Roast for 20 minutes. Remove from oven, cover with foil and allow to cool slightly. Peel off and remove skin and slice flesh into thick strips.

3   Preheat grill plate or barbecue grill to high. In a bowl, toss zucchini and eggplant with half the oil. Grill vegetables until soft.

4   Heat remaining oil in a large non-stick frying pan over high heat. Add garlic and onion and saute until soft.

5   Arrange vegetables, including tomato and basil, in layers in a non-stick baking dish, lightly seasoning every few layers. Crumble ricotta over the top and bake for 30 minutes. Allow to cool for 10 minutes before serving.

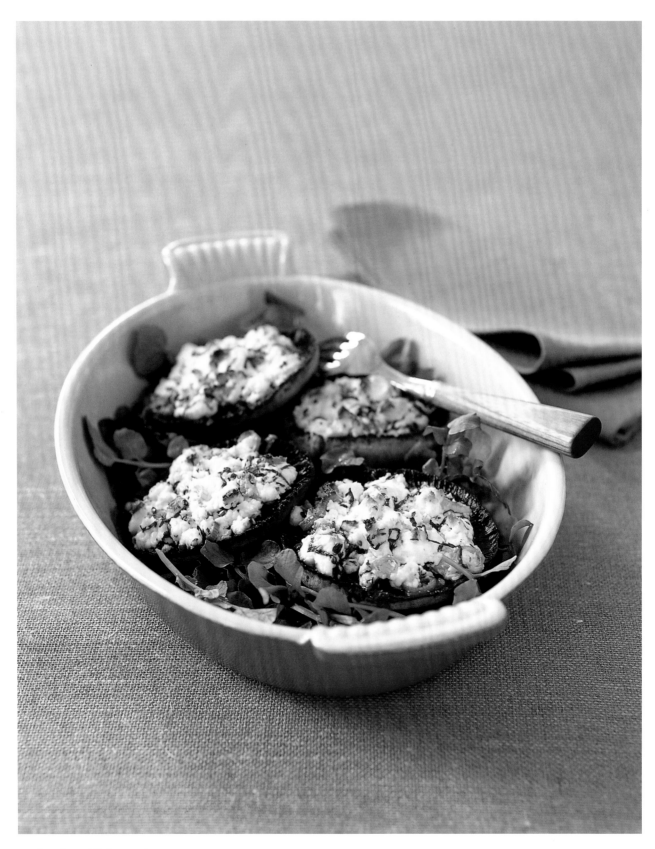

1 SERVE =
1 unit dairy
2 units vegetables
1 unit fats

Baked mushrooms with goat's cheese and watercress

SERVES 4 PREP 25 mins **COOK** 25 mins

8 large field mushrooms,
  stems removed
8 sprigs lemon thyme
1 cup (250 ml) white wine
100 g goat's cheese
4 spring onions (scallions),
  finely sliced
1 tablespoon chopped basil
1 tablespoon olive oil
2 teaspoons balsamic vinegar
1 bunch watercress, washed
  and trimmed

1 Preheat oven to 180°C.

2 Place mushrooms, underside up, in a baking dish. Add thyme, pour over wine and lightly season. Cover with foil and bake for 15 minutes.

3 In a bowl, mix goat's cheese, spring onion, basil and 1 teaspoon of the oil. Spoon mixture evenly onto mushrooms, then bake for a further 10 minutes.

4 Mix together balsamic vinegar and remaining oil. Serve mushrooms with a salad of watercress and balsamic dressing.

Lemon and chilli chicken skewers

SERVES 4 **PREP** 15 mins + marinating time **COOK** 8 mins

1 clove garlic, crushed
¼ cup (60 ml) lemon juice
1 green chilli, seeded
and finely chopped
½ cup (125 ml) buttermilk
400 g skinless chicken breast,
cut into 2 cm cubes

1 In a large bowl, combine garlic, lemon juice, chilli and buttermilk. Add chicken and turn to coat thoroughly. Cover bowl and allow chicken to marinate for 30 minutes.

2 If using bamboo skewers, soak them in hot water for 30 minutes before use.

3 Preheat a grill plate or barbecue grill to high.

4 Thread chicken pieces onto 8 skewers. Grill for 2 minutes each side – 8 minutes in total – or until cooked through.

5 Serve skewers with a large helping of your favourite salad or steamed vegetables.

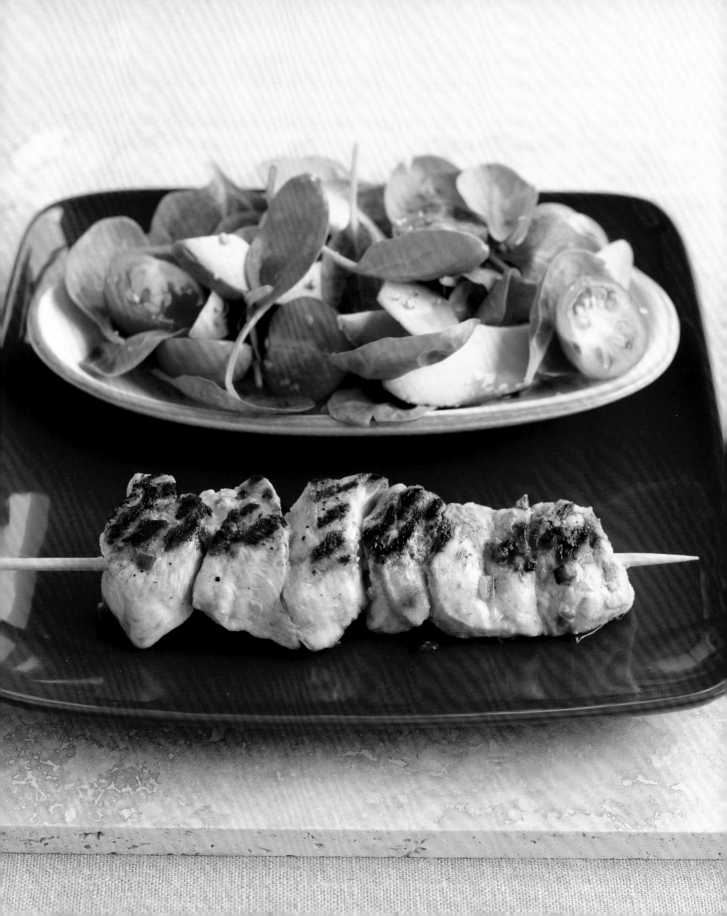

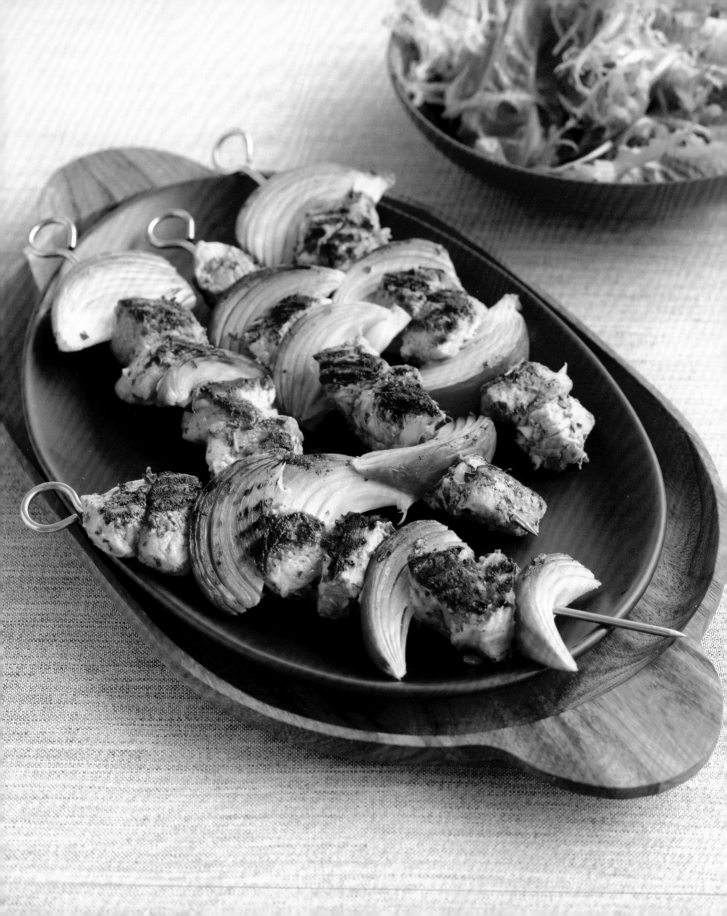

Pork and onion kebabs

SERVES 4   PREP 15 mins + marinating time   COOK 8 mins

400 g pork fillet, cut into 2 cm cubes
2 small red (Spanish) onions,
   cut into wedges

MARINADE
2 tablespoons finely chopped thyme
finely grated zest and
   juice of 1 orange
2 tablespoons olive oil
1 tablespoon honey
1 tablespoon lemon juice
1 clove garlic, roughly chopped

1 Place all marinade ingredients in a large bowl. Add pork and, using a wooden spoon, turn to coat thoroughly. Cover bowl and refrigerate for 1–2 hours.

2 If using bamboo skewers, soak them in hot water for 30 minutes before use.

3 Preheat a grill plate or barbecue grill to high.

4 Thread pork and onion onto 4 long skewers. Grill for 2 minutes each side – 8 minutes in total – or until cooked through. Serve with a mixed-leaf salad.

Vegetable curry

SERVES 4   PREP 10 mins   COOK 25 mins

2 teaspoons vegetable oil
1 onion, chopped
2 cloves garlic, crushed
1 × 3 cm piece ginger, finely grated
½ teaspoon chilli powder
1 teaspoon ground cumin
1 teaspoon ground coriander
1 teaspoon ground turmeric
3 cups (600 g) mixed vegetables,
   diced
1 × 400 g tin chopped tomatoes
1½ teaspoons garam masala
handful of baby spinach leaves
   (optional)
1 tablespoon lemon juice
curry leaves and roughly chopped
   coriander (cilantro), to serve
   (optional)

Serve this curry with grilled meat, poultry or fish from your daily protein allowance. If you opt for a vegetarian option, boost your protein intake by stirring in a 400 g tin of rinsed and drained chickpeas or 400 g diced tofu at step 4. Warm through and serve.

1 Heat the oil in a medium saucepan over medium heat and saute the onion, garlic, ginger, chilli powder, cumin, coriander and turmeric for about 3 minutes or until fragrant.

2 Add any harder vegetables you have selected to use (such as potato, carrot or pumpkin) and stir until combined with the spice mix. Stir in the chopped tomatoes and ½ cup (125 ml) water.

3 Cover and simmer for 10 minutes, then add any remaining softer vegetables (such as eggplant, capsicum, broccoli or zucchini) and cook for a further 10 minutes or until all the vegetables are tender.

4 Stir in the garam masala, spinach (if using) and lemon juice. Season to taste and serve with meat or fish from your daily protein allowance or rice from your daily bread allowance, garnished with curry leaves and coriander (if using).

TIP Select from the following vegetables to use in your curry: potato, cauliflower, pumpkin, beans, zucchini (courgette), eggplant (aubergine), mushrooms, capsicum (pepper), broccoli, peas and corn.

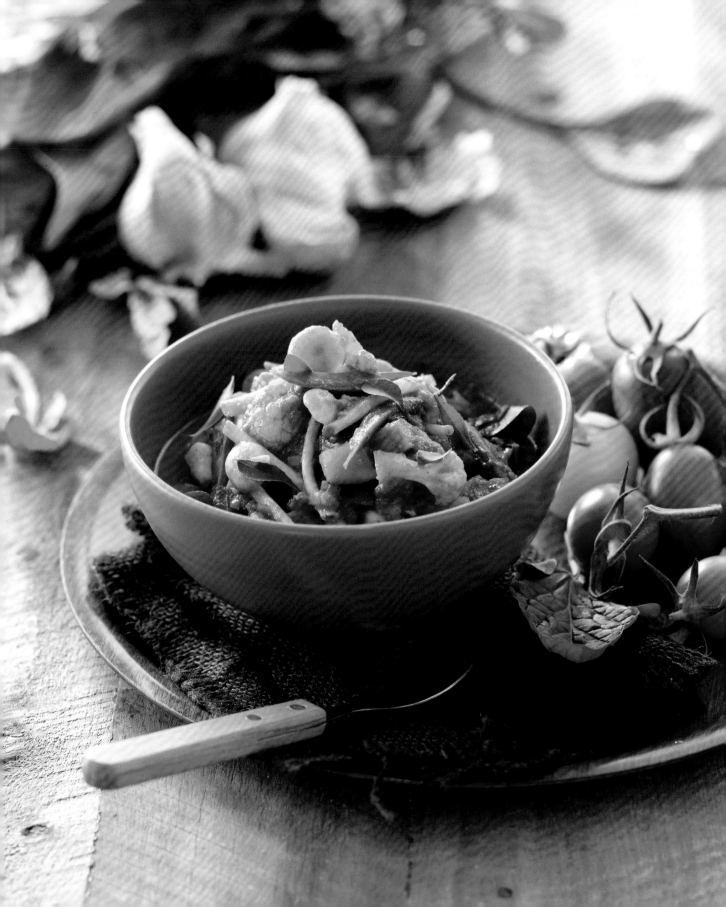

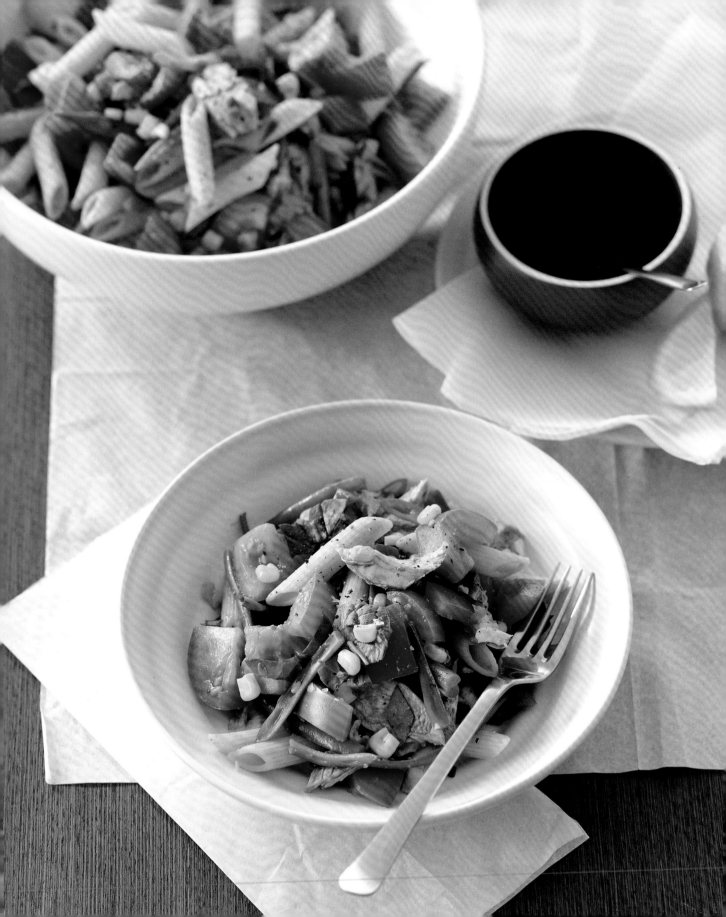

1 SERVE =
1 unit protein
1 unit bread
1 unit vegetables
1 unit fats

Chicken and vegetable pasta salad

SERVES 4   PREP 15 mins   COOK 20 mins

180 g penne (or other short pasta)
1 cup (160 g) frozen corn kernels
200 g green beans, sliced
3 tomatoes, chopped
1 red capsicum (pepper), diced
300 g cooked chicken, diced
2 handfuls of baby spinach leaves

DRESSING
1 teaspoon Dijon mustard
1 clove garlic, crushed
1 tablespoon lemon juice
1 tablespoon balsamic vinegar
1 tablespoon extra virgin olive oil

The dressing for this colourful salad provides a tangy kick that complements the tender chicken and crisp vegetables.

1 Cook the pasta according to the packet instructions. Drain and rinse under cold water to cool.

2 Bring a large saucepan of water to the boil. Add the corn and beans and cook for 1 minute. Drain and refresh under cold water.

3 In a large bowl combine the pasta, corn mix, tomato, capsicum, chicken and spinach leaves.

4 To make the dressing, combine the ingredients in a jar with a screw-top lid. Toss through the salad and serve.

TIP This salad is a great way to use up leftover chicken from a roast, but if you don't have any chicken, use shredded turkey or tinned tuna. It is a natural home for leftover pasta too, or try it with rice. Play around with the flavours and use whatever fresh vegetables you have on hand – peas, asparagus or broccoli are all delicious.

1 SERVE =
1 unit protein
1 unit vegetables
1 unit fats

Salmon salad with tarragon and caper dressing

SERVES 4   PREP 10 mins   COOK 5 mins

100 g green beans
1 × 400 g tin salmon
12 cherry tomatoes, halved
4 spring onions (scallions),
   finely sliced
1 cos (romaine) lettuce,
   torn into pieces

DRESSING
1 tablespoon capers,
   finely chopped
1 tablespoon tarragon,
   finely chopped
2 teaspoons lemon juice
1 tablespoon olive oil

1 Bring a small saucepan of lightly salted water to a boil. Blanch beans for 5 minutes. Drain and cool under cold running water.

2 In a small bowl, mix all dressing ingredients and season to taste.

3 Drain salmon and place in a salad bowl with beans, tomatoes, spring onion and lettuce. Pour dressing over salad, toss well and serve immediately.

VARIATIONS

Salmon goes with many ingredients. Try the following combinations of flavours, or make up your own: tinned salmon, red onion, capsicum, tomatoes and lettuce; tinned or smoked salmon with capers, red onion, asparagus and dill.

Tinned tuna also makes a quick and easy lunch when tossed with other salad ingredients. For example, toss together tinned tuna, celery, tomatoes, cucumber and lettuce and dress with oil-free salad dressing.

Roast beef and beetroot salad

SERVES 4 **PREP** 10 mins

4 cooked beetroots, peeled and quartered
50 g parmesan, shaved
400 g cold roast beef, finely sliced
generous amount of salad greens
   (baby spinach, rocket [arugula],
   cos [romaine], etc)
½ cup basil, torn

DRESSING
2 tablespoons olive oil
1 tablespoon balsamic vinegar
1 clove garlic, chopped
½ teaspoon Equal
1 teaspoon Dijon mustard

1 In a small bowl, whisk together all dressing ingredients.

2 Toss remaining ingredients together in a large bowl. Pour dressing over, toss and season to taste.

Prawn and avocado salad

SERVES 4 **PREP** 20 mins

perfectly for a long weekend lunch. The quantities can easily be doubled if you are feeding a crowd.

75 g mixed lettuce leaves
8 cherry tomatoes, quartered
80 g avocado, halved, seeded and sliced
400 g cooked medium prawns,
   peeled and deveined, tails intact

MUSTARD DRESSING
1 tablespoon extra virgin olive oil
2 tablespoons red wine vinegar
1 tablespoon seeded mustard

1 To make the dressing, combine all the ingredients in a screw-top jar and shake well to combine. Season with a pinch of salt and pepper.

2 Place the lettuce and tomato on serving plates and arrange the avocado slices and prawns on top. Drizzle with the dressing and serve.

TIP Other types of cooked seafood or chicken can be used in place of the prawns, if preferred.

1 SERVE =
1 unit protein
½ unit dairy
1½ units vegetables
1 unit fats

Rosemary lamb with olive and feta salad

SERVES 4   PREP 15 mins + resting time   COOK 10 mins

1 tablespoon chopped rosemary

1 clove garlic, crushed

3 teaspoons redcurrant jelly

400 g lamb fillets, trimmed
   of fat and sinew

1 tablespoon olive oil

12 green olives

100 g reduced-fat feta

2 baby cos lettuces, outer leaves
   discarded, leaves separated

1 bulb fennel, finely sliced

1½ tablespoons oil-free
   balsamic dressing

1 In a small bowl, mix rosemary, garlic and redcurrant jelly. Add lamb and toss to coat thoroughly.

2 Heat oil in a large non-stick frying pan over medium heat. Add lamb and cook for 3 minutes each side, or until done to your liking. Remove lamb from heat, cover with foil and set aside to rest for 5 minutes.

3 In a large bowl, combine olives, feta, cos leaves and fennel. Toss with balsamic dressing and divide among serving plates. Slice lamb thickly on the diagonal and arrange on top of salad.

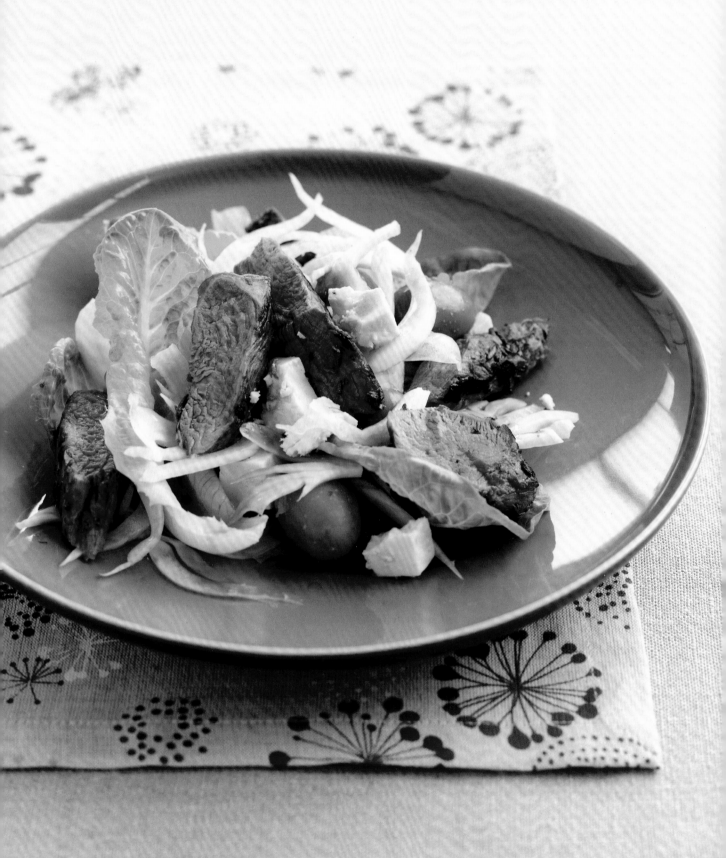

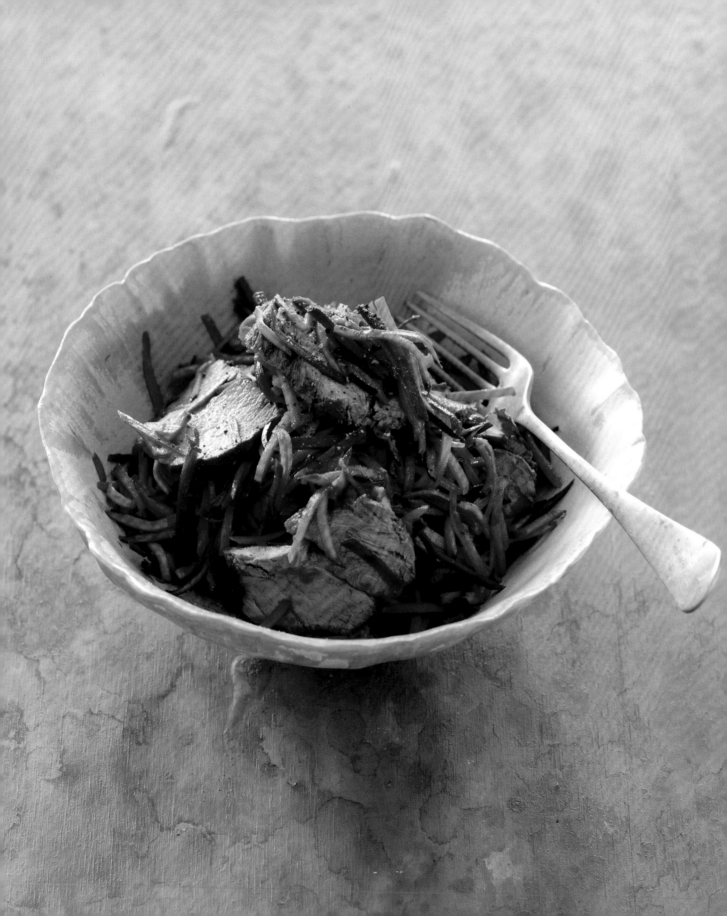

1 SERVE =
1 unit protein
½ unit fruit
2½ units vegetables
1 unit fats

Beef and 'raw energy' salad

SERVES 4   PREP 25 mins   COOK 15 mins

olive oil spray
1 × 400 g piece beef fillet,
    trimmed of fat
2 large beetroots, peeled
    and grated
2 carrots, grated
3 zucchini (courgettes),
    trimmed and grated

DRESSING
⅓ cup (55 g) currants
1 clove garlic, crushed
4 anchovy fillets, drained of oil
    and finely chopped
1 tablespoon Dijon mustard
¼ cup (60 ml) balsamic vinegar
1 tablespoon extra virgin olive oil

The combination of grated vegetables used in this salad makes for a crunchy and refreshing accompaniment to the meat. If you don't have time to cook, use 400 g thinly sliced cold cooked roast beef instead (or you could use cooked lamb, pork or chicken or tinned tuna or salmon).

1 Preheat the oven to 200°C. Spray a small ovenproof frying pan with olive oil and place over medium–high heat. Once hot, add the beef fillet and cook, turning often, for 3–4 minutes or until browned all over. Transfer the pan to the oven and cook for 12–15 minutes for medium–rare or until cooked to your liking. Remove from the oven and leave to cool to room temperature, then thinly slice the beef.

2 For the dressing, place the currants in a small bowl and pour over just enough boiling water to cover. Leave to stand for 20 minutes or until plump, then drain well. Place the currants, garlic, anchovy, mustard, and vinegar in a bowl and whisk to combine well. Add the oil and whisk again, then season to taste with salt and pepper and set aside.

3 Place the beetroot, carrot and zucchini in a large bowl and toss to combine well. Add the beef to the bowl, then drizzle over the dressing and toss to combine. Season to taste, divide among bowls and serve immediately.

1 SERVE =
1 unit protein
½ unit vegetables
1 unit fats

Tandoori chicken salad

SERVES 4 PREP 10 mins + marinating and resting time COOK 15 mins

1½ tablespoons tandoori paste
50 g reduced-fat natural yoghurt
400 g skinless chicken breast
100 g rocket (arugula) leaves
4 Roma (plum) tomatoes,
   thickly sliced
2 Lebanese (short) cucumbers,
   julienne
sprigs of coriander (cilantro)
lemon wedges

DRESSING
150 g reduced-fat natural yoghurt
2½ tablespoons mint sauce
1 tablespoon olive oil
2 tablespoons lemon juice

1 Mix tandoori paste and yoghurt in a bowl. Add chicken, turning to coat thoroughly. Cover and chill for anywhere from 30 minutes to overnight – the longer you leave it, the better the result.

2 Heat a grill plate or non-stick frying pan over high heat and cook chicken for 6 minutes each side, or until cooked through. Set aside for 5 minutes to rest. Cut into strips.

3 Mix all dressing ingredients in a small bowl. Place rocket, tomato and cucumber in a large salad bowl and top with chicken. Drizzle dressing over and serve with coriander sprigs and lemon wedges.

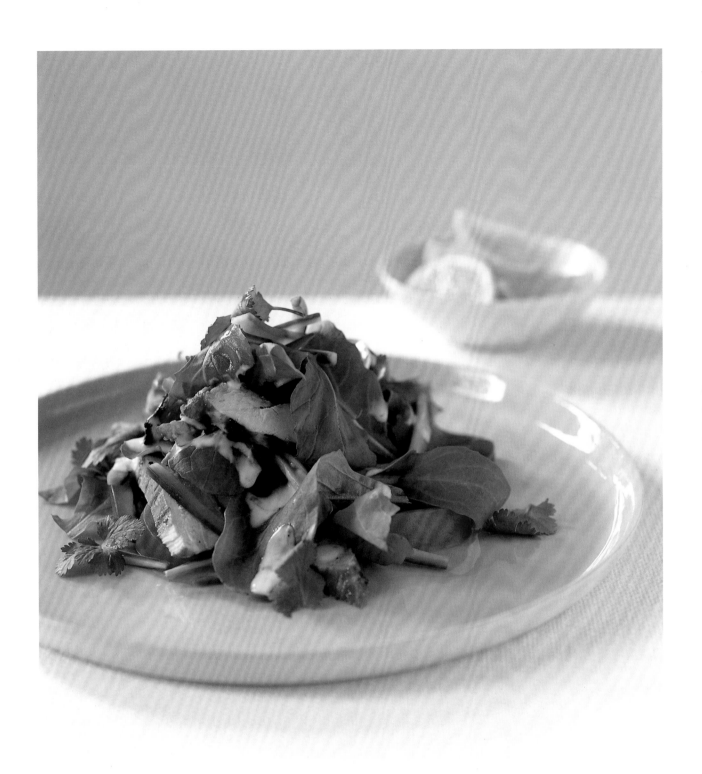

Chicken, corn and bamboo shoot san choy bau

SERVES 4   PREP 30 mins   COOK 15 mins

2 egg whites, beaten
2 teaspoons cornflour
2 × 200 g skinless chicken breast
   fillets, trimmed of fat,
   cut into 5 mm pieces
2 tablespoons salt-reduced
   light soy sauce
2 tablespoons oyster sauce
230 g baby corn, thinly sliced
1 × 3 cm piece ginger, peeled
   and finely chopped
2 cloves garlic, crushed
1 × 225 g tin bamboo shoots,
   drained
4 spring onions, trimmed
   and thinly sliced
3 teaspoons vegetable oil
2 cups (160 g) bean sprouts
iceberg lettuce leaves, to serve
coriander (cilantro) (optional),
   to serve

San choy bau is a classic Chinese dish traditionally featuring pork. Here it is served with chicken, but you could use any meat you like. The stir-fried meat and veg is spooned into the lettuce leaves and then eaten with your hands – the kids will love it! You can find tinned bamboo shoots in the Asian section of most supermarkets.

1 Place the egg white, cornflour and chicken in a bowl and mix with a fork to combine well. Add the soy and oyster sauce and stir to combine, then set aside.

2 Place the corn, ginger, garlic, bamboo shoots and spring onion in a bowl and toss together.

3 Heat a wok over high heat and, when hot, add half the oil and half the vegetable mixture. Stir-fry for 3 minutes or until the onion has just started to soften. Add half the chicken mixture and stir-fry for 4 minutes or until the chicken is cooked through (add a splash of water if the mixture gets a little dry).

4 Place the mixture on a warmed platter and cover loosely with foil to keep warm. Rinse the wok and repeat with the remaining oil, vegetable mixture and chicken mixture.

5 Gently stir the bean sprouts through the mixture, then spoon into lettuce leaves, top with coriander (if using) and serve.

TIP When stir-frying large amounts in a wok, work in batches to ensure that all the ingredients are cooked evenly and fry rather than stew.

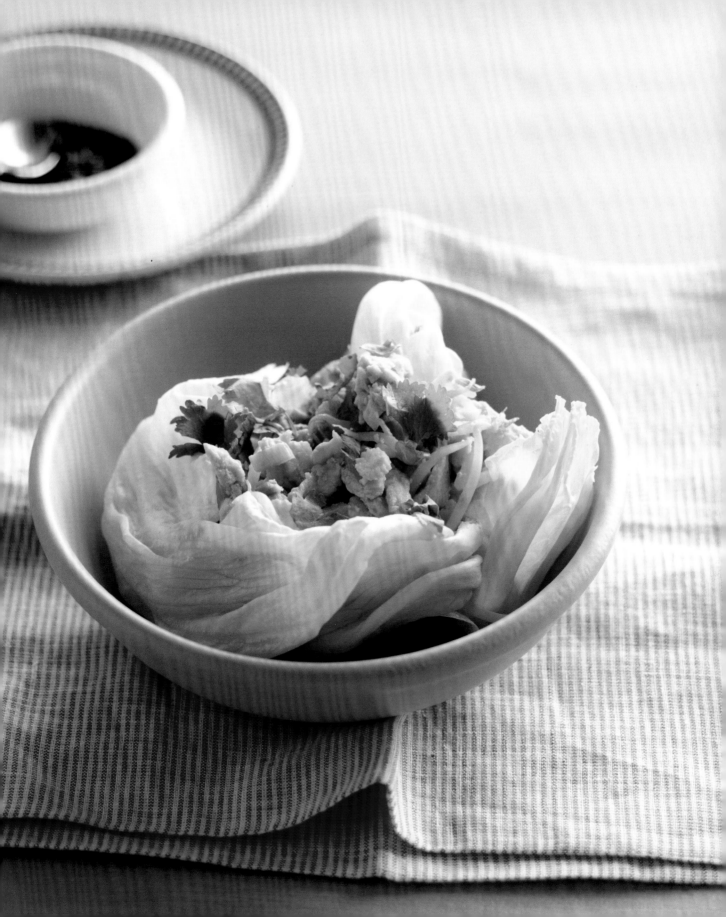

Roast vegetable and couscous salad

SERVES 4   PREP 20 mins   COOK 20 mins

1 cup (150 g) diced pumpkin (squash)
1 red capsicum (pepper), diced
1 zucchini (courgette), diced
1 small eggplant (aubergine), diced
1 tablespoon olive oil
1 cup (250 ml) salt-reduced
   chicken stock
1 cup (200 g) couscous
1 tablespoon lemon juice
3 tablespoons chopped flat-leaf
   (Italian) parsley

A North African staple, couscous is quick and easy to prepare. Store any leftovers in an airtight container in the fridge and enjoy them for lunch the next day.

1 Preheat the oven to 200°C and line a baking tray with baking paper.

2 Combine the pumpkin, capsicum, zucchini and eggplant in a bowl, drizzle with the olive oil and toss to coat. Spread the vegetables in a single layer on the prepared tray and bake for 20 minutes or until tender.

3 Meanwhile, bring the stock to the boil in a medium saucepan over medium heat. Place the couscous in a heatproof bowl and pour on the hot stock, then cover and set aside for 10 minutes. Fluff up the couscous with a fork and transfer to a large salad bowl.

4 Add the roast vegetables, lemon juice and parsley to the bowl and toss through the couscous. Serve warm.

> **TIP** You can easily vary the flavour with different herbs or spices. For instance, add a teaspoon ground cumin to the hot stock, and stir in 3 tablespoons chopped coriander just before serving.

1 SERVE =
1½ units protein
½ unit bread
1½ units vegetables
1 unit fats

Salad niçoise

SERVES 4 **PREP** 15 mins **COOK** 15 mins

300 g potatoes
100 g green beans, trimmed
1 clove garlic, cut in half
1 tablespoon extra virgin olive oil
2 teaspoons white wine vinegar
   or lemon juice
1 teaspoon Dijon mustard
100 g salad leaves
4 tomatoes, cut into wedges
1 × 425 g tin tuna in spring
   water, drained
4 hard-boiled eggs, shelled
   and quartered
50 g chargrilled capsicum
   (pepper), rinsed if in oil
4 tablespoons black olives

This is a simple take on the classic salad originating from the sunny South of France.

1 Boil the potatoes in a saucepan of boiling water for 15 minutes or until tender. Drain, cool then slice.

2 Meanwhile, steam the beans for 2–3 minutes or until tender but still bright green.

3 To prepare a dressing, rub the inside of a glass jar with the cut sides of the garlic clove. Add the olive oil, vinegar or lemon juice and mustard, season with salt and pepper and shake to combine.

4 Divide the salad leaves among four plates. Arrange the potato slices, beans, tomato, tuna, eggs, capsicum and black olives over the top. Drizzle with the dressing and serve immediately.

> **TIP** This is also delicious with seared or poached tuna or salmon. If you have used your bread quota for the day, leave out the potatoes.

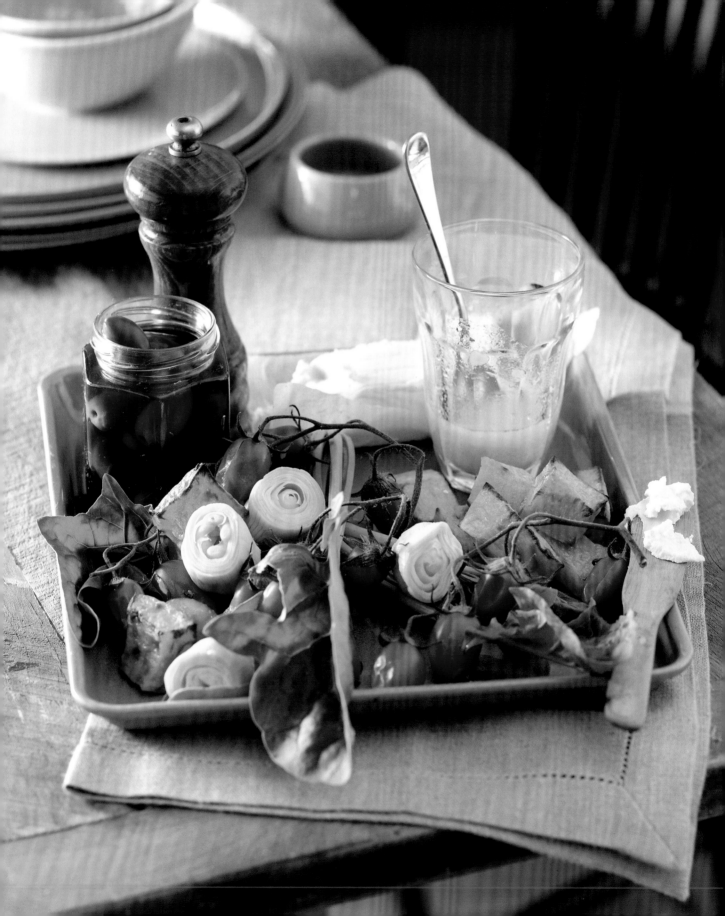

Antipasto salad

SERVES 4   PREP 15 mins   COOK 25 mins

200 g pumpkin (squash),
    peeled and diced
olive oil spray
150 g baby roma (plum)
    tomatoes on the vine
2 tablespoons lemon juice
1 tablespoon extra virgin olive oil
½ teaspoon Dijon mustard
1 clove garlic, crushed
150 g spinach leaves
100 g marinated artichoke hearts,
    drained of all oil
4 tablespoons black olives
100 g goat's cheese, crumbled

This innovative recipe brings together a variety of antipasto favourites, ready for a lunchbox or a comforting meal in a bowl.

1   Preheat the oven to 180°C and line a baking tray with baking paper. Place the pumpkin on the prepared tray and spray with olive oil. Roast for 25 minutes or until golden and cooked through. Add the tomatoes for the last 15 minutes of cooking.

2   Whisk together the lemon juice, olive oil, Dijon mustard and garlic.

3   Arrange the spinach leaves on a serving platter and top with the pumpkin, tomatoes, artichoke hearts, olives and goat's cheese. Pour the dressing over the salad and serve immediately.

TIP The roasted vegetables may be added to the salad when hot or cold.

Rocket, sweet potato and chickpea salad

SERVES 4   PREP 15 mins   **COOK** 25 mins

500 g sweet potato, peeled
   and cut into cubes
olive oil spray
1 tablespoon extra virgin olive oil
2 tablespoons orange juice
1 teaspoon grated orange zest
2 teaspoons white wine vinegar
1 teaspoon balsamic vinegar
1 × 400 g tin chickpeas, rinsed
   and drained
1 red capsicum (pepper), seeded
   and thinly sliced
100 g rocket leaves

This salad can be a fresh and satisfying lunch, and also makes an excellent accompaniment to a summer barbecue.

1   Preheat the oven to 180°C and line a baking tray with baking paper. Spray the sweet potato with olive oil, place on the tray and roast for 20–25 minutes or until golden and tender.

2   Meanwhile, whisk together the olive oil, orange juice, orange zest and both vinegars.

3   Combine the sweet potato, chickpeas, capsicum and rocket in a large bowl. Add the dressing and mix to combine. Season and serve.

TIP The sweet potato can be replaced with pumpkin, and if you don't have any rocket in the crisper, any type of salad leaves would work here.

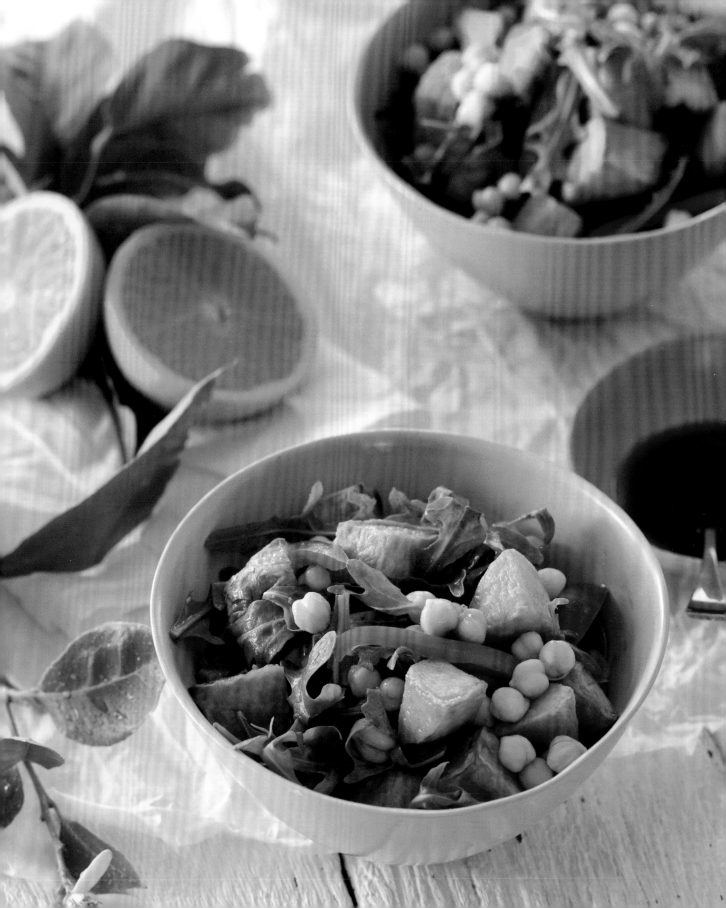

Spicy chicken noodle salad

SERVES 4   PREP 20 mins   COOK 15 mins

400 g chicken breast fillet
100 g rice vermicelli noodles
2 tablespoons lime juice
1 teaspoon brown sugar
1 tablespoon fish sauce
1 small red chilli, finely
  chopped (optional)
¼ Chinese cabbage,
  finely shredded
1 carrot, cut into matchsticks
1 red capsicum (pepper),
  cut into thin strips
1 cup (80 g) bean sprouts
½ cup (25 g) shredded mint
½ cup (25 g) shredded coriander
  (cilantro)
lime wedges, to serve

Spice up the middle of your day with this Asian-inspired concoction. The crisp vegetables add a pleasing crunch, while the herbs bring a freshness to every mouthful.

1 Place the chicken in a small saucepan and cover with water. Bring to the boil over medium heat, then reduce the heat to low and simmer for 10 minutes. Remove the pan from the heat and set aside to cool.

2 Meanwhile, prepare the noodles according to the packet instructions. Drain well.

3 Make a quick dressing by combining the lime juice, sugar, fish sauce and chilli (if using) in a bowl, stirring until the sugar has dissolved.

4 Finely shred the cooled chicken and combine in a large bowl with the noodles, Chinese cabbage, carrot, capsicum, bean sprouts, mint and coriander. Pour the dressing over the top and serve with lime wedges.

TIP If you are taking the salad to school or work for lunch, pack the dressing separately and add it just before eating. This is another great way to use up leftover cooked chicken, or try it with pork.

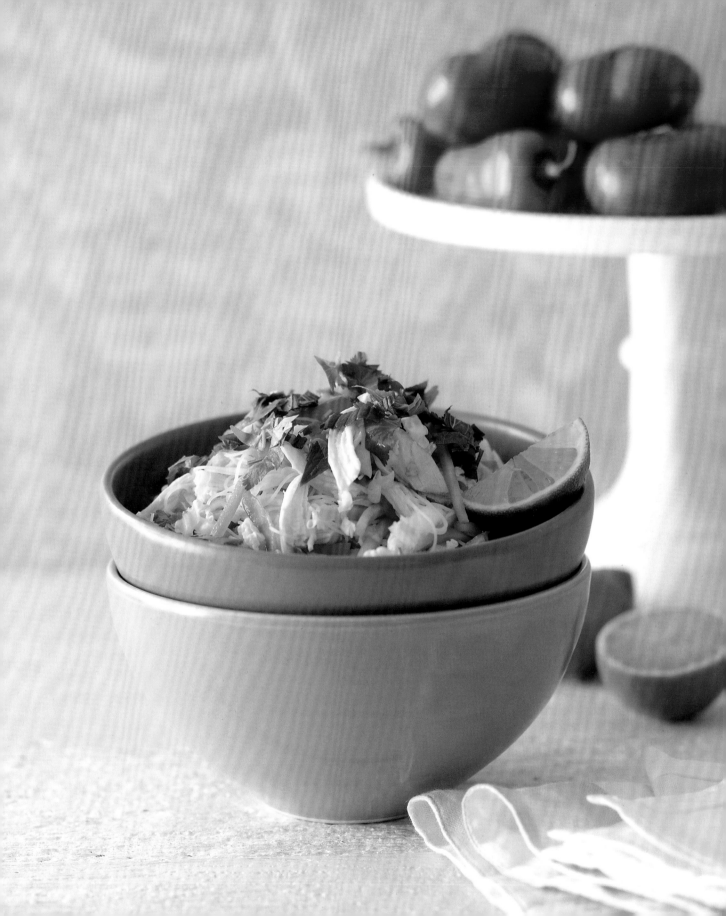

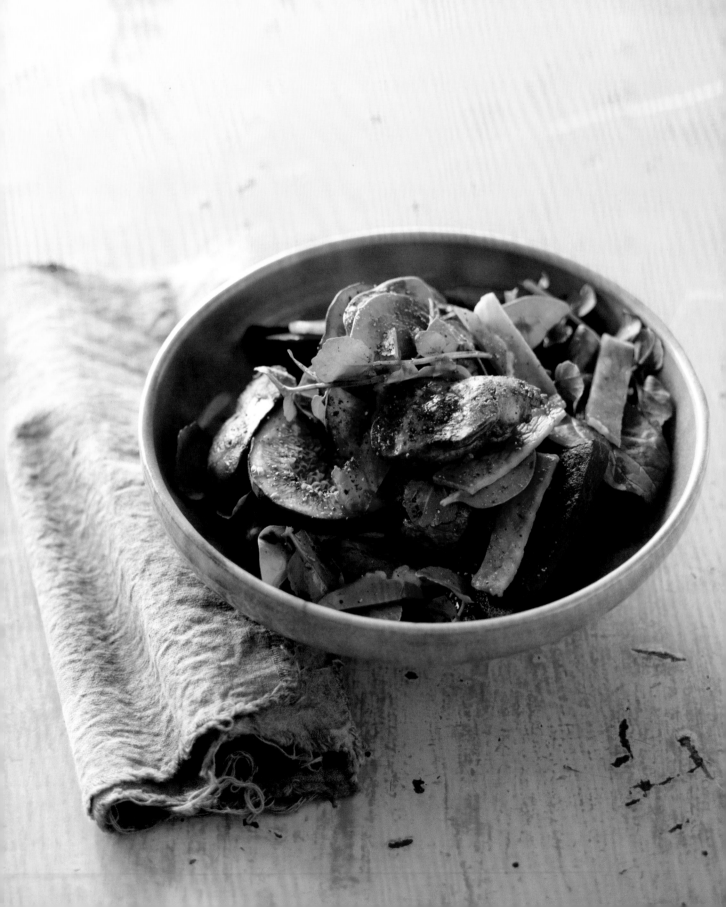

1 SERVE =
1 unit protein
1 unit fruit
1½ units vegetables
1 unit fats

Chicken liver, beetroot, fig and spinach salad

SERVES 4   PREP 15 mins   COOK 10 mins

olive oil spray
100 g lean rindless bacon
300 g chicken livers, trimmed
    and halved
1 × 440 g tin baby beetroot,
    drained and sliced
8 large ripe figs, cut into
    5 mm thick slices
large handful baby spinach leaves
handful watercress sprigs
2½ tablespoons balsamic vinegar
1 tablespoon extra virgin olive oil

Brighten up your lunchtime with this flavoursome salad. Chicken livers are lean, highly nutritious (they are especially high in iron), low in fat and economical – not to mention delicious! The trick is not to overcook them; they should still be a little pink in the middle. Use lean beef or lamb if you prefer. Drained, tinned beetroot is a good substitute for fresh beetroot when time is tight.

1 Heat a large frying pan over medium heat. Once hot, spray with olive oil and add the bacon. Cook, turning once, for 3–4 minutes or until cooked through, then remove from the pan and set aside.

2 Increase the heat to medium–high, add the chicken livers and cook, turning occasionally, for 4–5 minutes or until cooked through but still a little pink in the middle.

3 Cut the bacon into strips, then combine all the ingredients in a large bowl, toss to combine well, and serve.

TIP If you can't get fresh figs, used halved seedless grapes or sliced peaches instead.

1 SERVE =
1 unit protein
1 unit dairy
1 unit fruit
1½ units vegetables
¼ unit fats

Pork and grape waldorf salad

SERVES 4   PREP 20 mins   COOK 20 mins + standing time

olive oil spray
1 × 400 g piece pork fillet,
   trimmed of fat
4 sticks celery, cut into
   thin matchsticks
600 g seedless green grapes, halved
100 g gruyere, cut into small pieces
2 tablespoons reduced-fat
   mayonnaise
2 tablespoons lemon juice
large handful watercress

This salad is a great all-rounder and perfect for when you are having guests for lunch. You could use celeriac instead of celery, when it is in season in winter. Peel the celeriac and cut into very thin matchsticks just before you intend to serve it, as it will discolour quickly.

1 Preheat the oven to 180°C.

2 Heat a non-stick ovenproof frying pan over medium–high heat, then spray the pan with olive oil and add the pork. Cook, turning often, for 3–4 minutes or until golden all over. Transfer the pan to the oven and cook for 7–8 minutes or until the pork is cooked through but still a little pink in the middle. Remove from the oven and leave to cool to room temperature, then slice.

3 Toss the pork in a bowl with all the remaining ingredients. Divide among plates and serve immediately.

Chicken and mango salad

SERVES 4   PREP 15 mins   COOK 10 mins

400 g chicken breast fillet
100 g salad leaves
1 mango, peeled and sliced
1 Lebanese (small) cucumber,
    halved and sliced
½ red (Spanish) onion, thinly sliced
1 tablespoon extra virgin olive oil
2 tablespoons lime juice
½ teaspoon grated ginger
1 teaspoon soy sauce
chopped chilli, to taste (optional)
3 tablespoons roughly chopped
    coriander (cilantro)

The Asian flavours in the dressing bring to life the gently poached chicken and sweet slices of mango.

1 Place the chicken in a small saucepan and cover with water. Bring to the boil over medium heat, then reduce the heat to low and simmer gently for 10 minutes. Remove the pan from the heat and set aside to cool, then shred the meat.

2 Arrange the salad leaves on a serving platter or indivdual plates and top with the chicken, mango, cucumber and onion.

3 Whisk together the olive oil, lime juice, grated ginger, soy sauce and chilli (if using). Pour the dressing over the salad and sprinkle with coriander.

1 SERVE =
1 unit protein
1 unit bread
2 units dairy
1 unit vegetables
½ unit fats

Chicken caesar salad

SERVES 4   PREP 15 mins   COOK 16 mins + standing time

olive oil spray
2 × 200 g skinless chicken
   breast fillets
140 g day-old baguette,
   very thinly sliced
4 baby cos lettuces, tough outer
   leaves removed
200 g parmesan, shaved
16 anchovy fillets, drained of oil
½ cup (125 ml) reduced-fat
   mayonnaise

A delicious version of a classic recipe that makes for a wonderful light lunch. Use cooked turkey or prawns instead of chicken if you like.

1   Preheat the oven to 200°C.

2   Heat a non-stick ovenproof frying pan over medium–high heat. Once hot, spray with olive oil, add the chicken breasts and cook for 1 minute. Turn the chicken breasts over, add 2 tablespoons water to the pan, then cover tightly with foil and transfer to the oven to cook for 15 minutes. Remove the pan from the oven and leave to stand, covered, for 30 minutes or until the chicken has cooled to room temperature. Using your fingers, coarsely shred the meat or cut into bite-sized pieces, then set aside.

3   Meanwhile, lower the oven temperature to 180°C. Place the baguette slices in a single layer on a baking tray and bake for 10 minutes or until golden and crisp. Remove from the oven and set aside. When cool enough to handle, use your hands to break the toast into smaller pieces.

4   Combine the chicken, lettuce, two-thirds of the parmesan, the anchovy, mayonnaise and toast pieces in a large bowl. Using your hands, gently mix to combine well. Divide among bowls, scatter over the remaining parmesan and serve immediately.

TIP Halve the amount of parmesan if you want to use just 1 unit of dairy here.

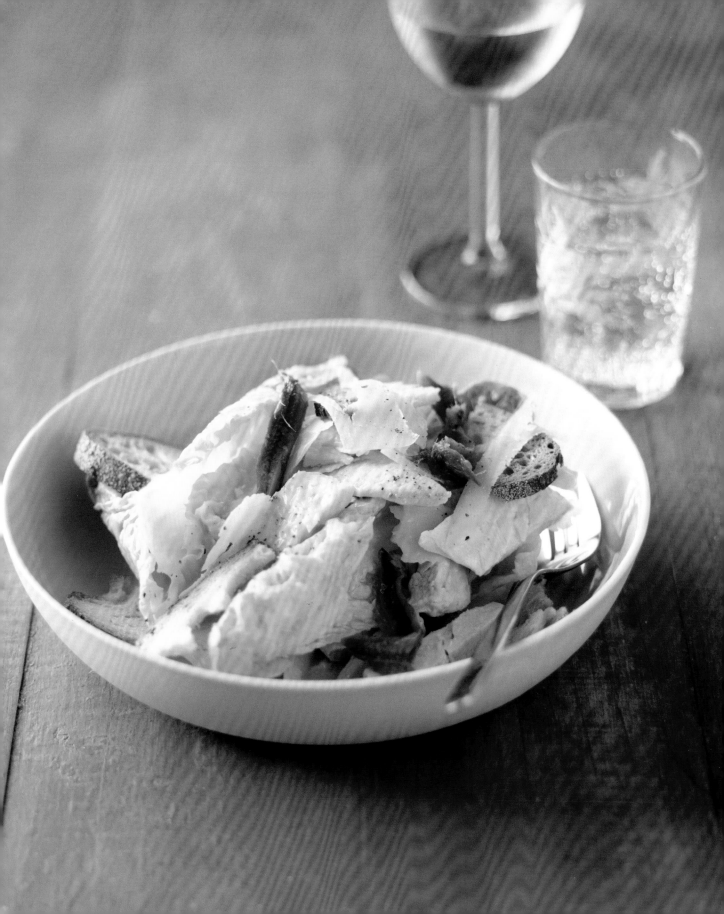

1 SERVE =
1 unit protein
¼ unit dairy
1½ units vegetables

Warm lamb salad with yoghurt dressing

SERVES 4   PREP 15 mins   COOK 6 mins

400 g lamb backstraps, trimmed
olive oil spray
200 g reduced-fat Greek-style yoghurt
grated zest and juice of ½ lemon
1 clove garlic, crushed
1 tablespoon finely chopped mint
250 g grape or cherry tomatoes,
   halved
100 g rocket leaves
1 roasted red capsicum
   (pepper), sliced

Enjoy all the flavours of traditional Greek cuisine in one easy-to-prepare salad.

1 Heat a chargrill or frying pan over high heat. Season the lamb backstraps and spray with olive oil. Cook for 3 minutes each side or until cooked to your liking, then set aside to rest.

2 Whisk together the yoghurt, lemon zest and juice, garlic and mint until smooth. Season to taste.

3 Combine the tomatoes, rocket and capsicum on a large serving platter. Slice the lamb and toss through the salad. Serve with the yoghurt dressing.

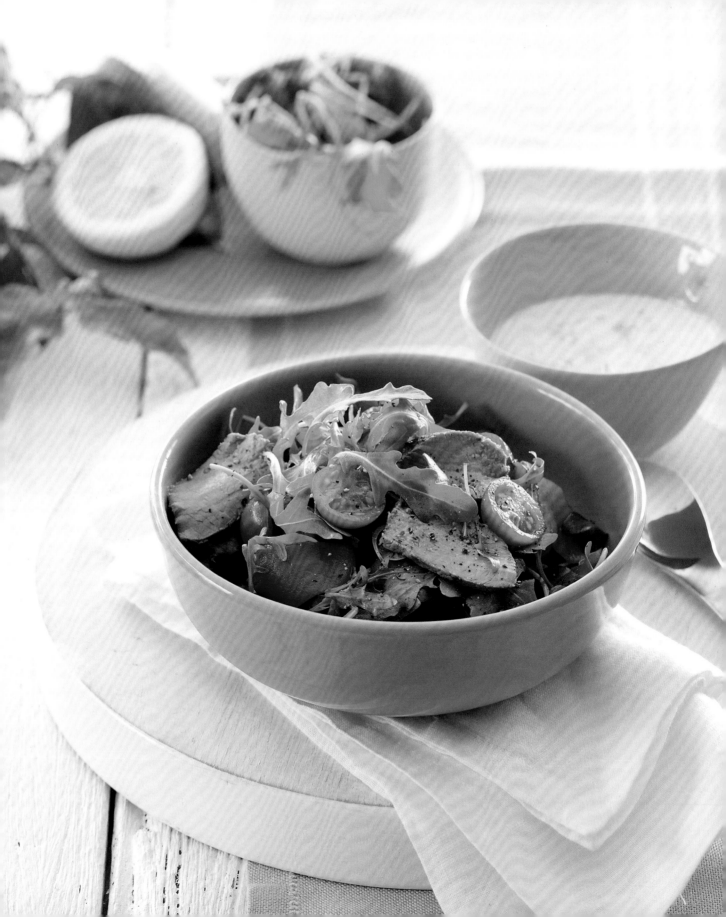

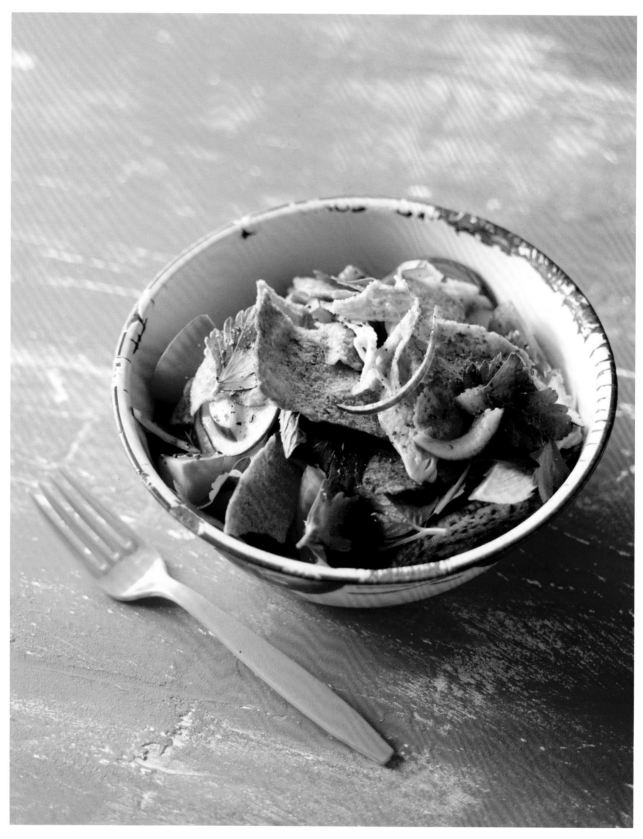

Chicken fattoush

SERVES 4   PREP 20 mins   COOK 15 mins + standing time

olive oil spray
2 × 200 g skinless chicken
    breast fillets
4 × 35 g Lebanese breads
300 g cherry tomatoes, halved
1 large cucumber, halved lengthways,
    then each half thinly sliced
1 red (Spanish) onion, thinly sliced
1 bunch radishes, trimmed
    and thinly sliced
large handful mint leaves (optional)
large handful flat-leaf (Italian)
    parsley leaves (optional)
¹/₃ cup (80 ml) lemon juice
1 tablespoon extra virgin olive oil
1 teaspoon dried chilli flakes,
    or to taste

Fattoush is a Middle Eastern salad that is light and refreshing for lunch and very quick to make. It's also a great way to use up slightly stale Lebanese bread.

1   Preheat the oven to 200°C.

2   Heat a non-stick ovenproof frying pan over medium–high heat. Once hot, spray with olive oil, add the chicken breasts and cook for 1 minute. Turn the chicken breasts over, add 2 tablespoons water to the pan, then cover tightly with foil and transfer to the oven to cook for 15 minutes. Remove the pan from the oven and set aside for 30 minutes or until the chicken has cooled to room temperature.

3   Meanwhile, using a large serrated knife or your hands, open out each piece of bread and split into two rounds. Place the eight rounds on baking trays and bake for 20 minutes or until crisp. When cool enough to handle, break into large pieces and place in a bowl with the tomato, cucumber and onion. Toss to mix well.

4   Slice the chicken on the diagonal into thin slices, then add to the bowl. Add the remaining ingredients, toss to combine well, then divide among bowls and serve immediately.

TIP If you want to make this salad even more substantial, add 100 g crumbled reduced-fat feta from your dairy allowance.

1 SERVE =
1 unit protein
1 unit bread
1½ units vegetables
1 unit fats

Pumpkin, lentil, rocket and beef salad

SERVES 4   PREP 15 mins   COOK 30 mins

1 kg pumpkin (squash),
   peeled, seeded and cut
   into bite-sized pieces
2 × 200 g beef steaks, such
   as sirloin, trimmed of fat
1 × 400 g tinned lentils, drained
small handful basil leaves
large handful baby spinach leaves
2 tablespoons balsamic vinegar
1 tablespoon extra virgin olive oil
2 tablespoons tapenade

This earthy salad has something to please everyone and is a great lunch option. Use pitted black olives instead of the tapenade if you like.

1 Preheat the oven to 180°C. Spray a roasting tin with olive oil, toss in the pumpkin pieces and roast for 30 minutes or until tender and golden. Set aside to cool slightly.

2 Meanwhile, heat a chargrill plate or heavy-based frying pan over medium–high heat. Spray the steaks lightly with olive oil, then cook for 3 minutes on each side for medium–rare or until cooked to your liking. Remove from the heat and leave to rest, covered, for 5 minutes, before slicing thickly.

3 Place all the ingredients, except the tapenade, in a large bowl and toss gently to combine well. Divide among bowls or plates, then add a spoonful of tapenade and serve immediately.

TIP Add 75–100 g blanched green beans per person to increase the vegetable content.

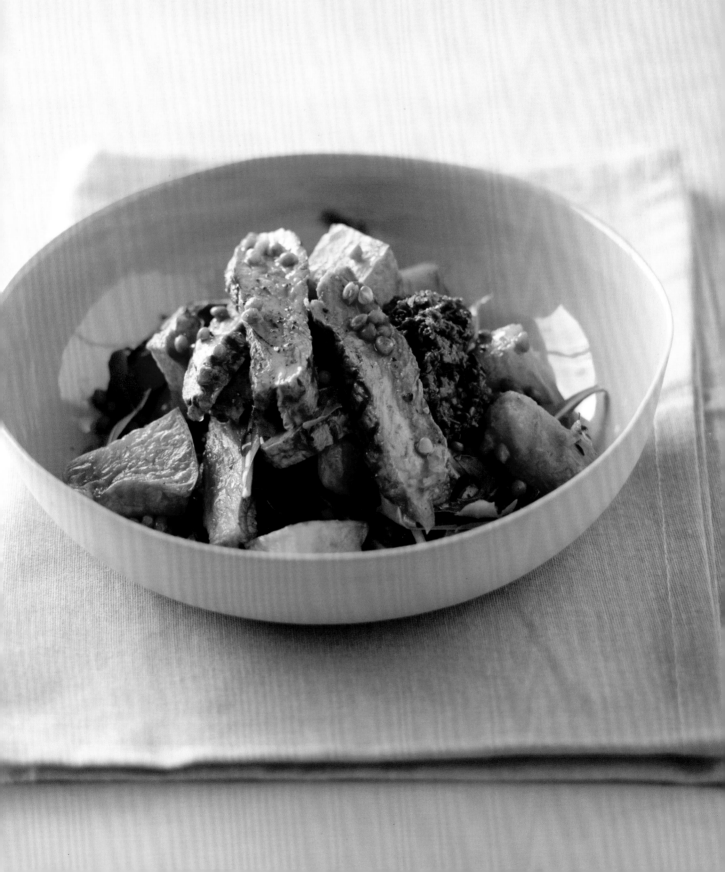

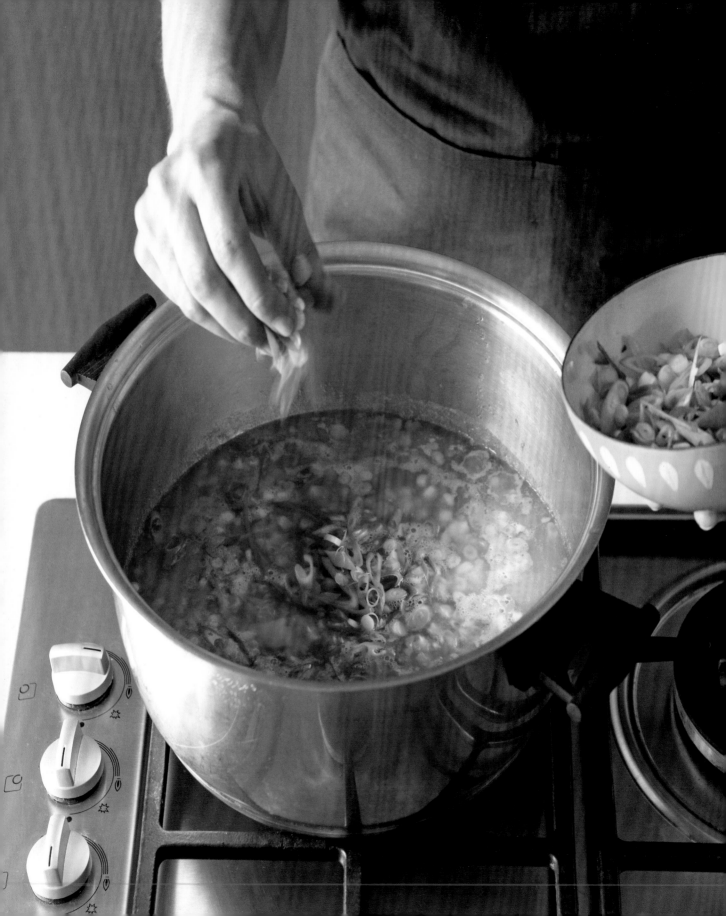

soups

Chinese master stock

MAKES 2 LITRES **PREP** 10 mins **COOK** 35 mins

1 cup (250 ml) light soy sauce
1 cup (250 ml) Chinese cooking wine
3 cloves garlic, peeled
1 × 4 cm piece ginger, julienne
3 spring onions
2 sticks cinnamon
4 star anise
2 tablespoons brown sugar
3 strips orange zest

This is a very handy base to have on hand in your freezer. It can be used repeatedly for poaching meat – just follow the instructions in step 3 to keep the stock fresh and flavoursome for each use.

1 Combine all the ingredients in a large saucepan with 2 litres water. Bring to the boil, then reduce the heat and simmer for 30 minutes.

2 The stock can now be used to poach a whole chicken or cuts such as chicken thigh or leg.

3 After every use bring the stock to the boil, then strain and allow to cool. Freeze in an airtight container. When you're ready to use it again, allow it to thaw then top it up to 2 litres with water. Add fresh garlic, ginger and spring onions each time you reuse the stock, and fresh spices every second time.

TIP To poach a whole chicken or chicken pieces, bring the stock to a simmer and gently drop the chicken into the liquid. Bring to the boil, then reduce heat to a simmer and cook for 20 minutes or until chicken is cooked through. Remove from the heat then cover and allow the chicken to cool in the stock. Strip the chicken from the bone and serve cold in a salad or hot with steamed Asian greens.

1 SERVE =
2 units protein
½ unit bread
1 unit vegetables*
* or 2 units with serving suggestion

Scotch broth

SERVES 4   **PREP** 20 mins   **COOK** 2 hours

½ cup (100 g) pearl barley
1 kg lamb neck chops, trimmed of fat
2 cups (500 ml) salt-reduced
   beef stock
1 onion, chopped
1 leek, white part only,
   finely sliced and washed
1 carrot, diced
1 parsnip, peeled and diced
1 swede, peeled and diced
1 cup (80 g) shredded cabbage
½ cup (60 g) frozen peas
roughly chopped flat-leaf (Italian)
   parsley, to serve

With no fat units, and filled with tasty vegetables, this hearty and healthy meal is just the thing when you're trying to be extra good.

1 Place the barley in a large bowl, cover with cold water and set aside to soak.

2 Place the lamb in a large saucepan with 1.5 litres water. Bring to the boil, then reduce the heat and simmer, uncovered, for 45 minutes, skimming the surface as required.

3 Drain the barley and add to the lamb with the stock, onion, leek, carrot, parsnip and swede. Cover and simmer for 45 minutes.

4 Remove the lamb with a pair of tongs and add the cabbage and peas to the broth. Cook for a further 10 minutes. When the lamb has cooled slightly, remove the meat from the bones, then roughly chop it and return it to the broth (discard the bones). Stir in the parsley, season to taste and serve with extra steamed vegetables.

TIP This will be more than enough broth for four people and can yield eight lunch-sized servings, so freeze any leftovers in meal-sized portions for a later date.

Vietnamese beef broth

SERVES 4 **PREP** 15 mins **COOK** 20 mins

1 litre salt-reduced beef stock

2 slices ginger

1 clove garlic, sliced

1 stalk lemongrass, lightly
  crushed with a knife

4 star anise

1 cinnamon stick

1 tablespoon fish sauce,
  plus extra to serve

1 tablespoon lime juice

1 teaspoon sugar

1 onion, thinly sliced

1¹/₃ cups (200 g) cooked rice noodles

400 g rump steak, trimmed of fat
  and thinly sliced

4 spring onions, finely sliced

½ cup (40 g) bean sprouts

large handful of Vietnamese mint
  or mint leaves

large handful of coriander
  (cilantro) leaves

lime wedges, to serve (optional)

Also known as beef pho, this broth packs in a lot of flavour. The stock is hot enough to cook the thinly sliced beef in the serving bowls, so there is no need to cook it separately.

1 Combine the stock, ginger, garlic, lemongrass, star anise, cinnamon, fish sauce, lime juice, sugar and onion in a saucepan and bring to the boil. Reduce the heat and simmer gently for about 15 minutes. Strain the broth, discarding the spices.

2 Divide the noodles among four serving bowls and top with the beef slices. Pour over the hot broth, then add the spring onion, bean sprouts and herbs. Serve with extra fish sauce and lime wedges, if you like.

TIP Vietnamese mint has a strong peppery flavour and is widely available. If you can't find it, use regular mint instead. You can replace the rice noodles with any other type of thin noodles; for example, egg noodles.

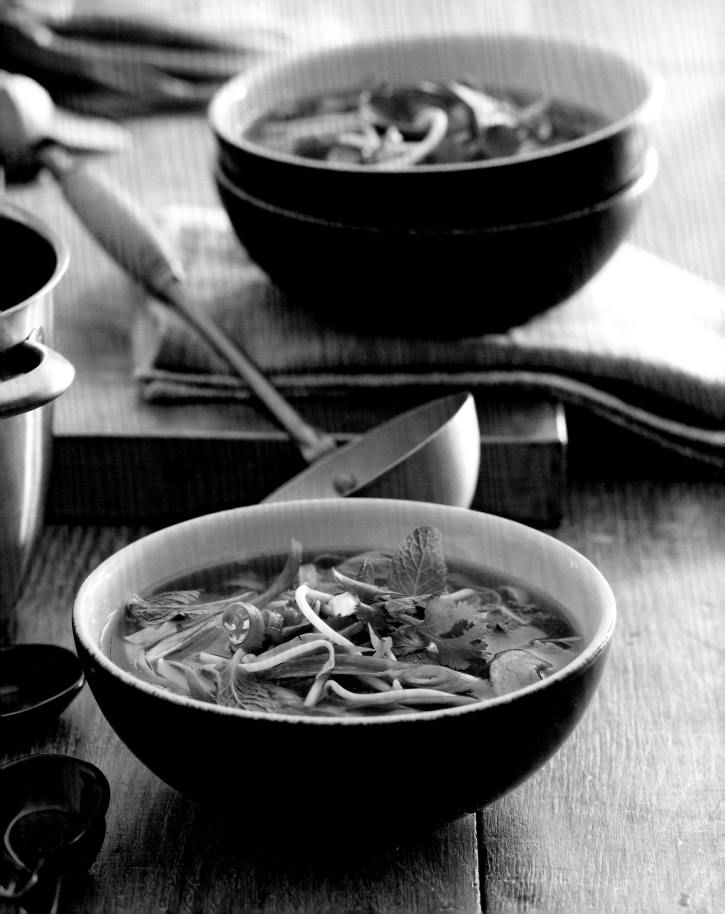

Light vegetable soup

SERVES 4 **PREP** 10 mins **COOK** 30 mins

1 litre good-quality vegetable stock
2 carrots, sliced
2 sticks celery, chopped
1 onion, chopped
¼ cup roughly chopped parsley
1 × 400 g tin crushed tomatoes
¼ cup finely shredded basil
1 tablespoon rosemary, finely chopped

1 Bring stock to a boil in a large saucepan. Add carrot, celery, onion, parsley and tomato and simmer gently for 30 minutes.

2 Stir through basil and rosemary and season to taste.

BEEF SOUP

1 SERVE = 1 unit protein, 1 unit vegetables

To make beef soup, add 400 g diced beef with the vegetables, parsley and tomato. Simmer for 1 hour, or until beef is tender.

Spiced red lentil and vegetable soup

SERVES 4 **PREP** 10 mins **COOK** 40 mins

2 teaspoons olive oil
1 carrot, roughly chopped
1 onion, roughly chopped
2 sticks celery, roughly chopped
1 clove garlic, crushed
1 tablespoon freshly grated ginger
1 cup (200 g) dried red lentils
2 teaspoons garam masala
½ teaspoon chilli powder
1 × 400 g tin tomatoes
1 litre water
freshly ground black pepper
⅓ cup chopped coriander (cilantro)
⅓ cup chopped flat-leaf (Italian) parsley
⅓ cup (95 g) reduced-fat natural yoghurt

1 Heat oil in a heavy-based saucepan over medium heat. Add carrot, onion and celery and cook for 5 minutes, or until vegetables are soft. Add garlic, ginger, lentils and spices and stir to combine. Add tomatoes and water and bring to a boil. Reduce heat and simmer for 30 minutes, or until lentils are soft. Season with pepper and stir through coriander and parsley. Spoon into bowls and serve with a dollop of yoghurt.

Mushroom, spinach and white bean soup

SERVES 4   PREP 20 mins   COOK 25 mins

1 tablespoon olive oil
1 onion, finely chopped
2 cloves garlic, crushed
600 g field mushrooms,
    finely chopped
3 sprigs thyme
large pinch ground nutmeg
2 cups (500 ml) salt-reduced
    chicken or vegetable stock
1 × 400 g tin cannellini beans,
    rinsed and drained
100 g baby spinach leaves,
    chopped
2 tablespoons chopped
    chives (optional)

This is a great soup for lunch on a winter's day. You could use drained tinned lentils instead of white beans, or you could omit the pulses altogether if you'd prefer not to dip into your bread allowance – the recipe will work just as well.

1   Heat the olive oil in a large saucepan over medium heat. Add the onion and garlic and cook, stirring, for 5 minutes or until softened. Add the mushrooms and thyme, then cover and cook, stirring occasionally, for 10 minutes or until the mushrooms are very soft. Add the nutmeg and stock and bring to simmering point, then reduce the heat to low–medium and cook for 2–3 minutes. Discard the thyme sprigs.

2   Puree the soup in a blender or food processor, or in the pan with a stick blender, then return to the stove over low–medium heat. Stir in the cannellini beans and spinach and season to taste, then cover and cook for 3–4 minutes or until the spinach has wilted and the beans have heated through.

3   Divide the soup among warmed bowls, sprinkle with chives (if using) and serve immediately.

TIP For a smoother soup, add the beans before you puree the mixture.

Tomato and watermelon gazpacho with mint and feta

SERVES 4   PREP 10 mins + refrigerating time

2 large tomatoes, chopped
1 red capsicum (pepper), trimmed,
    seeded and chopped
½ red (Spanish) onion, chopped
600 g peeled and chopped
    seedless watermelon
2½ teaspoons red wine vinegar,
    or to taste
½ cup (100 g) reduced-fat feta,
    crumbled
ice cubes, to serve (optional)
mint leaves, to garnish (optional)
crispbread, to serve

This is extremely quick and easy, and makes a fabulous lunch served with 100 g per person grilled lean chicken or pork, or cold meat alongside.

1 Working in batches if necessary, combine the vegetables and watermelon in a blender or food processor and process until smooth.

2 Transfer to a bowl, then stir in the vinegar. Season to taste, adding more vinegar if desired, then refrigerate until well chilled.

3 Divide the soup among bowls. Add the feta and ice cubes (if using), then season with pepper and scatter with mint leaves (if using). Serve with crispbread alongside.

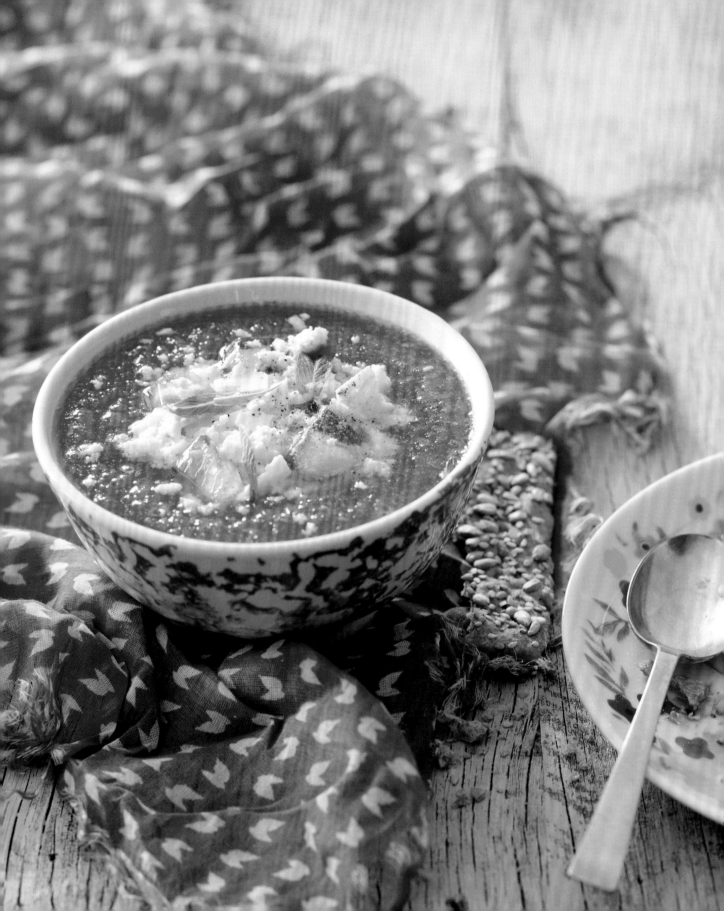

Roast red capsicum and tomato soup

SERVES 4 **PREP** 20 mins **COOK** 45 mins

2 red capsicums (peppers),
   halved and seeded
2 tablespoons olive oil
1 large onion, finely sliced
2 cloves garlic, crushed
1 tablespoon tomato paste
750 g ripe tomatoes,
   roughly chopped
2 cups (500 ml) vegetable stock
1 tablet Equal (optional)
1 handful basil, torn

1 Preheat oven to 180°C.

2 Place capsicums in a shallow baking dish skin-side up and drizzle with half the oil. Roast for 25 minutes, or until softened. Remove from oven, then cover with foil and allow to cool slightly. Peel off and discard skin and roughly chop flesh.

3 Heat remaining oil in a large saucepan over medium heat. Add onion and saute until soft. Add garlic and tomato paste and cook for 2 minutes, stirring constantly. Add capsicum, tomato and stock, then cover and simmer for 15 minutes.

4 Allow to cool slightly, then puree using a blender or hand-held processor. Season to taste. For a sweeter soup add Equal.

5 Reheat soup and serve sprinkled with basil.

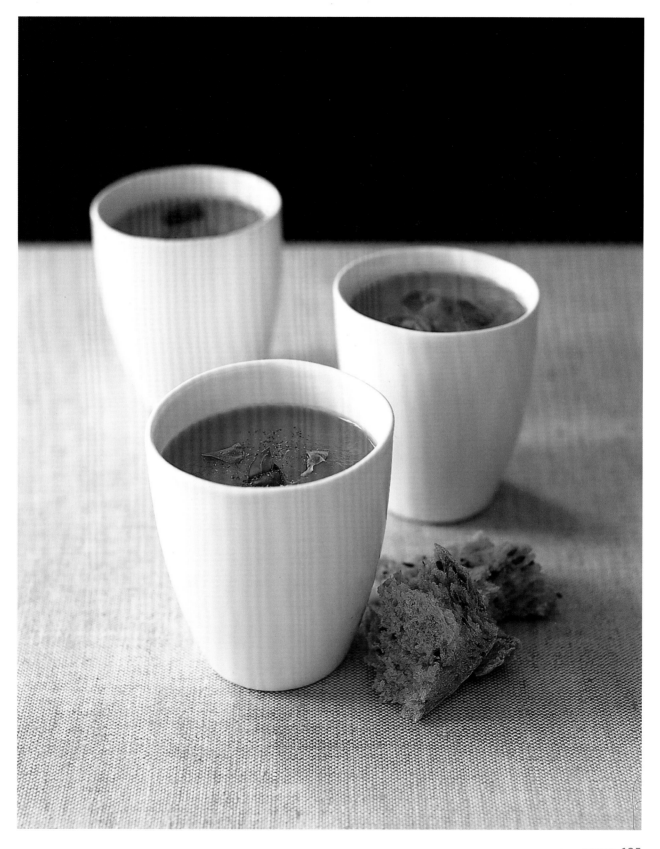

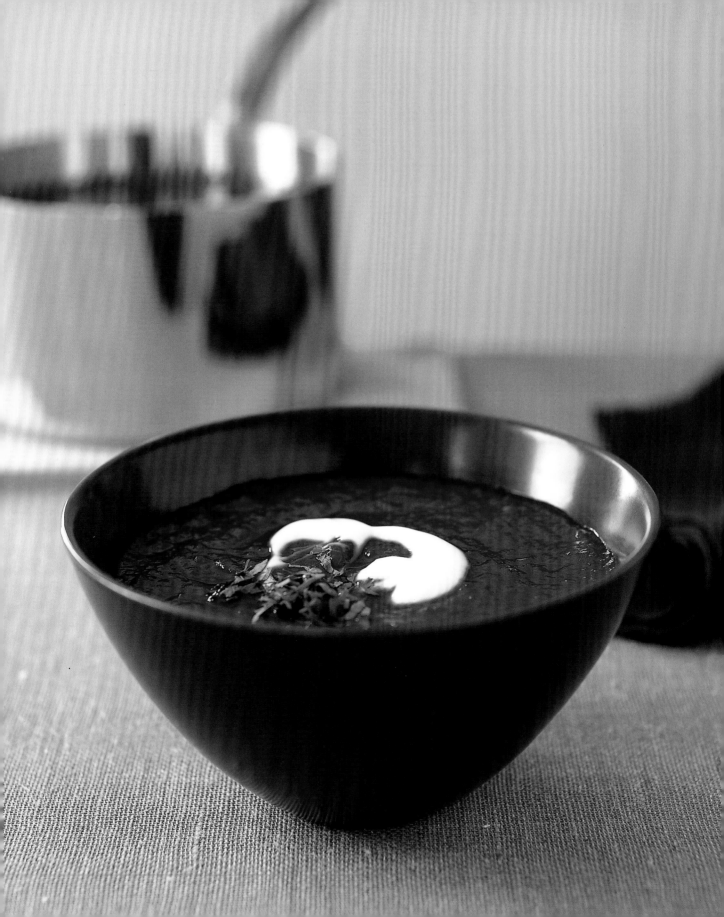

Beautiful borscht

SERVES 4   PREP 15 mins   COOK 50 mins

4 beetroots, peeled and quartered
1 carrot, roughly chopped
1 parsnip, roughly chopped
1 leek, roughly chopped and washed
1 onion, roughly chopped
3 bay leaves
½ teaspoon allspice
½ cup (125 ml) lemon juice
1.5 litres vegetable stock
2 tablespoons reduced-fat
  natural yoghurt
1 handful flat-leaf (Italian) parsley,
  roughly chopped

1 Bring vegetables, bay leaves, allspice, lemon juice and stock to
   a boil in a large saucepan. Reduce heat and simmer for 45 minutes.

2 Allow to cool slightly, then remove bay leaves and puree using
   a blender or hand-held processor. Season to taste.

3 Gently reheat soup and serve with a dollop of reduced-fat yoghurt
   and a sprinkling of parsley. This soup can also be served cold.

Tomato, carrot and mint soup

SERVES 4   PREP 15 mins   COOK 40 mins

To make this refreshing soup a bit more hearty, add some meat from your daily protein allowance. Cooked chunks of lamb stirred through right at the end would work well.

1 tablespoon olive oil
2 cloves garlic, crushed
1 onion, coarsely chopped
600 g carrots, sliced
1 large red capsicum (pepper),
   trimmed, seeded and chopped
1 tablespoon tomato paste (puree)
400 g tomatoes, chopped
3 teaspoons dried mint
2 cups (500 g) salt-reduced chicken
   or vegetable stock
small handful torn mint leaves
   (optional), to serve

1 Heat the olive oil in a large saucepan over medium heat. Add the garlic and onion and cook, stirring, for 5 minutes or until softened. Add the carrot and capsicum, then cover and cook, stirring occasionally, for 15 minutes or until the vegetables are just tender. Add the tomato paste and cook, stirring constantly, for 2 minutes.

2 Add the tomato, dried mint and stock and bring to simmering point, then cook for 20 minutes or until the tomato has softened.

3 Puree the soup in a blender or food processor, or in the pan with a stick blender, then return to the stove and gently reheat.

4 Divide the soup among warmed bowls, scatter with torn mint leaves (if using) and serve immediately.

Carrot and parsnip soup

SERVES 4   PREP 15 mins   COOK 45 mins

Double the quantities for this warming soup and save it for an evening when you don't have time to cook.

1 tablespoon extra virgin olive oil
1 onion, chopped
1 clove garlic, crushed
300 g carrots, sliced
300 g parsnips, peeled and sliced
150 g pumpkin, peeled and sliced
1 litre salt-reduced chicken
   or vegetable stock
1 cup (250 ml) reduced-fat milk
roughly chopped flat-leaf (Italian)
   parsley, to serve

1 Heat the olive oil in a large saucepan over medium heat and saute the onion, stirring, for 4–5 minutes or until softened. Add the garlic, carrot, parsnip and potato and cook, stirring, for a further minute, then pour in the stock and bring to the boil.

2 Reduce the heat and simmer for 30 minutes or until the vegetables are soft. Allow to cool slightly, then puree the soup with a stick blender or in a food processor. Return to the saucepan, add the milk, season and heat through.

3 Serve sprinkled with chopped parsley and, if liked, bread from your daily allowance.

Celeriac and pea soup with lemon cream

SERVES 4   PREP 25 mins   COOK 30 mins

1 tablespoon olive oil
1 celeriac (about 600 g), peeled
    and cut into small pieces
1 large onion, coarsely chopped
1 stick celery, coarsely chopped
2 cloves garlic, crushed
2 cups (240 g) fresh podded
    or frozen peas
3 cups (750 ml) salt-reduced
    chicken or fish stock
½ cup (125 ml) reduced-fat
    evaporated milk, chilled
1½ teaspoons finely grated
    lemon zest

Celeriac tastes milder and slightly sweeter than celery and is wonderful both cooked or grated raw into salads. For a more substantial meal, serve this with grilled fish or chicken pieces or steamed mussels from your daily protein allowance.

1   Heat the olive oil in a large saucepan over medium heat, then add the celeriac, onion, celery and garlic and cook, stirring often, for 5 minutes or until the vegetables are starting to soften. Cover and cook for 25 minutes, stirring occasionally, or until the vegetables are tender. Add the peas and stock and bring to simmering point, then cover and cook over medium–high heat for 5 minutes or until the peas are tender.

2   Puree the soup in a blender or food processor, or in the pan with a stick blender, then return to the stove and gently reheat.

3   Combine the milk and lemon zest in a bowl and whisk until thick. Divide the soup among warmed bowls, spoon over the lemon cream and serve immediately.

TIP Make sure you prepare the celeriac just before cooking or it will discolour.

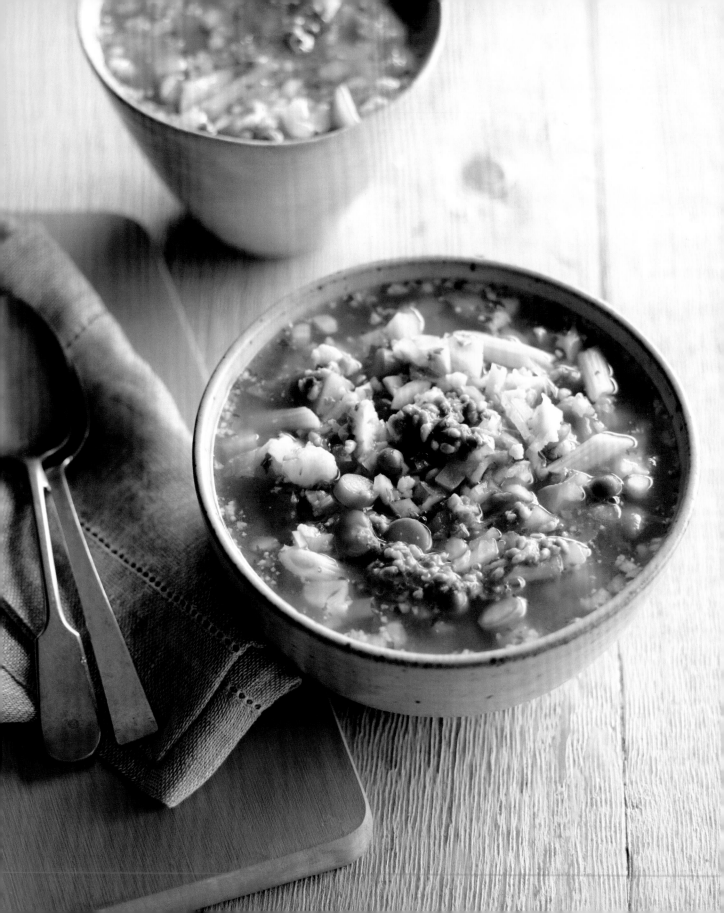

Spring minestrone

SERVES 4   PREP 20 mins   COOK 15 mins

1 cup (150 g) fresh podded
   or frozen broad beans
1 tablespoon olive oil
1 onion, finely chopped
2 cloves garlic, crushed
1 small bulb fennel, trimmed
   and cut into 1 cm pieces
1 choko, peeled and finely chopped
   or 1 head broccoli, trimmed and
   cut into 1 cm pieces
¼ head cauliflower, trimmed
   and cut into 1 cm pieces
1.5 litres salt-reduced chicken stock
1 bay leaf
½ cup (60 g) dried mini penne rigate,
   ditali or other small pasta shapes
1 bunch asparagus, trimmed and
   thinly sliced
1 cup (120 g) fresh podded
   or frozen peas
1 tablespoon pesto

This classic soup makes for a quick and tasty lunch, and the pesto adds a burst of flavour.

1 Cook the broad beans in a saucepan of boiling water for 3–4 minutes or until tender. Drain well, reserving the cooking water, then plunge them into a bowl of cold water to cool. Drain again, then peel and set aside.

2 Heat the olive oil in a large saucepan over medium heat, then add the onion, garlic, fennel, choko or broccoli and cauliflower and cook, stirring, over medium heat for 5 minutes or until the vegetables have softened. Add the stock and bay leaf, then bring to simmering point.

3 Meanwhile, bring a small saucepan of water to the boil, add the pasta and cook for 7–8 minutes or until al dente, then drain well.

4 Add the asparagus and peas to the vegetables in the saucepan, bring to simmering point and cook for 4–5 minutes or until the vegetables are tender. Add the pasta and broad beans and season to taste with salt and pepper, then remove the bay leaf. Divide among warmed bowls, top with a teaspoonful of pesto and serve immediately.

Moroccan-spiced pumpkin soup

SERVES 4 PREP 20 mins COOK 25 mins

1 tablespoon olive oil
1 onion, coarsely chopped
2 cloves garlic, crushed
1–1½ tablespoons Moroccan
    spice mix
800 g pumpkin (squash), peeled,
    seeded and chopped
2 parsnips, peeled and chopped
300 ml orange juice
1¼ cups (310 ml) salt-reduced
    chicken or vegetable stock,
    plus extra if needed
80 g reduced-fat Greek-style
    yoghurt
12 semi-dried tomatoes,
    drained well
crusty bread, to serve

This is a sweet, spicy twist on classic pumpkin soup. Serve it with 100 g cooked fish per person for a satisfying lunch.

1 Heat the olive oil in a large heavy-based saucepan over medium heat. Add the onion and garlic and cook, stirring often, for 5–6 minutes or until softened. Add the spice mix and cook for 2 minutes or until fragrant. Add the pumpkin, parsnip, orange juice and stock, stir to combine, then bring to simmering point. Reduce the heat to low–medium and cook for 15 minutes or until the vegetables are very tender.

2 Puree the soup in a blender or food processor, or in the pan with a stick blender, then return to the stove to heat through. Season with salt and pepper and add a little more stock or water to thin the soup, if desired. Divide the soup among warmed bowls, top each with a spoonful of yoghurt and the tomatoes, then serve with bread from your daily allowance.

TIP Moroccan spice mix can be added to casseroles and salads and used as a rub for grilled meats. It's available from the spice section of most supermarkets.

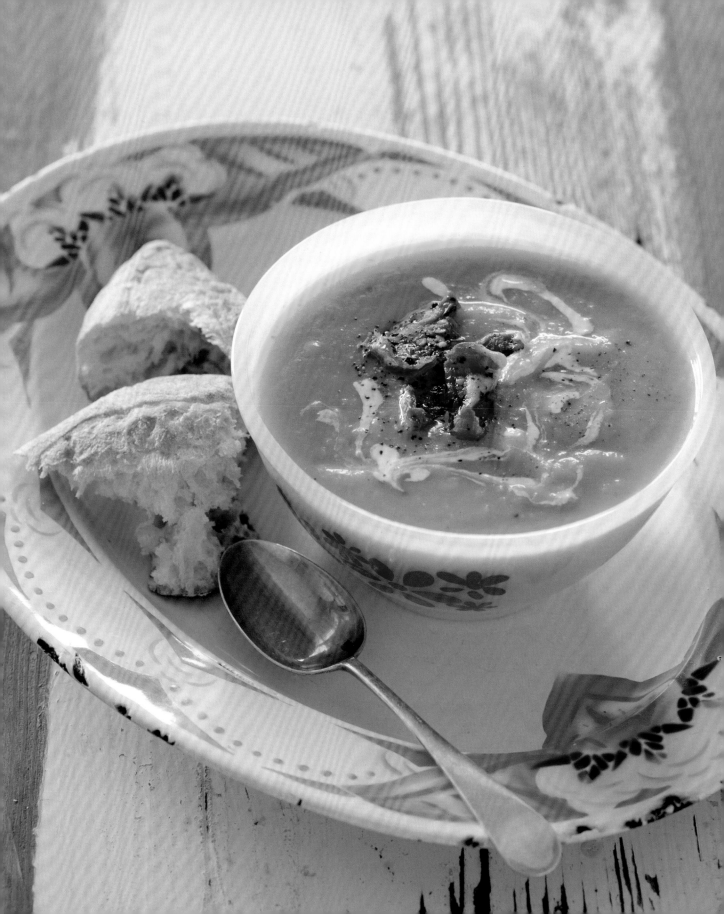

Cauliflower, lentil and tomato soup

SERVES 4   PREP 15 mins   COOK 30 mins

1 tablespoon extra virgin olive oil
1 large onion, finely chopped
2 carrots, diced
1 stick celery, diced
2 cloves garlic, crushed
1 teaspoon grated ginger
2 teaspoons curry powder
600 g cauliflower, cut into
   small florets
1.5 litres salt-reduced chicken
   or vegetable stock
½ cup (100 g) red lentils
1 × 400 g tin chopped tomatoes
2 tablespoons lemon juice
roughly chopped chives, to serve
reduced-fat yoghurt, to serve

**Thick and hearty, this curried soup will warm you inside and
out. The serves are generous so there will probably be leftovers,
which you can enjoy the next day.**

1 Heat the olive oil in a large saucepan over medium heat and saute the
   onion, carrot, celery, garlic and ginger for 5 minutes. Add the curry
   powder and cook for a further minute or until fragrant.

2 Stir in the cauliflower, stock, lentils and chopped tomatoes. Bring to
   the boil, then reduce the heat and simmer, covered, for 20 minutes
   or until the vegetables and lentils are tender.

3 Puree the soup in a blender, or in the pan with a stick blender, then
   return to the heat. Stir in the lemon juice and season to taste. Finish
   with a dollop of reduced-fat yoghurt, some chopped chives and
   a grinding of black pepper.

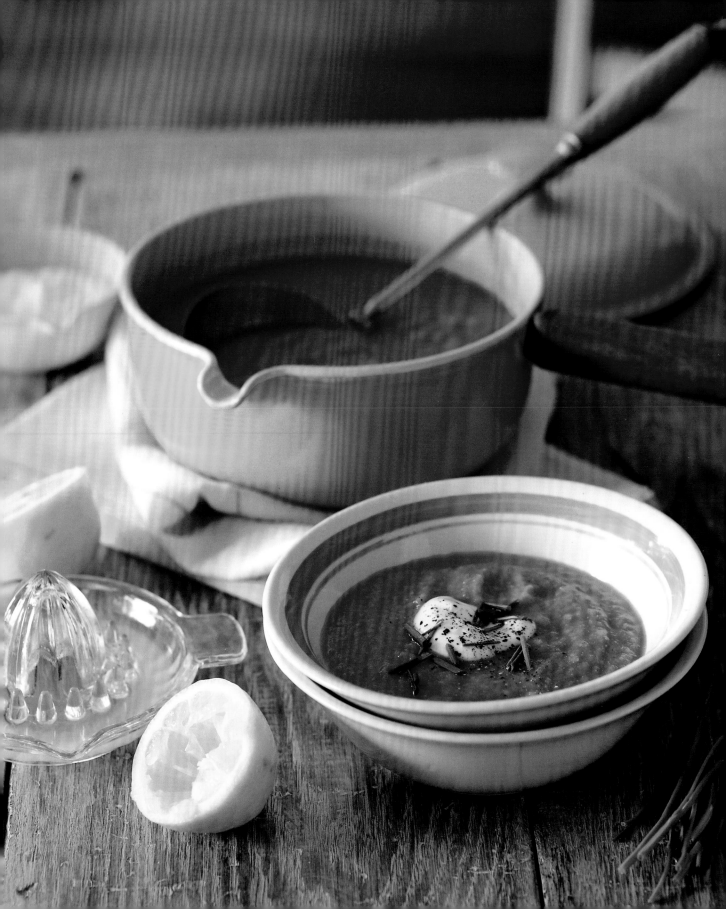

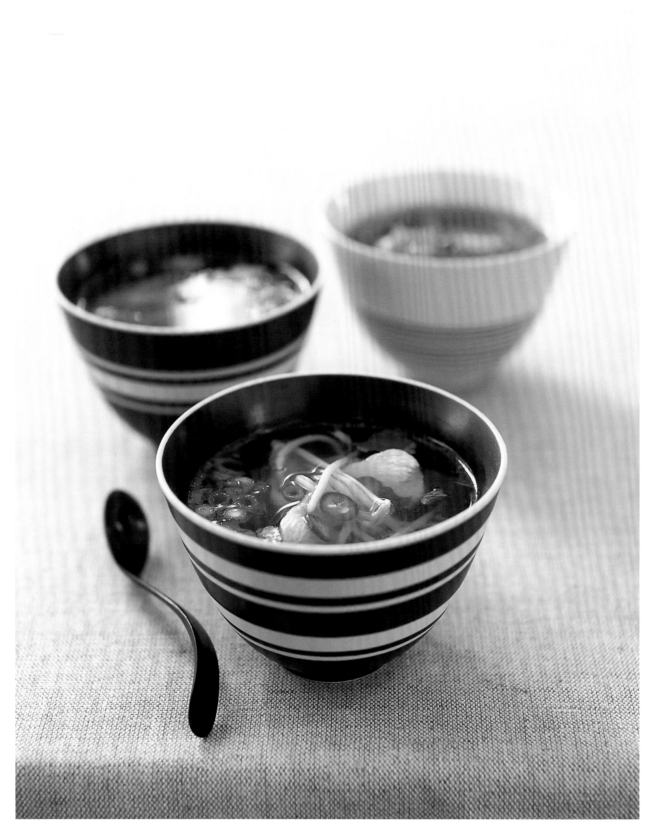

Oriental chicken soup

SERVES 4   PREP 10 mins   COOK 15 mins

2 teaspoons peanut oil
2 stalks lemongrass, chopped
   (or 2 teaspoons lemongrass paste)
4 spring onions (scallions), chopped
1 red chilli, sliced
1 litre good-quality chicken stock
1 tablespoon fish sauce
1 tablespoon soy sauce
400 g chicken breast, thinly sliced
2 cups (160 g) bean sprouts
1 teaspoon Equal
chopped coriander (cilantro) and mint

1 Heat oil in a small frying pan over medium heat. Add lemongrass, spring onion and chilli and cook, stirring, for 2 minutes. Remove from heat and set aside.

2 In a medium saucepan, bring stock to a boil. Add lemongrass mixture, fish sauce, soy sauce and chicken, then reduce heat and simmer for 10 minutes, or until chicken is cooked.

3 Add bean sprouts and stir to heat through. Season to taste with Equal – the sweetness will balance out the flavours of the soup. Serve topped with coriander and mint.

Corn, ginger and spring onion soup

SERVES 4   PREP 10 mins   COOK 25 mins

1 tablespoon vegetable oil
1 onion, chopped
1 stick celery, chopped
2½ tablespoons chopped ginger
1 sweet potato (about 350 g),
   peeled and chopped
½ cup (125 ml) dry sherry
1 litre salt-reduced chicken or
   vegetable stock
4 cups (640 g) corn kernels
   (tinned or frozen)
2 spring onions, trimmed, white
   part thinly sliced, green part
   sliced on the diagonal

A delicious, warming lunch, with a hint of ginger and the sweetness of sherry. Make more than you need and freeze the leftovers for another time.

1   Heat the vegetable oil in a large saucepan over medium heat, add the onion, celery, ginger and sweet potato, then cover and cook, stirring occasionally, for 10 minutes or until the vegetables are starting to soften. Add the sherry, then bring to the boil and cook for 5 minutes or until the sherry reduces a little. Add the stock, bring to simmering point, then cook for 10 minutes or until the vegetables are very soft.

2   Puree the soup in a blender or food processor, or in the pan with a stick blender, then return to the stove and gently reheat.

3   Meanwhile, cook the corn kernels in a saucepan of boiling water for 5–6 minutes or until tender. Drain, then add to the saucepan along with the thinly sliced white part of the spring onion and bring to simmering point.

4   Divide the soup among warmed bowls, then sprinkle with the reserved spring onion before serving.

TIP If you prefer not to use the sherry, simply replace it with ½ cup (125 ml) salt-reduced stock and omit the step of reducing.

1 SERVE =
2 units protein
1½ units bread
1½ units vegetables
1 unit fats

Chicken noodle soup

SERVES 4   PREP 15 mins   COOK 30 mins

1 tablespoon olive oil
1 onion, chopped
2 carrots, diced
2 sticks celery, diced
2 potatoes, peeled and diced
3 cloves garlic, sliced
1 teaspoon dried thyme
2 litres salt-reduced chicken stock
800 g chicken breast fillets, diced
120 g thin noodles or spaghettini
1 cup (200 g) corn kernels (tinned
   or frozen)
3 tablespoons chopped
   flat-leaf (Italian) parsley

This classic soup is a favourite with all ages.

1 Heat the olive oil in a large saucepan. Add the onion, carrot, celery and potato and cook, stirring, for 5 minutes or until the vegetables are starting to soften. Stir in the garlic and thyme. Add the stock and chicken and simmer for 15 minutes or until the vegetables are soft.

2 Add the noodles and corn and cook for 10 minutes or until cooked through. Add 1–2 cups (250–500 ml) water if the soup is too thick. Stir in the parsley and serve immediately.

TIP If you want to make a big batch of this soup to freeze some for later, stop at the end of step 1. The noodles and corn can be added when you are reheating the soup. Other pastas, such as macaroni or spirals, can be used in place of the spaghetti, and try adding other vegetables too.

Hot and sour soup

SERVES 4   PREP 20 mins   COOK 20 mins

3 teaspoons vegetable oil

400 g field mushrooms, thinly sliced

1.5 litres salt-reduced chicken stock

1 × 4 cm piece ginger, peeled and
cut into fine matchsticks

2 cloves garlic, finely sliced

2½ tablespoons salt-reduced
light soy sauce

¼ cup (60 ml) dry sherry

2 tablespoons cider vinegar

1 × 600 g piece pork fillet, trimmed
of fat, cut into thin slices,
then cut into matchsticks

1 × 75 g tin bamboo shoots,
rinsed and drained

200 g firm tofu, cut into 1 cm pieces

2 spring onions, trimmed and sliced
on the diagonal

2 tablespoons cornflour (cornstarch)

1 teaspoon sesame oil (optional)

The classic Chinese flavours of this soup are wonderful for dinner.

1   Heat the vegetable oil in a large saucepan over medium heat, then add the mushroom and cook, stirring often, for 5–6 minutes or until tender.

2   Add the stock, ginger, garlic, soy sauce, sherry, vinegar and 1 teaspoon freshly ground black pepper. Bring to simmering point, then reduce the heat to low, cover and cook for 10 minutes to allow the flavours to develop. Add the pork and bamboo shoots, stirring the mixture to separate the pork slices, and cook for 1 minute. Add the tofu and most of the spring onion, reserving a small handful for the garnish, and bring to simmering point.

3   Meanwhile, combine the cornflour with ¼ cup (60 ml) water in a small bowl to form a smooth paste. Add the paste to the soup mixture, then cook, stirring, over medium heat for 2–3 minutes or until the liquid boils and thickens slightly. Stir in the sesame oil (if using), then divide the soup among warmed bowls, scatter over the reserved spring onion and serve.

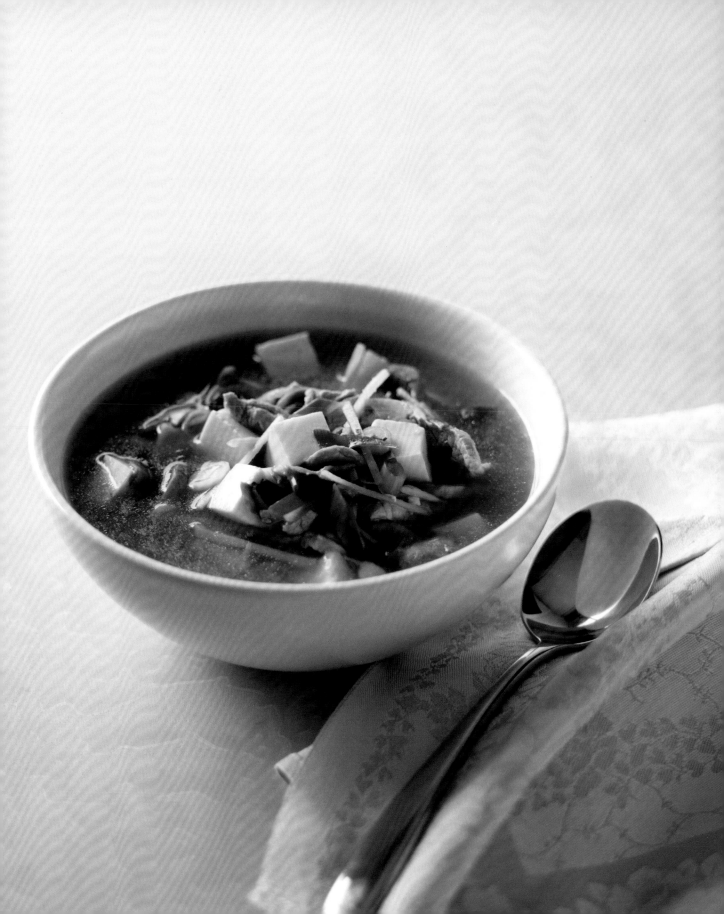

1 SERVE =
1 unit protein
½ unit vegetables
1 unit fats

Sweet corn and crab soup

SERVES 4   PREP 15 mins   COOK 15 mins

1 tablespoon vegetable oil
1 onion, finely chopped
1 stick celery, finely diced
1 clove garlic, crushed
2 teaspoons freshly grated ginger
1 × 125 g tin corn, or 2 cooked corn
  cobs, kernels removed
1 litre salt-reduced chicken stock
¼ cup (60 ml) soy sauce
3 × 170 g tins crab meat, drained
4 spring onions (scallions),
  finely sliced
¼ cup roughly chopped
  coriander (cilantro)

1 Heat oil in a heavy-based saucepan over medium heat. Add onion, celery, garlic and ginger and cook for 3 minutes, or until soft. Add corn and chicken stock and bring to a boil. Reduce heat and simmer for 10 minutes. Remove from heat and allow to cool.

2 Transfer to a food processor and blend, leaving soup slightly chunky. Return soup to the saucepan and add soy sauce, crab meat, spring onions and coriander.

3 Serve sprinkled with a little extra chopped coriander, if desired.

VARIATION

You can easily use chicken instead of crab meat. Simply follow the recipe above, but add 400 g chicken mince when you add the corn and chicken stock, and omit the crab meat.

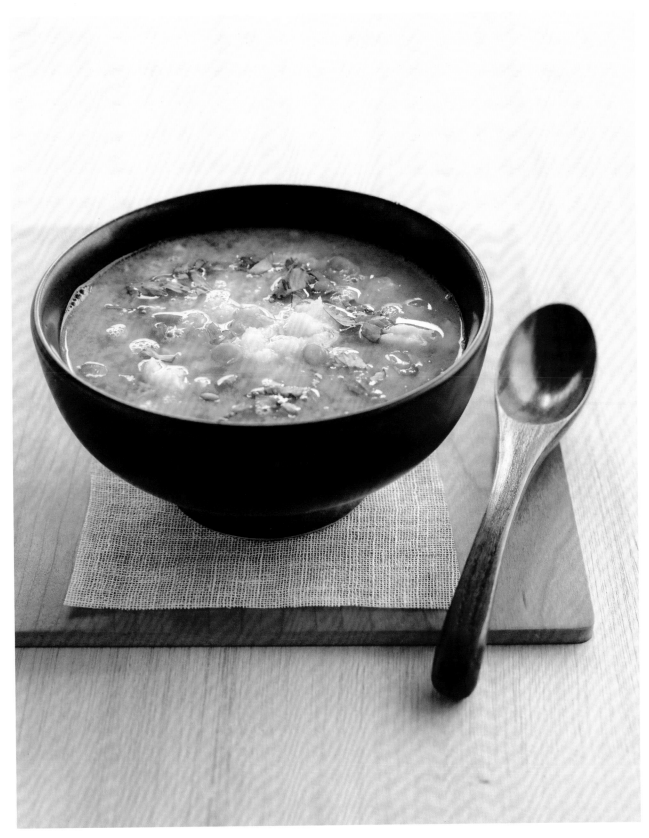

Fish chowder

SERVES 4 PREP 20 mins COOK 30 mins

1 tablespoon olive oil
1 onion, finely chopped
2 cloves garlic, crushed
2 sticks celery, diced
1 carrot, diced
2 potatoes, diced
1 bay leaf
½ teaspoon dried basil
½ teaspoon dried thyme
1 × 400 g tin chopped tomatoes
2 cups (500 ml) salt-reduced
   chicken stock
1 zucchini (courgette), diced
400 g fish fillets, skin and bones
   removed, cut into large dice
roughly chopped flat-leaf (Italian)
   parsley, to serve
Tabasco sauce, to serve (optional)

This soup is packed with vegetables, herbs and, of course, tempting chunks of fish. Hearty and nourishing, it needs no accompaniment.

1 Heat the olive oil in a large saucepan over medium heat. Add the onion, garlic, celery and carrot and cook for 5 minutes or until the onion has softened.

2 Add the potato, bay leaf, basil, thyme, chopped tomatoes, stock, zucchini and 1 cup (250 ml) water and bring to the boil. Reduce the heat and simmer, covered, for 15 minutes or until all the vegetables are tender.

3 Add the fish pieces, then cover and simmer for a further 5–6 minutes or until just cooked through. Sprinkle with parsley and serve with a few drops of Tabasco sauce (if using).

TIP For a bit of variety, the fish can be replaced with your choice of seafood – try prawns, scallops or a marinara mix.

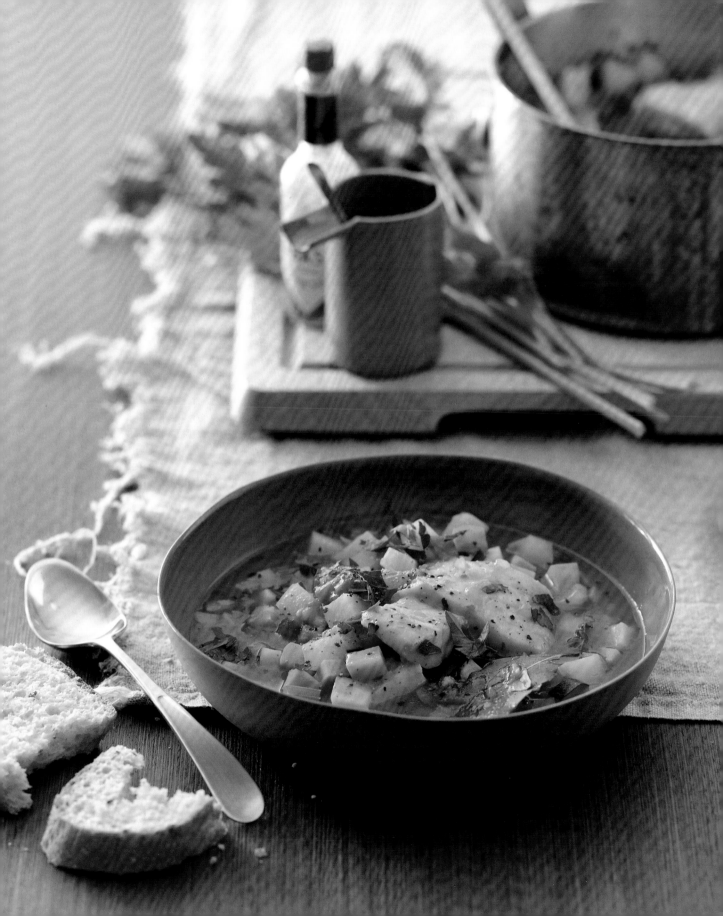

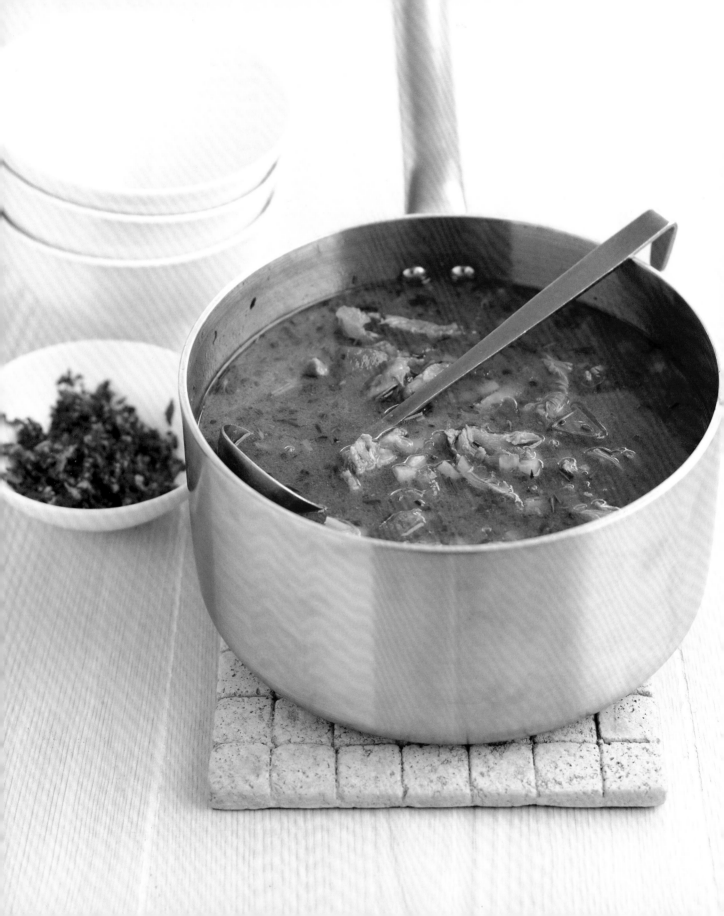

1 SERVE =
1 unit protein
½ unit vegetables
½ unit fats

Lamb shank soup with gremolata

SERVES 4   PREP 20 mins + cooling time   COOK 1 hour

2 teaspoons canola oil
3 lamb shanks (900 g with bone:
   100 g meat per person), excess
   fat removed
1 onion, chopped
2 carrots, chopped
1 stick celery, chopped
1 tablespoon chopped rosemary
1 clove garlic, chopped
2 large tomatoes, diced
1 litre salt-reduced beef stock
2 cups (500 ml) water
freshly ground black pepper
1 tablespoon finely grated
   lemon zest
2 tablespoons finely chopped
   flat-leaf (Italian) parsley

1   Heat oil in a heavy-based saucepan over medium heat. Add lamb shanks and cook, turning occasionally, for 10 minutes, or until golden. Remove shanks from pan and set aside. Add onion, carrots and celery to pan and cook for 5 minutes, or until soft. Return shanks to pan, add rosemary, garlic, tomatoes, stock and water, and bring to a boil. Reduce heat and simmer for 40 minutes, or until meat is almost falling off the bone.

2   Using a large spoon, skim off any foam, then remove shanks from soup. Allow to cool a little, then pull meat off the bone and chop roughly. Return meat to the soup, season with pepper and serve sprinkled with lemon zest and parsley.

Minestrone with meatballs

SERVES 4   PREP 20 mins   COOK 45 mins

MEATBALLS

½ **onion, finely chopped**
400 g lean minced (ground) beef
2 tablespoons finely chopped
  flat-leaf (Italian) parsley
1 clove garlic, crushed
2 teaspoons olive oil

SOUP

2 teaspoons olive oil
1 clove garlic, crushed
½ **onion, chopped**
1 stick celery, chopped
1 carrot, chopped
2 × 400 g tins chopped tomatoes
1 cup (250 ml) beef stock
½ **cup basil, chopped**

1 To make meatballs, mix all ingredients except oil in a large bowl. Roll tablespoonfuls of mixture into balls and set aside. Heat oil in a large frying pan over high heat. Carefully add half the meatballs and cook, turning occasionally, for 8–10 minutes, or until browned. Remove from pan and drain on paper towel. Repeat with remaining uncooked meatballs. Do not overcrowd pan when cooking or meatballs will stew.

2 For the soup, heat oil in a large saucepan over medium heat. Add garlic, onion, celery and carrot and cook, stirring constantly, until onion is soft. Add tomato and stock and bring to a boil. Reduce heat and simmer, covered, for 10 minutes.

3 Add meatballs to soup and simmer, uncovered, for 3 minutes, or until meatballs are heated through. Stir through basil and season to taste.

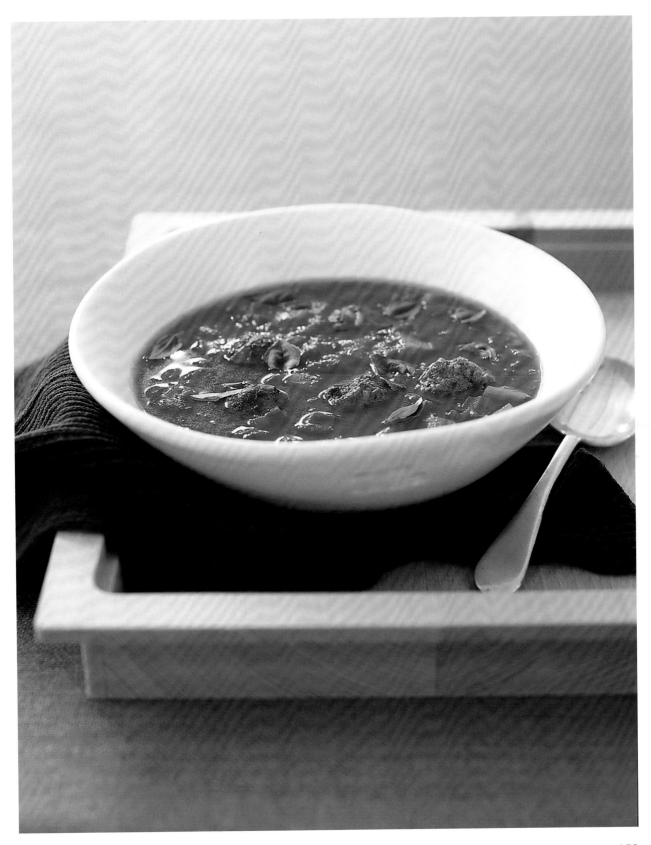

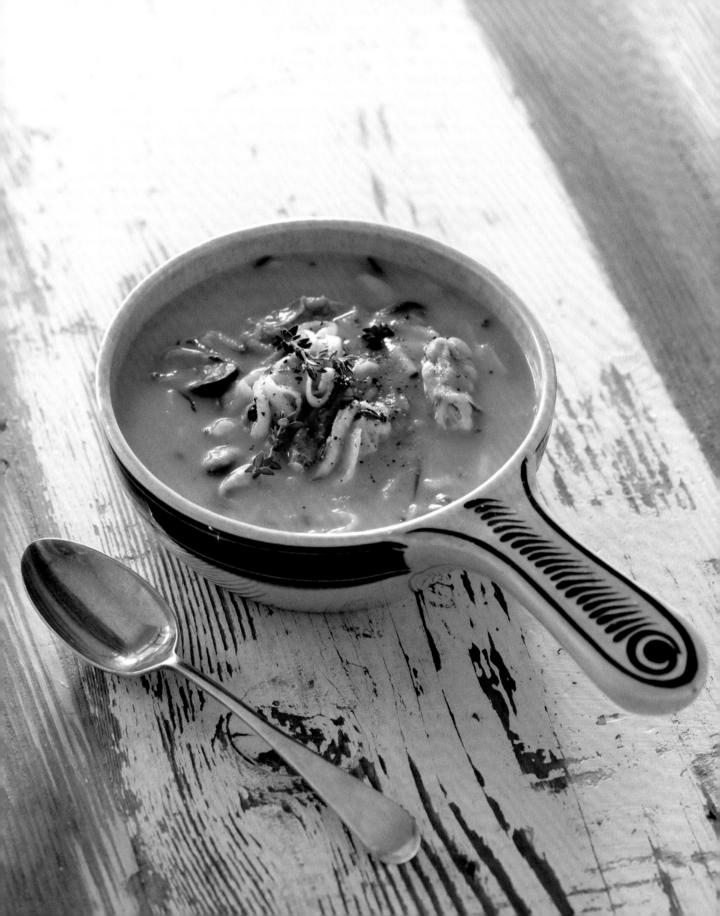

Zucchini, potato and mussel soup

SERVES 4   PREP 30 mins   COOK 30 mins

2 kg mussels, scrubbed
   and debearded
1 tablespoon olive oil
1 large onion, coarsely chopped
1 stick celery, coarsely chopped
600 g potatoes, chopped
1.25 litres salt-reduced fish
   or chicken stock
3 zucchini (courgettes), trimmed
   and finely grated
4 sprigs thyme, torn

Mussels are delicious for lunch and so easy to cook. Use swede instead of potatoes here if you want to enjoy this for dinner.

1   Bring 2 cups (500 ml) water to the boil in a large saucepan. Add half the mussels, cover the pan then cook, shaking the pan often, for about 3 minutes or until the mussels have opened. Transfer the cooked mussels to a bowl with a slotted spoon, then repeat with the remaining mussels. Reserve the cooking liquid. Remove the mussels from their shells and set aside, discarding the shells.

2   Heat the oil in a large heavy-based saucepan over medium heat, then add the onion, celery and potato. Cook, stirring often, for 10 minutes or until the vegetables have softened. Add the reserved cooking liquid and the stock, bring the mixture to simmering point, then cook over low–medium heat for 20 minutes or until the potato is tender. Puree the soup in a blender or food processor, or in the pan with a stick blender, then return to the stove.

3   Add the zucchini, cover and cook for 2 minutes or until the zucchini is tender. Season, then stir in the mussels. Cook for 1–2 minutes or until warmed through, then divide among warmed bowls and serve immediately with thyme sprinkled over.

TIP 2 kg small black mussels in their shells yield about 100 g mussel meat.

Mulligatawny

SERVES 4   PREP 15 mins   COOK 45 mins

1 tablespoon vegetable oil
1 onion, chopped
2 cloves garlic, crushed
1 × 3 cm piece ginger, grated
2 carrots, diced
1 stick celery, diced
1 tablespoon curry paste
   (or to taste)
1.5–2 litres salt-reduced beef stock
$^1/_3$ cup (65 g) red lentils
700 g lean lamb,
   trimmed of fat and finely diced
6 curry leaves or 2 bay leaves
2 teaspoons garam masala
$^1/_3$ cup (65 g) basmati rice
2 medium potatoes,
   peeled and diced
juice of 1 lemon
¼ cup (60 ml) reduced-fat coconut-
   flavoured evaporated milk
   (optional)
roughly chopped coriander
   (cilantro), to serve (optional)

This flavoursome soup is traditionally served in India and Sri Lanka. Translated from Tamil, mulligatawny literally means 'pepper water', although pepper is not an essential ingredient. Make it a day ahead and refrigerate until you're ready to heat it through and serve.

1 Heat the oil in a large saucepan over medium heat. Add the onion, garlic, ginger, carrot and celery and gently cook for 5 minutes or until softened.

2 Stir in the curry paste, then add the stock, lentils, lamb, curry or bay leaves and garam masala and stir to combine. Bring to the boil, then reduce the heat and simmer, covered, for 25 minutes. Add the rice and potato and cook for a further 15 minutes. Stir in the lemon juice and evaporated milk (if using) until heated through, then serve, sprinkled with coriander if liked.

TIP For a different take on this dish, use chicken instead of lamb, and chicken stock in place of the beef stock. There will almost certainly be leftovers, so have them for lunch the next day.

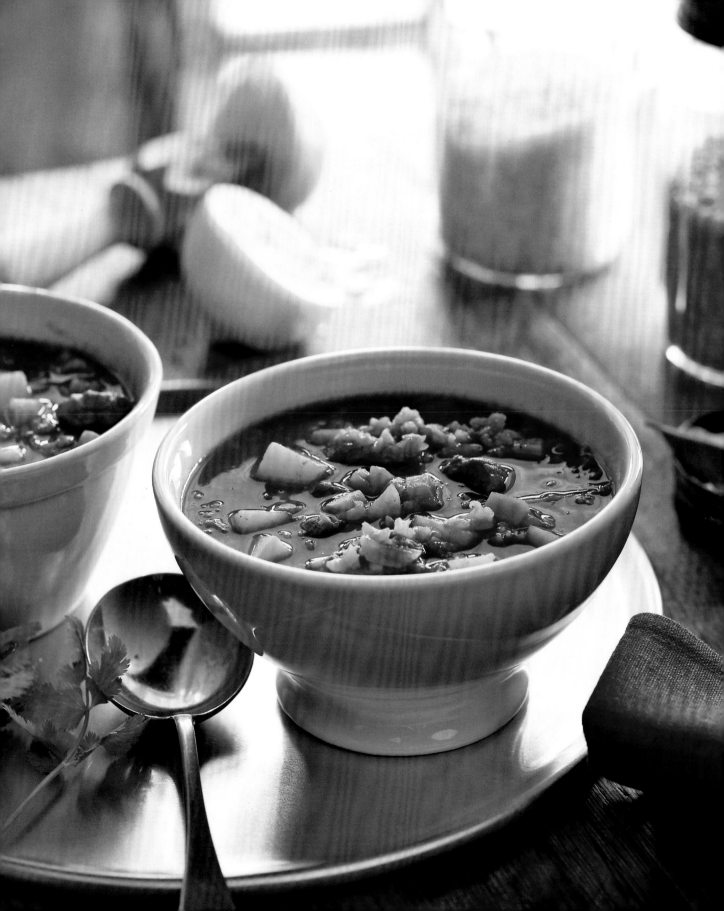

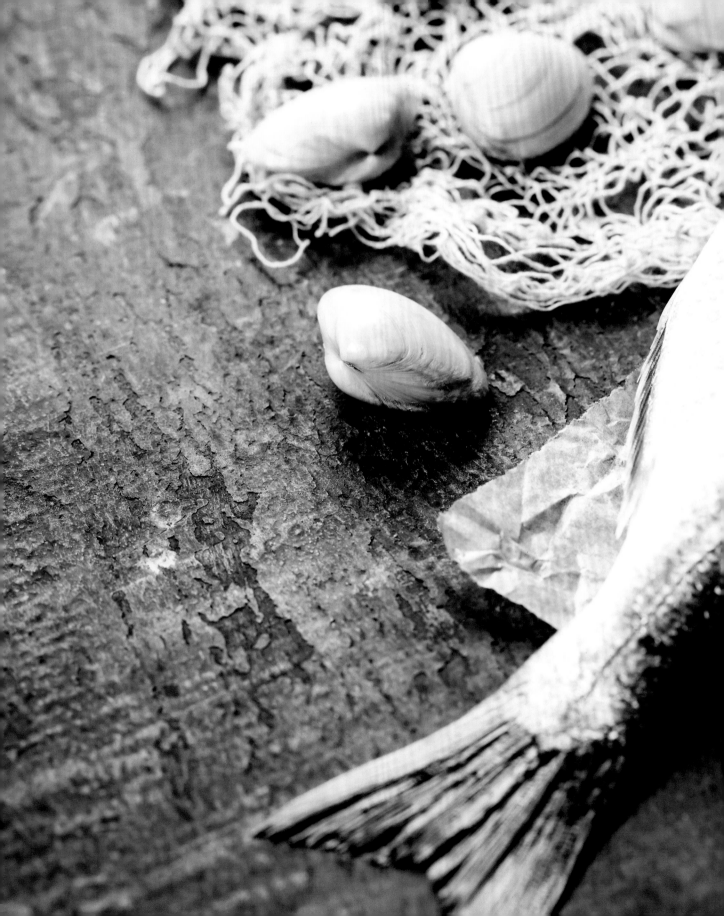

seafood

Char-grilled salmon with parsley relish, asparagus and pumpkin

SERVES 4   **PREP** 10 mins   **COOK** 20 mins

400 g butternut pumpkin,
   peeled and thickly sliced
1 tablespoon olive oil
4 × 200 g salmon fillets
16 spears asparagus
¹/₃ cup (110 g) Parsley Relish
   (see page 534)
lime wedges

1 Preheat oven to 180°C.

2 Place pumpkin in a bowl with half the oil and toss to coat. Transfer to a baking dish and lightly season. Bake for 20 minutes, or until soft and golden.

3 Meanwhile, heat a non-stick grill plate or barbecue grill to high. Lightly brush salmon fillets with remaining oil. Place salmon on grill, flesh-side down, and cook for 4 minutes. Turn salmon and cook for a further 4 minutes. Remove from heat and set aside, covered.

4 Bring a saucepan of lightly salted water to a boil. Add asparagus and blanch for 2 minutes, then drain. Arrange salmon on pumpkin slices, then top with parsley relish and add asparagus spears. Serve with lime wedges.

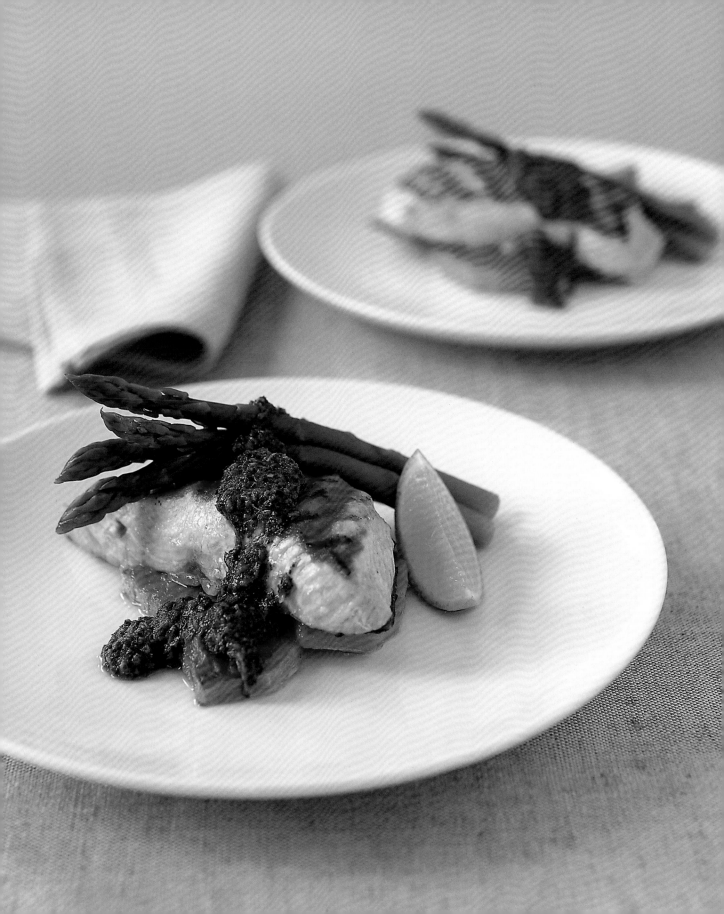

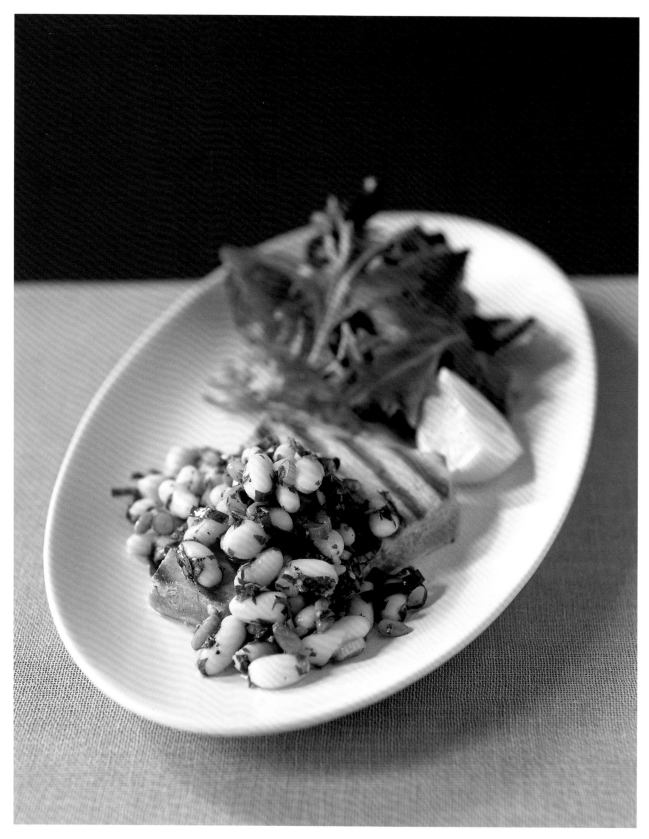

Tuna with cannellini bean and basil salad

SERVES 4   **PREP** 10 mins   **COOK** 10 mins

1 tablespoon pine nuts
4 × 100 g tuna steaks
olive oil spray
1 tablespoon lemon juice
1 tablespoon olive oil
½ clove garlic, crushed
1 × 400 g tin white cannellini beans,
    drained and rinsed
½ cup basil, finely sliced
¹/₃ cup flat-leaf (Italian) parsley,
    finely chopped
¼ cup finely sliced spring onions
    (scallions)

1   Heat a small non-stick frying pan over medium heat. Add pine nuts and toss for 5 minutes, or until toasted and golden. Set aside.

2   Lightly spray tuna steaks with oil spray. Heat a large non-stick frying pan or grill plate over high heat until almost smoking. Add tuna and cook for 2 minutes each side – the tuna should still be pink and 'glassy' in the middle (don't be tempted to cook the tuna any longer or it will be dry and unpleasant). Allow to cool slightly.

3   Place remaining ingredients and pine nuts in a bowl and gently toss. Season to taste.

4   Serve tuna with bean salad on the side.

Thai salmon and green bean salad with coconut dressing

SERVES 4   PREP 25 mins   COOK 12 mins

400 g green beans, trimmed
2 bunches asparagus, trimmed
    and cut into 5 cm lengths
2 cups (160 g) bean sprouts
1¹/₃ cups (200 g) fresh rice noodles
1 × 400 g salmon or ocean trout fillet,
    skin-on, pin-boned
2 large handfuls cress (optional)
lime wedges (optional), to serve

COCONUT DRESSING
1 stalk lemongrass, trimmed
    and finely chopped
2½ tablespoons lime juice
¹/₃ cup (100 g) sweet chilli sauce
2 teaspoons fish sauce
½ cup (125 ml) reduced-fat coconut-
    flavoured evaporated milk

This is a refreshing light lunch, or you could double the amount of fish and serve this for dinner. Use tofu, cooked chicken, lean beef or pork in place of fish if you like.

1   To make the dressing, whisk all the ingredients together in a small bowl and set aside.

2   Bring a saucepan of water to the boil. Add the beans and asparagus and cook for 2–3 minutes or until just tender. Remove using a slotted spoon or tongs and drain well, then place on paper towel to remove any remaining water. Add the bean sprouts to the pan and cook for 30–40 seconds or until just wilted, then drain well. Bring another saucepan of water to the boil, add the noodles and cook for 5 minutes or according to the directions on the pack, until tender. Drain well.

3   Heat a heavy-based frying pan over medium–high heat, add the fish and cook for 3 minutes. Turn the fish over and cook for another 2–3 minutes or until cooked through but still a little pink in the middle. Remove from the pan and cool slightly then, using your fingers, remove the skin and break the fish into large flakes.

4   Combine the fish with the cooked vegetables in a large bowl. Pour over the dressing and toss gently to combine. Divide the noodles among bowls, then place the cress (if using) on top. Serve immediately with lime wedges to the side, if using.

TIP The easiest way to remove the pin bones from fish fillets such as salmon is to pull them out with a pair of clean tweezers.

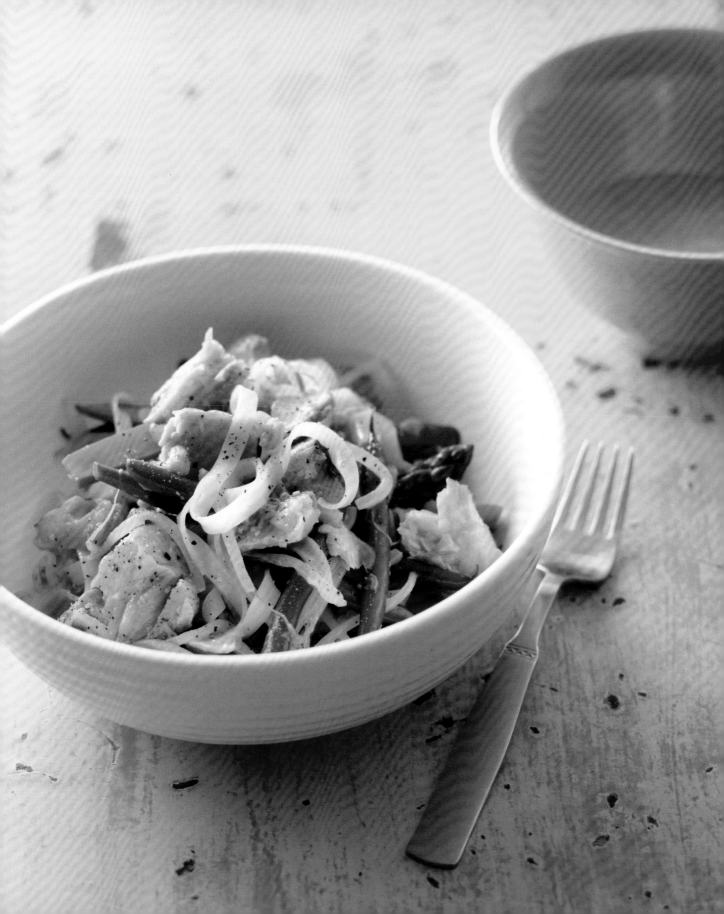

1 SERVE =
2 units protein
1 unit vegetables
1½ units fats

Swordfish steaks with warm zucchini and olive salad

SERVES 4 **PREP** 10 mins **COOK** 10 mins

4 × 200 g swordfish steaks
1 tablespoon olive oil
freshly ground black pepper
lemon wedges

SALAD

2 teaspoons olive oil
2 tablespoons lemon juice
½ red (Spanish) onion, finely sliced
12 kalamata olives
1 tablespoon baby capers
3 small zucchini (corgette),
    thickly sliced
½ cup roughly chopped flat-leaf
    (Italian) parsley

1   To make the salad, combine oil, lemon juice, onion, olives and capers in a bowl.

2   Steam zucchini until tender but not mushy. Transfer immediately to onion mixture and toss to coat.

3   Heat a non-stick frying pan over medium heat. Brush swordfish steaks with oil and pan-fry for 2 minutes each side.

4   Toss parsley through zucchini salad and spoon onto serving plates. Top with swordfish and season with pepper. Serve with a wedge each of lemon.

Stir-fried king prawns

SERVES 4 **PREP** 20 mins **COOK** 5 mins

1 green chilli, roughly chopped
¼ cup (60 ml) lime juice
1 tablespoon fish sauce
1 stalk lemongrass, white part only,
   roughly chopped
2 cloves garlic, roughly chopped
1 tablespoon vegetable oil
1 kg large uncooked prawns (shrimp)
   (200 g meat per person),
   peeled and de-veined
1 red capsicum (pepper), seeded and sliced
2 bunches bok choy (pak choi), chopped
2 cups (160 g) bean sprouts
4 spring onions (scallions), finely sliced
¹⁄₃ cup roughly chopped coriander (cilantro)

1 Place chilli, lime juice, fish sauce, lemongrass and
   garlic in a food processor and blend to a rough paste.

2 Heat a wok or large frying pan over high heat. Add oil
   and, when smoking, add prawns. Stir-fry for 2 minutes,
   or until prawns have just begun to change colour.
   Add capsicum, bok choy and chilli paste and stir-fry
   for a further 3 minutes.

3 To serve, toss through bean sprouts, spring onion
   and coriander.

Moroccan snapper fillets

SERVES 4 **PREP** 15 mins **COOK** 15 mins

4 × 200 g snapper fillets
1 tablespoon olive oil
freshly ground black pepper
1 teaspoon ground cumin
1 teaspoon ground coriander
½ teaspoon ground cardamom
½ teaspoon ground cinnamon
1 clove garlic, chopped
¼ cup chopped coriander
   (cilantro) leaves
¼ cup chopped flat-leaf
   (Italian) parsley
juice and finely grated zest of 1 lemon

1 Preheat oven to 180°C.

2 Pat fish dry with paper towel. Brush with half the oil
   and season with pepper. Arrange fish in a single layer
   in a baking dish.

3 In a bowl, mix remaining ingredients to a loose paste.
   Spread paste evenly over top of fish. Seal baking dish
   with foil. Bake for 10–15 minutes, or until cooked –
   when cooked, the flesh will flake away easily when
   pressed with a fork.

4 Serve with green vegetables or salad.

Steamed mussels with spaghetti

SERVES 4   PREP 15 mins   COOK 20 mins

200 g spaghetti
750 g tomato passata
1 cup (250 ml) white wine
2 cloves garlic, crushed
2 kg mussels, cleaned and debearded
$^1/_3$ cup roughly chopped basil,
   plus extra leaves to garnish
Tabasco sauce, to serve (optional)

This speedy dish is ready in the time it takes to cook the spaghetti. To reduce your prep time, buy mussels that have already been cleaned (available in cryovac packs from fishmongers and some supermarkets).

1   Cook the spaghetti according to the packet instructions. Drain.

2   Meanwhile, place the passata, wine and garlic in a wide saucepan or deep frying pan and bring to the boil over high heat.

3   Add the mussels and cover with a tight-fitting lid. Cook for 3–4 minutes or until all the mussels have opened (discard any that do not open). Remove from the heat and stir in the basil and spaghetti. Garnish with extra basil leaves and serve hot with Tabasco, if desired, and salad.

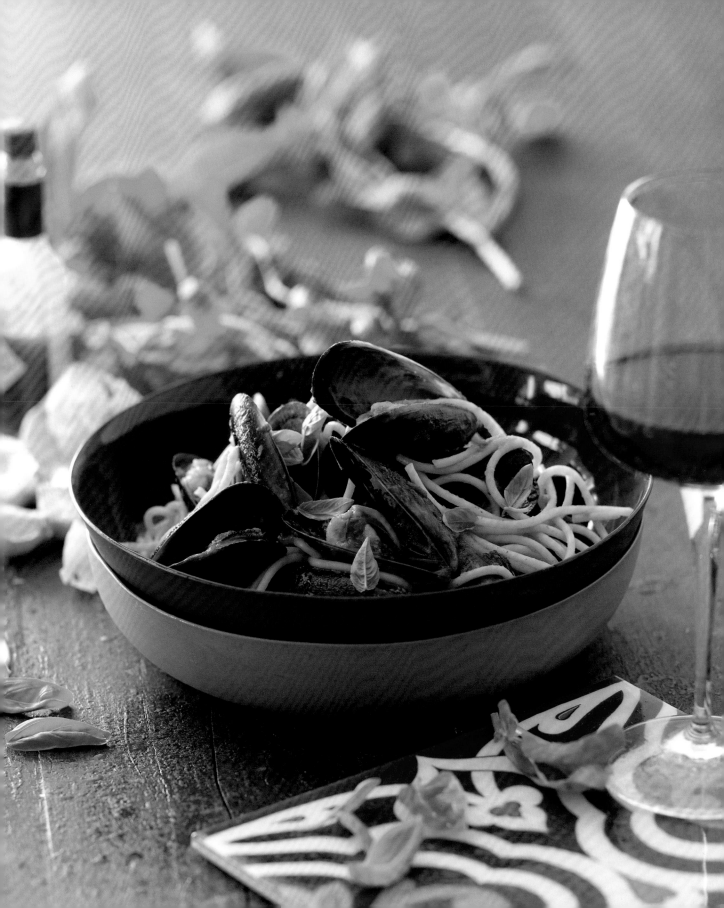

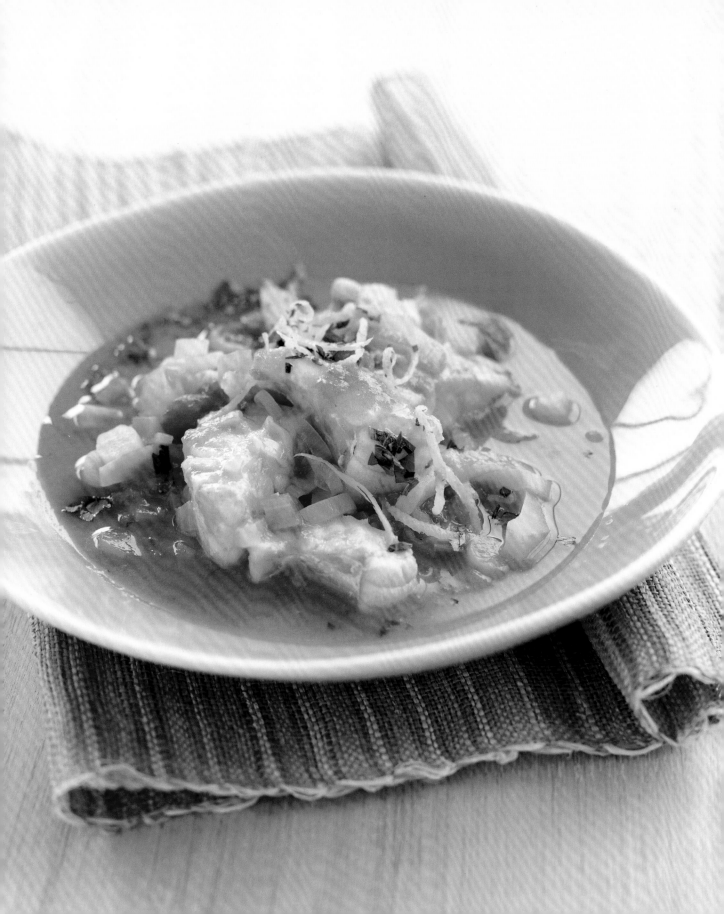

1 SERVE =
2 units protein
1 unit vegetables
1 unit fats

Fish stew with tomato and basil

SERVES 4   **PREP** 15 mins   **COOK** 40 mins

1 tablespoon olive oil
1 leek, white part only, finely
  sliced and washed
2 sticks celery, sliced
2 cloves garlic, crushed
1 bulb fennel, finely sliced
1 × 400 g tin chopped tomatoes
1 cup (250 ml) white wine
2 cups (500 ml) fish stock or
  chicken stock
800 g fish fillets (blue-eye, flathead
  or ling), cut into 4 cm pieces
¼ cup roughly chopped basil
finely grated zest of 1 lemon
  and 2 tablespoons juice

1   Heat oil in a heavy-based saucepan over medium heat. Add leek, celery, garlic and fennel and cook for 10 minutes, or until vegetables are soft. Add tomatoes, wine and stock and bring to a boil. Reduce heat and simmer for 20 minutes. Add fish and simmer for a further 10 minutes. Gently stir through basil, lemon zest and lemon juice, reserving a little basil and zest to garnish, if desired. Season to taste.

2   Serve with a big green salad and crusty bread from your daily bread allowance.

1 SERVE =
2 units protein
1 unit vegetables
1 unit fats

Mediterranean baked salmon with rocket salad

SERVES 4   PREP 15 mins   COOK 15 mins

2 tomatoes, seeded and chopped
2 teaspoons capers, rinsed
   and drained
1 red (Spanish) onion,
   finely chopped
2 cloves garlic, crushed
1 teaspoon grated lemon zest
olive oil spray
4 × 200 g salmon fillets, skin
   and bones removed
truss cherry tomatoes, to serve
lemon wedges, to serve

ROCKET SALAD
150 g baby rocket leaves
1 tablespoon lemon juice
1 tablespoon olive oil
3 tablespoons finely
   shredded basil

These salmon parcels are so simple to prepare. For a rustic presentation, serve the salmon still in the foil and let everyone open their own parcels.

1 Preheat the oven to 200°C.

2 In a medium bowl, combine the tomato, capers, onion, garlic and lemon zest.

3 Spray four 30 cm square sheets of foil with olive oil and place a salmon fillet on each. Top with the tomato mixture, then bring the edges of the foil together and fold to enclose the fish securely. Place the fish parcels on a baking tray and bake for 10–15 minutes or until the fish is cooked through.

4 Meanwhile, to make the rocket salad, toss together all the ingredients in a bowl and divide among four serving plates.

5 Remove the cooked fish from the foil parcels and serve with the salad, cherry tomatoes and lemon wedges.

TIP You can also make this dish with white fish fillets.

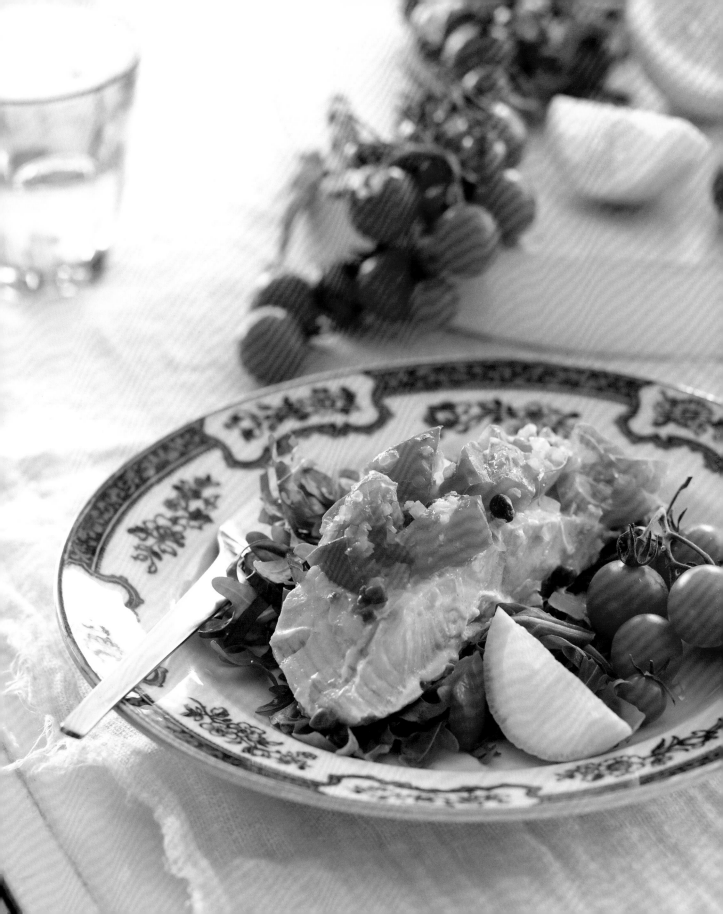

1 SERVE =
2 units protein
½ unit vegetables
½ unit fats

Japanese-style grilled fish with Asian greens

SERVES 4   PREP 15 mins   **COOK** 10 mins

2 tablespoons white miso
2 tablespoons mirin, plus
  extra to serve
2 teaspoons olive oil
800 g white fish fillets, skin
  and bones removed
400 g Asian greens, such as
  pak choy or choy sum
4 spring onions, sliced
light soy sauce, to serve

Lovely and light, this dish is based on the unique flavours of miso and mirin. The method is simplicity itself, but the results are spectacular.

1   Combine the miso, mirin and olive oil in a small bowl. Rub the miso mixture over the fish fillets.

2   Preheat the oven grill to high. Place the fillets on a baking tray, then cook under the grill for 5–7 minutes or until just cooked through.

3   Meanwhile, steam the Asian greens until tender.

4   Sprinkle the fish with spring onion and drizzle with a little light soy sauce and extra mirin. Serve with the steamed Asian greens.

> **TIP** Miso is a Japanese condiment made from fermented soy beans. It is sold in tubs or sachets and is available from the Asian section of your local supermarket. Mirin is a sweet Japanese rice wine only used in cooking. It's often used as a glaze or as part of a dipping sauce and can be added to stir-fries and marinades. Look for it in the Asian section of your local supermarket, or at an Asian grocery store. This is lovely with all types of white fish – try whiting, gemfish, snapper or flathead.

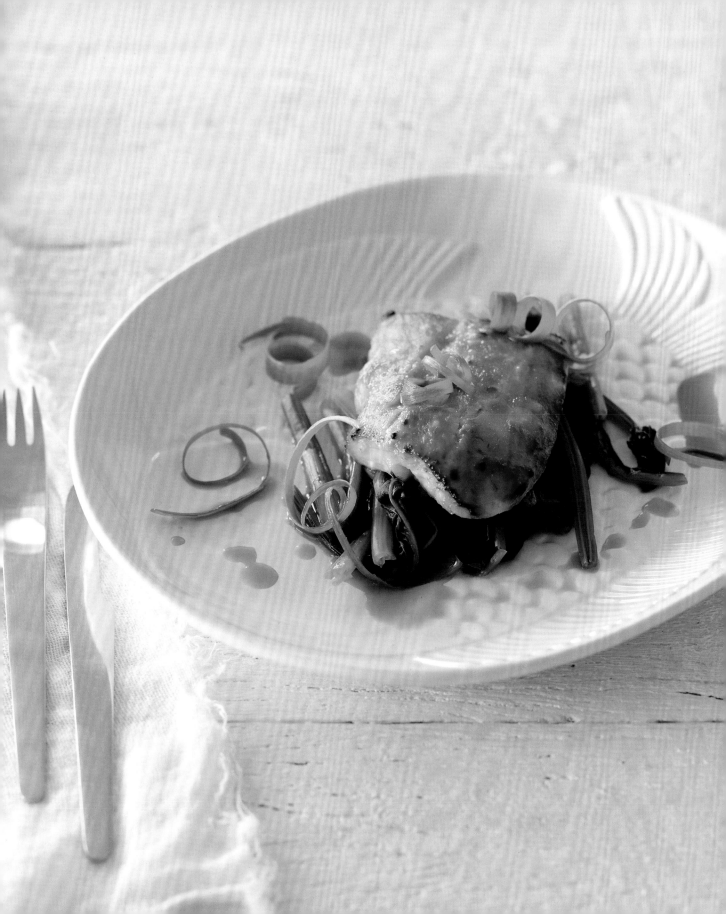

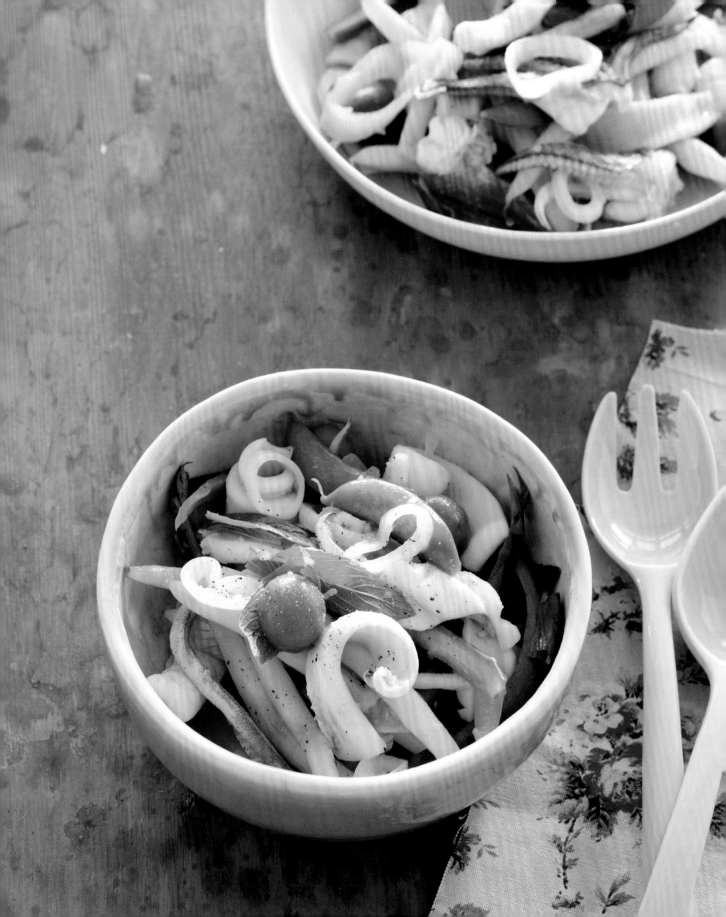

Spring vegetable and calamari saute

SERVES 4   PREP 20 mins   COOK 12 mins

150 g asparagus, trimmed

150 g yellow or green beans, trimmed

150 g sugar snap peas, trimmed

1 tablespoon olive oil

2 cloves garlic, crushed

3 spring onions, trimmed and thinly sliced

1 yellow banana capsicum (pepper), trimmed, seeded and cut into rings *or* 1 small yellow capsicum (pepper), trimmed, seeded and halved lengthways, then sliced

1.2 kg calamari, cleaned and cut into 1 cm wide pieces, tentacles reserved

2½ tablespoons lemon juice

2 teaspoons finely grated lemon zest

¼ cup (60 ml) salt-reduced chicken stock or water

½ cup (60 g) pitted green olives (optional)

large handful mint leaves (optional), to serve

The delicate flavour and tender texture of sauteed calamari is perfectly matched by the crunch of the spring vegetables here. This is a light yet satisfying meal, ideal for when the weather starts to warm up.

1 Bring a large saucepan of water to the boil, add the asparagus and beans and cook for 2 minutes, then add the sugar snaps and cook for 1 minute. Drain well and set aside.

2 Heat the oil in a large heavy-based frying pan over medium–high heat. Add the garlic, spring onion and capsicum and cook, stirring, for 3 minutes or until the vegetables start to soften. Add the calamari, lemon juice, zest and stock or water and cook, stirring often, for 2–3 minutes or until the calamari is just cooked. Add the reserved vegetables, olives and mint (if using) and toss together for 1 minute to warm through. Divide among bowls and serve immediately.

TIP Substitute the calamari with peeled raw prawns, if preferred.

Squid salad with rocket and chickpeas

SERVES 4   PREP 20 mins   COOK 5 mins

800 g squid hoods, cleaned,
   cut into pieces and scored
2 teaspoons olive oil
½ teaspoon chilli flakes (optional)
100 g baby rocket leaves
1 × 400 g tin chickpeas,
   rinsed and drained
2 tomatoes, diced
½ red (Spanish) onion, thinly sliced
1 Lebanese (small) cucumber, diced
½ cup (10 g) torn flat-leaf (Italian)
   parsley

DRESSING
¼ cup (60 ml) lemon juice
2 teaspoons olive oil
1 clove garlic, crushed

The chickpeas may seem like an unusual ingredient here, but they add a mealy texture that contrasts well with the crispness of the salad.

1 To make the dressing, place all the ingredients in a screw-top jar and shake to combine.

2 Season the squid with salt and pepper and place in a bowl with the olive oil and chilli (if using). Gently toss to coat. Heat a non-stick frying pan over medium–high heat and cook the squid for 2 minutes each side or until just cooked (you may need to do this in batches).

3 While still hot, toss the squid in the dressing.

4 Divide the rocket among four plates, top with the chickpeas, tomato, onion, cucumber and parsley, and finish with the squid and dressing. Serve immediately.

TIP Squid can be purchased already cleaned, but if you prefer to do this yourself, simply grasp the body with one hand and the head with another and gently pull apart. Discard the quill and insides and peel off the outer skin. You can also buy squid as rings, and these are fine to use in the recipe. Prawns may be used in place of the squid.

1 SERVE =
2 units protein
2½ units vegetables

olive oil spray

4 × 200 g salmon fillets, skin-on and pin-boned

TOMATO-BRAISED LEEKS

4 leeks, trimmed, washed and split lengthways, leaving root end intact

2 cups (500 ml) salt-reduced chicken stock

1 × 400 g tin crushed tomato

finely grated zest of 1 lemon

2 sprigs rosemary

Salmon with tomato-braised leeks

SERVES 4   PREP 15 mins   COOK 45 mins

Another delicious dinner dish that looks impressive and takes no time at all to prepare. You could use white fish, such as blue eye or barramundi, instead of salmon if you like.

1   For the tomato-braised leeks, preheat the oven to 180°C and place the leeks in a large baking dish.

2   Place the stock, tomato and lemon zest in a saucepan and bring to simmering point. Pour this mixture over the leeks in the dish and season to taste with salt and pepper. Add the rosemary sprigs, then cover the dish tightly with foil and bake for 40 minutes or until tender. Remove the rosemary and season the leeks to taste.

3   Heat a chargrill plate or large heavy-based frying pan over medium heat. Once hot, spray with olive oil. Add the salmon, skin-side down, and cook for 5 minutes or until the skin is crisp and golden, then turn the fish over. Cook for 2 minutes or until cooked through but still a little pink in the middle.

4   Divide the braised leeks and cooking liquid among warmed plates, then top with a salmon fillet and serve.

Stir-fried chilli plum calamari with crunchy vegetable salad

SERVES 4 **PREP** 10 mins + marinating time **COOK** 5 mins

800 g calamari rings
4 spring onions (scallions),
  cut into 4 cm lengths
2 teaspoons peanut oil
2 limes, cut into wedges
handful picked coriander
  (cilantro) leaves

MARINADE
2 tablespoons plum sauce
2 tablespoons sweet chilli sauce
1 teaspoon sesame oil
1 tablespoon oyster sauce
1 tablespoon lime juice

CRUNCHY VEGETABLE SALAD
¹/₃ cup torn Thai basil
¹/₃ cup roughly chopped
  coriander (cilantro)
¹/₃ cup roughly chopped mint
2 carrots, sliced and cut
  into matchsticks
2 cups (160 g) bean sprouts
100 g snowpea sprouts

1 Place all marinade ingredients in a bowl. Add calamari and spring onions, and toss to coat thoroughly. Cover bowl and refrigerate for 20 minutes.

2 Meanwhile, make the salad by tossing together all the ingredients in a large bowl.

3 Heat peanut oil in a large heavy-based frying pan or wok over very high heat. When the oil is smoking, tip in the calamari mixture and stir-fry for 5 minutes, or until cooked. Serve salad topped with calamari, with lime wedges on the side, and scattered with coriander.

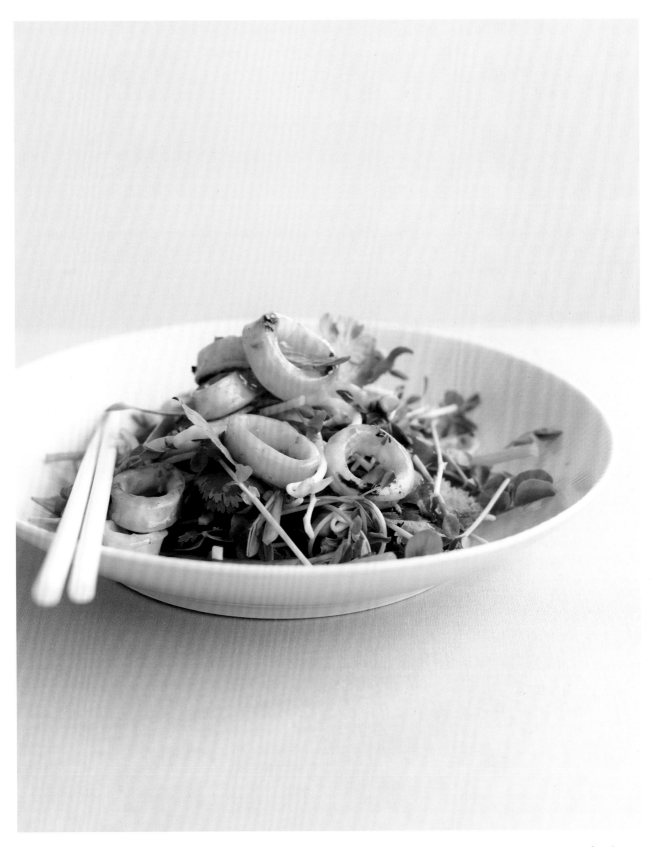

Salmon cooked in paper with vegetables, lime and ginger

SERVES 4   PREP 20 mins   COOK 15 mins

4 × 200 g salmon fillets, skin
   removed, pin-boned
1 × 2 cm piece ginger, peeled
   and finely chopped
1 stalk lemongrass, trimmed
   and thinly sliced
250 g snowpeas (mange-tout),
   trimmed
200 g baby corn, halved lengthways
16 spears asparagus, trimmed
2 limes, 1 halved, 1 thinly sliced
mixed green leaves, to serve

Wrapping fish in a parcel and cooking it in the oven allows it to steam delicately, and is a great way to infuse it with flavour. You'll have an aromatic dinner on the table in no time at all.

1   Preheat the oven to 200°C.

2   Cut four 40 cm × 30 cm pieces of baking paper and, working with one piece of paper at a time, place a piece of fish in the middle of the paper. Scatter a quarter of the ginger and lemongrass over each, then season to taste with salt and pepper. Divide the vegetables among the parcels, placing them on top of the fish.

3   Squeeze some lime juice over the fish and vegetables, then divide the lime slices among the parcels, placing them on top of the vegetables.

4   Bring the edges of the paper together and fold to enclose the ingredients securely. Place the parcels on a baking tray and bake for 12–15 minutes or until the fish is just cooked through.

5   Serve each fish parcel on a plate with some mixed green leaves alongside.

TIP Serve the parcels intact so they can be opened at the table – all those delicious cooking juices will be retained and the aroma will be irresistible.

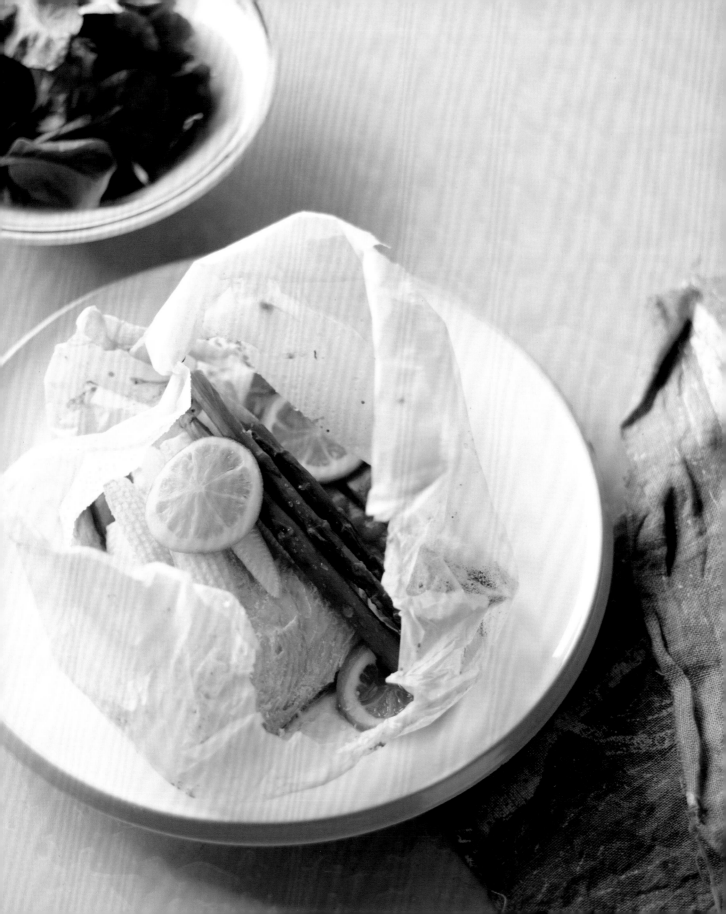

Hearty seafood, fennel and chickpea cioppino

SERVES 4   PREP 25 mins   COOK 25 mins

1 tablespoon olive oil
1 onion, finely chopped
2 cloves garlic, thinly sliced
2 sticks celery, finely chopped
3 carrots, thinly sliced
1 bulb fennel, trimmed, halved
   and thinly sliced
2 teaspoons dried oregano
1 tablespoon tomato paste (puree)
2 cups (500 ml) white wine
1 × 400 g tin chopped tomato
1 × 400 g tin chickpeas, drained
   and rinsed
200 g squid tubes,
   cut into 5 cm pieces
300 g uncooked king prawns,
   peeled and deveined
300 g white fish fillets,
   skin removed, flesh thinly sliced
flat-leaf (Italian) parsley
   (optional), to serve

Cioppino is an Italian-style fish stew. Depending on what you feel like for dinner, you can use any seafood or fish you like here – try steamed mussels or scallops instead of the prawns, or different varieties of fish.

1 Heat the oil in a large saucepan over medium heat, then add the onion, garlic, celery, carrot and fennel and cook, stirring often, for 10 minutes or until the vegetables have softened. Add the oregano and tomato paste and cook, stirring, for 1 minute. Add the wine and bring to the boil. Cook for 1–2 minutes.

2 Add the tomato and bring to simmering point, then reduce the heat to low and cook for 10 minutes or until the vegetables are tender. Stir in the chickpeas, seafood and fish, then cook, stirring often, for 3–4 minutes or until the seafood and fish is cooked through. Divide among bowls and serve immediately, topped with parsley (if using).

TIP Leave out the chickpeas if you prefer.

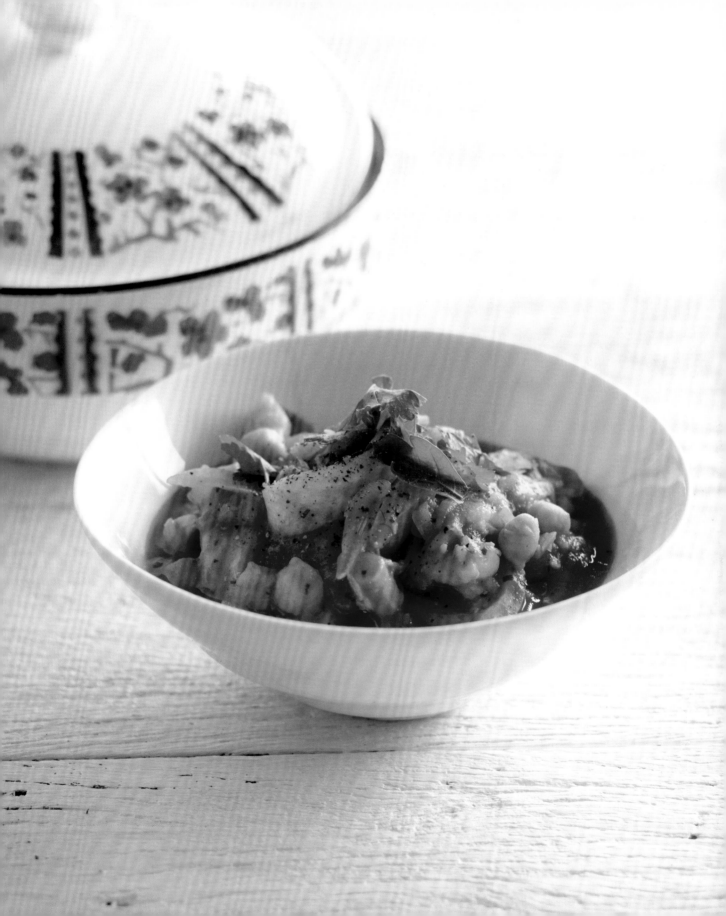

Poached blue-eye with peperonata and basil

SERVES 4   PREP 10 mins   COOK 15 mins

3 lemons
1 litre chicken stock or fish stock
2 sprigs flat-leaf (Italian) parsley
5 black peppercorns
1 bay leaf
4 × 200 g fillets blue-eye trevalla

PEPERONATA

2 tablespoons olive oil
2 red capsicums (peppers),
    seeded and sliced
1 red (Spanish) onion,
    finely chopped
2 cloves garlic, finely chopped
1 cup torn basil
freshly ground black pepper

1   Cut 1 lemon into slices and place in a deep frying pan along with stock, parsley, peppercorns and bay leaf, and bring to a boil. Reduce heat and simmer for 3 minutes. Add fish and simmer very gently for 8 minutes. Remove pan from heat and allow fish to rest in the liquid.

2   Meanwhile, heat a large saucepan over medium heat. Add oil and capsicum and cook for 5 minutes, or until the capsicum starts to soften. Add onion and garlic and cook for a further 5 minutes. Stir in basil and season well with pepper. Spoon this peperonata onto serving plates and top with fish. Serve with lemon wedges and your favourite steamed greens.

1 SERVE =
1 unit protein
½ unit bread
¼ unit dairy
1 unit vegetables

Salmon fishcakes with lemon yoghurt sauce

SERVES 4   PREP 25 mins + refrigerating time   COOK 10 mins

1 × 800 g tin salmon, drained,
    bones and skin removed
    and mashed (this will yield
    approximately 400 g salmon)
2 spring onions, finely chopped
1 teaspoon finely grated lemon zest
1 tablespoon finely chopped
    flat-leaf (Italian) parsley
½ teaspoon Worcestershire sauce
1 teaspoon Dijon mustard
2 eggs
80 g dried breadcrumbs
1 teaspoon olive oil

LEMON YOGHURT SAUCE
200 g reduced-fat yoghurt
2 teaspoons lemon juice
1 teaspoon finely grated
    lemon zest

MIXED LEAF AND TOMATO SALAD
100 g mixed salad leaves
1 punnet (250 g) grape
    tomatoes, halved
1 Lebanese (small) cucumber,
    thinly sliced
¼ red (Spanish) onion,
    thinly sliced
1 teaspoon capers,
    rinsed and drained
1 tablespoon lemon juice

Simple but delicious, the fresh flavours in this meal should ideally be enjoyed outside on a warm evening.

1 To make the fishcakes, combine all the ingredients, except for the breadcrumbs and olive oil, in a large bowl. Form into 12 patties with clean hands. Cover with plastic wrap and refrigerate for 1 hour.

2 To make the lemon yoghurt sauce, combine all the ingredients in a small bowl and mix well.

3 To make the mixed leaf and tomato salad, gently toss together all the ingredients.

4 Place the breadcrumbs in a small bowl and dip the fishcakes in, coating on all sides.

5 Heat the olive oil in a large frying pan over medium heat and cook the patties for 2 minutes each side, or until golden (you may need to do this in batches). Serve the fishcakes with a dollop of sauce and the salad to the side.

TIP If preferred, the lemon yoghurt sauce can be replaced with reduced-fat mayonnaise.

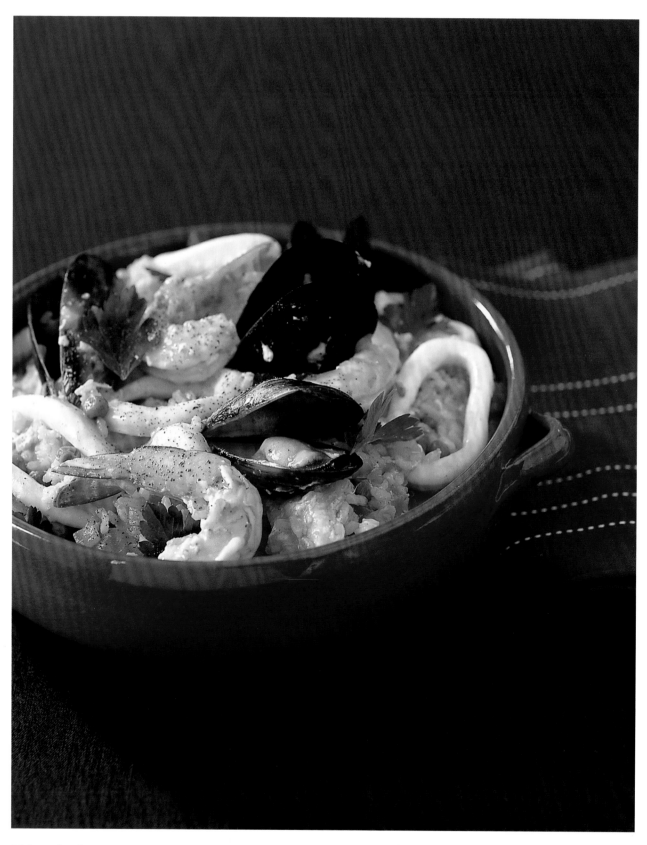

Seafood paella

SERVES 4   PREP 20 mins   COOK 50 mins

1 teaspoon saffron
1 teaspoon paprika
¼ cup (60 ml) boiling water
2 tablespoons olive oil
2 cloves garlic, crushed
1 onion, finely chopped
3 tomatoes, roughly chopped
200 g short-grain rice
1 litre chicken stock
400 g flathead fillets
150 g uncooked (green) prawns
    (shrimp), peeled
200 g mussels, bearded
    and washed
150 g calamari
150 g peas
½ cup flat-leaf (Italian) parsley,
    roughly chopped
freshly ground black pepper
lemon wedges

1 In a small non-stick frying pan, lightly toast saffron. Transfer to a cup, then crush and add paprika and boiling water. Stir to dissolve and set aside

2 Heat oil in a large heavy-based frying pan over medium heat. Add garlic and onion and cook for 5 minutes, or until soft. Add tomato and cook for 3 minutes. Add rice and cook, stirring to combine, for a further 5 minutes.

3 Meanwhile, bring stock to a boil in a saucepan. Add stock and saffron liquid to rice mixture, stirring well to combine. Simmer, uncovered, for 15 minutes. Place fish, prawns, mussels and calamari on top of rice. Cover frying pan with foil and cook for a further 10 minutes. Add peas, re-cover pan, and cook for a final 5 minutes. Sprinkle paella with parsley and season with pepper. Serve with wedges of lemon and offer a green salad on the side.

Steamed salmon with Thai sauce

SERVES 4   PREP 15 mins   COOK 15 mins

4 × 200 g salmon fillets
1 clove garlic, finely sliced
1 × 2 cm piece fresh ginger,
   finely chopped
1 stalk lemongrass, white part only,
   finely sliced
4 kaffir lime leaves, finely sliced
2 tablespoons fish sauce
1 teaspoon sesame oil
4 spring onions (scallions),
   finely sliced
4 slices lime
$^1/_3$ cup roughly chopped
   coriander (cilantro)
1 large red chilli, finely sliced
lime wedges

1   Place a bamboo steamer in a large frying pan or wok, then pour a little water into the pan. (The water level should not reach the middle of the steamer.) Bring the water to a boil.

2   Meanwhile, place fish on a small plate that fits into the steamer (you may need to cook the fish in 2 batches, depending on the size of the steamer). In a small bowl, mix garlic, ginger, lemongrass, lime leaves, fish sauce, sesame oil and half the spring onion. Spoon the mixture over the fish, then lay the lime slices on top. Carefully transfer the plate with the fish to the steamer and steam, covered, for 10 minutes. Remove from heat, transfer fish to serving plates and spoon over cooking juices. Garnish with coriander, chilli, lime wedges and the remaining spring onion, and serve with steamed mixed vegetables.

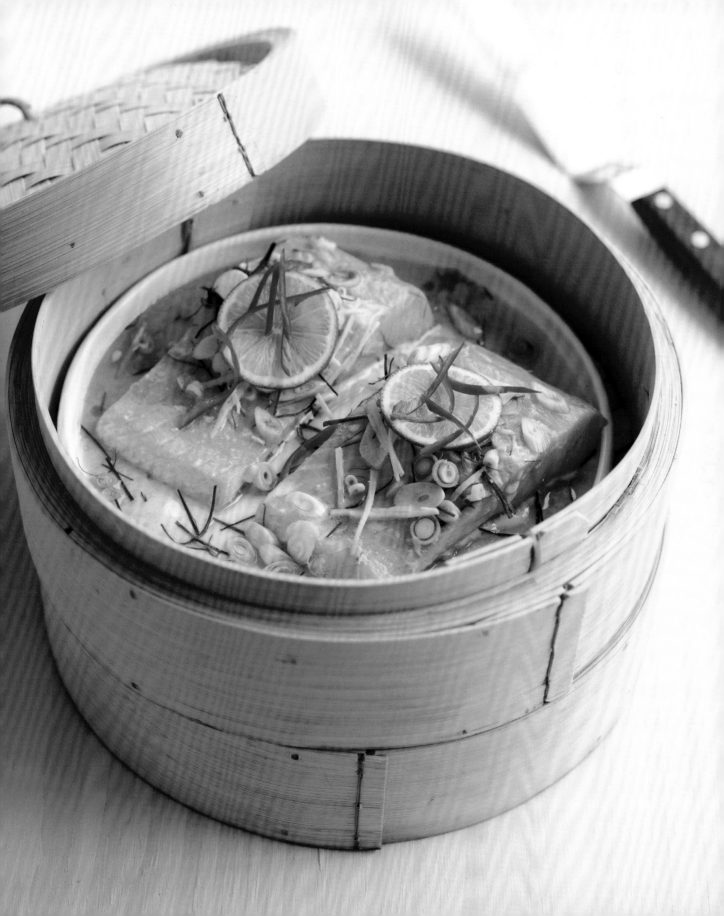

Tuna conchiglie bake

SERVES 4   **PREP** 15 mins   **COOK** 45 mins

200 g conchiglie (shell pasta)
1 teaspoon olive oil
100 g button mushrooms, sliced
1 clove garlic, crushed
2 zucchini (courgettes), diced
1 tablespoon olive oil, extra
2 tablespoons plain flour
2½ cups (625 ml) reduced-fat milk
75 g reduced-fat cheddar, grated
1 × 425 g tin tuna in spring water,
   drained and flaked
¼ cup chopped flat-leaf (Italian)
   parsley
50 g grated parmesan

A pasta bake has to come close to being the ultimate in comfort food. This clever recipe shows how you can still enjoy it without letting your diet halo slip.

1   Preheat the oven to 180°C.

2   Cook the pasta according to the packet instructions until al dente. Drain.

3   Meanwhile, heat the olive oil in a large frying pan over medium heat. Add the mushrooms and cook for 2–3 minutes until golden. Add the garlic and zucchini and cook until the zucchini has softened. Remove from the heat and transfer to a large bowl.

4   Heat the extra olive oil in a medium saucepan. Add the flour and stir until combined and just starting to bubble. Whisk in the milk and continue whisking until the sauce has thickened. Stir in the cheddar until melted and combined.

5   Add the cheese sauce to the cooked vegetables, then stir in the tuna, parsley and drained pasta. Stir to combine, then pour into a 1.5 litre baking dish. Sprinkle with the parmesan and bake for 20–25 minutes or until golden. Serve with a salad.

TIP The tuna can be replaced with shredded cooked chicken or tinned salmon.

1 SERVE =
1 unit protein
½ unit vegetables
1 unit fats

Scallops with prosciutto and cauliflower puree

SERVES 4   PREP 20 mins   COOK 20 mins

5 slices prosciutto
500 g cauliflower, cut into florets
2–3 tablespoons reduced-fat milk
1 tablespoon extra virgin olive oil
1 tablespoon lemon juice
20 scallops, roe removed
2 tablespoons baby herbs
   or snowpea sprouts
balsamic vinegar, to serve

Scallops add a touch of luxury to any occasion. Take care not to overcook them – they only need a minute each side in a hot pan.

1 Preheat the oven to 180°C and line a baking tray with baking paper. Lay the prosciutto on the tray and bake for 10 minutes or until crisp. Cool then break into crumbs with your hands. Set aside until serving.

2 Meanwhile, cook the cauliflower in a saucepan of boiling water for 15 minutes or until tender. Transfer to a food processor, gradually add the milk (you may not need all of it) and puree until smooth. Season to taste.

3 Combine the olive oil, lemon juice and a pinch of salt and pepper in a bowl. Add the scallops and stir to coat. Drain. Heat a non-stick frying pan over high heat and cook the scallops for 1 minute each side.

4 Spoon the cauliflower puree onto four serving plates and top with the scallops. Crumble the prosciutto over the scallops and finish with a handful of salad leaves. Drizzle with a little balsamic vinegar, then serve immediately.

TIP When buying scallops, look for moist, glossy flesh with a fresh sea smell. They can be purchased either shucked or still enclosed in their shell. Store them in the fridge and use within 24 hours.

1 SERVE =
2 units protein
2 units vegetables
1 unit fats

Fish with eggplant puree and braised capsicum

SERVES 4   PREP 25 mins   COOK 30 mins

2 eggplants (aubergines)
1 clove garlic, crushed
small handful flat-leaf (Italian)
    parsley, chopped (optional)
olive oil spray
4 × 200 g barramundi or other
    firm white fish fillets
rocket leaves and lemon wedges,
    to serve

BRAISED CAPSICUM
1 tablespoon olive oil
1 onion, sliced
2 cloves garlic, thinly sliced
2 large red capsicums (peppers),
    trimmed, seeded and sliced
1 tablespoon tomato paste (puree)
1 cup (250 ml) salt-reduced fish
    or chicken stock
1½ tablespoons red wine vinegar
small handful basil (optional)

Eggplant and capsicum are a classic Mediterranean combination, and here they really enhance the subtle flavour of the fish.

1   To make the braised capsicum, heat the oil in a saucepan over medium heat. Add the onion, garlic and capsicum, then cook, stirring often, for 5–6 minutes or until the vegetables have softened. Add the tomato paste and cook for 1 minute, then add the stock and vinegar. Bring to simmering point, then cover and cook for 15 minutes over low–medium heat or until the vegetables are very tender. Add the basil (if using) and stir through just to wilt.

2   Meanwhile, place each eggplant directly over a medium gas flame on your stovetop and cook, turning often, for 10 minutes or until the skin is blackened and the eggplant is very soft. (Alternatively, bake the eggplants in a preheated 200°C oven for 20 minutes or until soft). When the eggplants are cool enough to handle, peel them, taking care to get rid of as much charred skin as possible, then combine the flesh with the garlic and parsley in a bowl. Use a fork to mash to a coarse puree, then season to taste with salt and pepper.

3   Place a large heavy-based frying pan over medium heat. Once hot, spray the pan with olive oil and cook the barramundi, skin-side down, for 3–4 minutes, then turn and cook for 2–3 minutes or until cooked through.

4   Divide the braised capsicum among bowls or plates and serve with the fish and the eggplant puree, some rocket leaves to the side and lemon wedges to squeeze over.

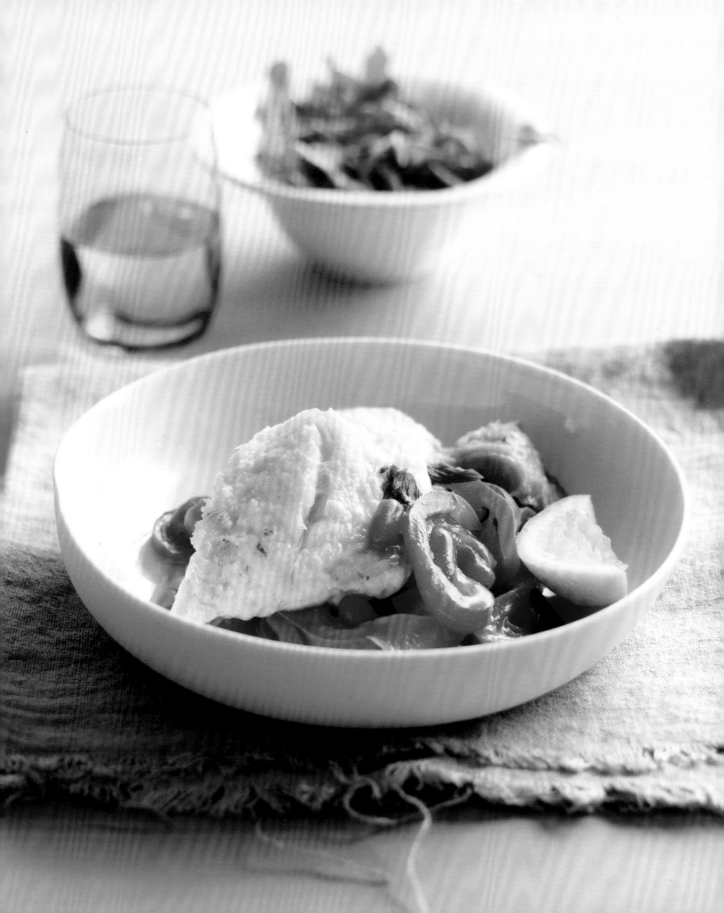

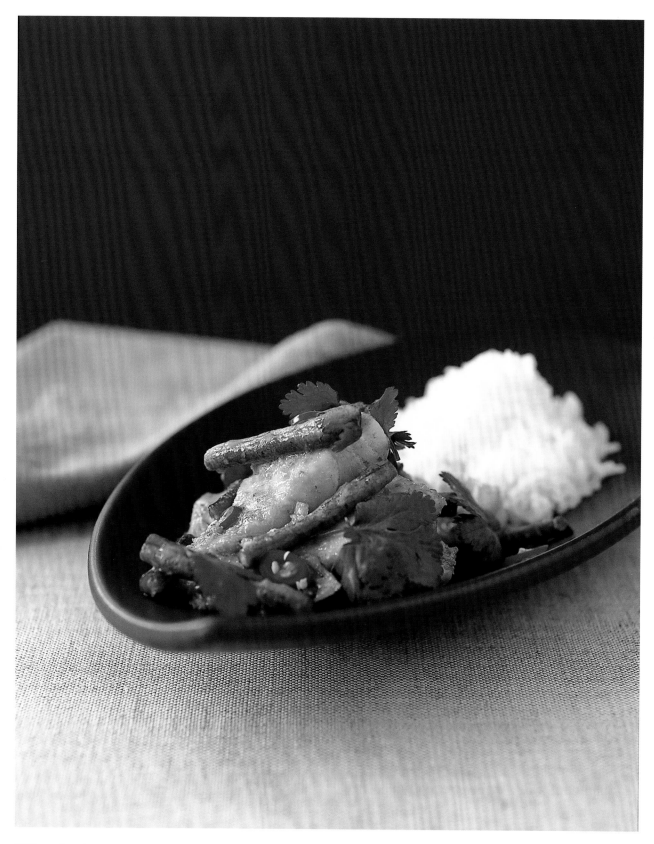

1 SERVE =
2 units protein
½ unit vegetables
1 unit fats

Barramundi curry with snake beans

SERVES 4   PREP 20 mins   COOK 10 mins

1 tablespoon peanut oil
800 g barramundi fillets,
   cut into chunks
1 teaspoon sugar
½ cup (125 ml) chicken stock
1 tablespoon fish sauce
200 g snake beans, cut
   into 5 cm lengths
coriander (cilantro) leaves

CURRY PASTE
1 red chilli, roughly chopped
1 stalk lemongrass, finely chopped
1 tablespoon chopped spring
   onion (scallion)
1 clove garlic, roughly chopped
2 teaspoons finely grated ginger
2 teaspoons chopped coriander
   (cilantro) root
1 teaspoon shrimp paste
2 kaffir lime leaves

1 Place all curry paste ingredients in a food processor and blend to a fine paste.

2 Heat oil in a large non-stick frying pan or wok over medium heat. Add curry paste and fish and stir-fry for 3 minutes, turning fish carefully to coat lightly with paste. Add sugar, chicken stock, fish sauce and beans and cook for a further 5 minutes. Remove from heat and sprinkle with coriander. Serve with rice from your daily bread allowance and steamed vegetables.

Poached salmon with lemon, olive and parsley relish and bean salad

SERVES 4   PREP 20 mins   COOK 14 mins

300 g green or yellow beans, trimmed

2 cups (300 g) fresh podded or frozen broad beans, peeled (see page 476)

1 bunch radishes, trimmed and thinly sliced

2½ tablespoons lemon juice

4 × 200 g salmon fillets, skin-on, pin-boned

lemon wedges (optional), to serve

LEMON, OLIVE AND PARSLEY RELISH

1 lemon, peeled with all white pith removed

handful flat-leaf (Italian) parsley leaves, thinly sliced

100 g pitted green olives, chopped

1 tablespoon extra virgin olive oil

Use this refreshing relish to dress up poached, steamed or barbecued chicken or white fish fillets such as snapper.

1   To make the relish, use a small sharp knife to remove the segments of the lemon, cutting between the membranes. Chop the lemon flesh, then combine in a small bowl with the remaining ingredients. Season with salt and pepper and set aside.

2   Bring a saucepan of water to the boil, then add the green beans and cook for 2 minutes. Add the broad beans and cook for another 1–2 minutes or until the vegetables are just tender. Drain the vegetables well, reserving the cooking water, then transfer to a large bowl. Add the radish and lemon juice and toss to combine, then set aside.

3   Place the reserved cooking water in a deep frying pan large enough to hold the fish. Bring the liquid to simmering point, then add the fish, skin-side down, adding a little more boiling water if necessary to just cover the fish. Simmer over low heat for 8–10 minutes or until the fish is cooked through but still a little pink in the middle.

4   Divide the salad mixture among four plates, then place a piece of fish alongside. Spoon over the relish, then serve immediately with lemon wedges (if using).

> **TIP** To increase your vegetable units for the day, add a handful of rocket or baby spinach leaves to the salad. Use shaved cucumber instead of radish, if preferred.

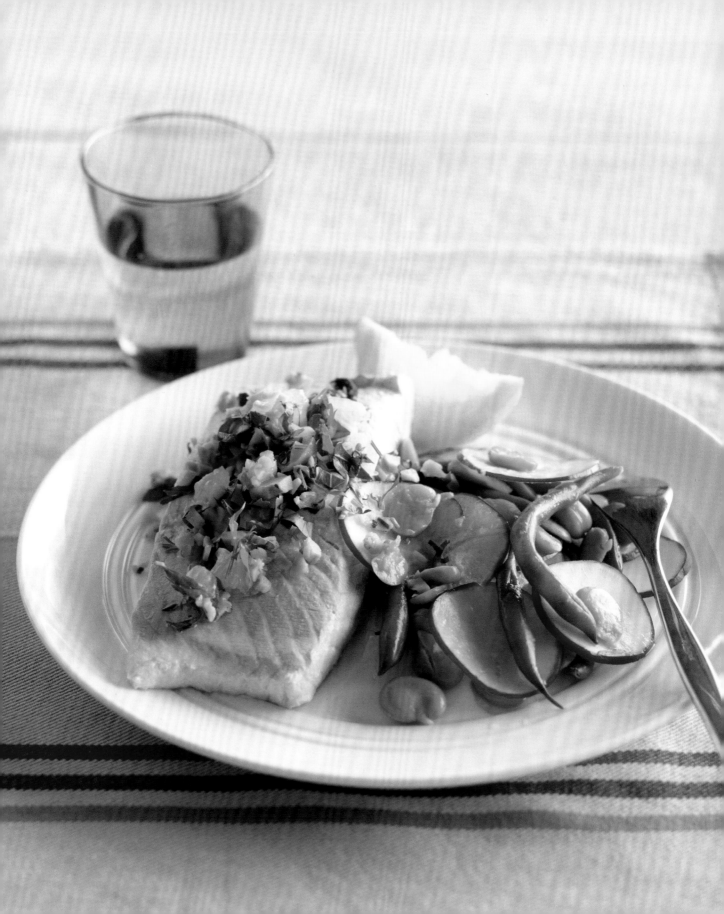

1 SERVE =
2 units protein
½ unit fruit
2½ units vegetables
1 unit fats

Fish tagine

SERVES 4 PREP 20 mins COOK 20 mins

1 tablespoon olive oil
1 onion, chopped
2 cloves garlic, crushed
1½ teaspoons each ground sweet
   paprika, cumin and coriander
1 teaspoon chilli powder
$^1/_3$ cup (50 g) raisins
400 g carrots, cut into batons
1 × 690 ml bottle salt-reduced
   tomato passata
200 g grape tomatoes, halved
1 tablespoon finely grated
   lemon zest
800 g boneless snapper or other
   white fish fillets, skin removed,
   pin-boned and cut into 1 cm
   wide strips
lemon wedges, to serve
Oven-steamed Vegetables
   (see page 519), to serve

CHILLI YOGHURT
3 teaspoons chilli paste
140 g reduced-fat Greek-style
   yoghurt

This quick tagine is healthy and full of flavour. Serve with a portion of couscous (see page 518) if you have a bread unit saved for the day.

1 Heat the olive oil in a large heavy-based saucepan over medium heat. Add the onion and garlic and cook, stirring, for 5 minutes or until softened. Add the spices and cook, stirring, for another minute or so until fragrant. Add the raisins, carrot and passata and bring to simmering point. Cover and cook over low heat for 10–15 minutes or until the carrot is tender. Add the tomato, lemon zest and fish, then cook over medium heat for 5 minutes or until the fish is cooked through.

2 Meanwhile, combine the chilli paste and yoghurt in a small bowl.

3 Serve the tagine with the chilli yoghurt and steamed vegetables alongside.

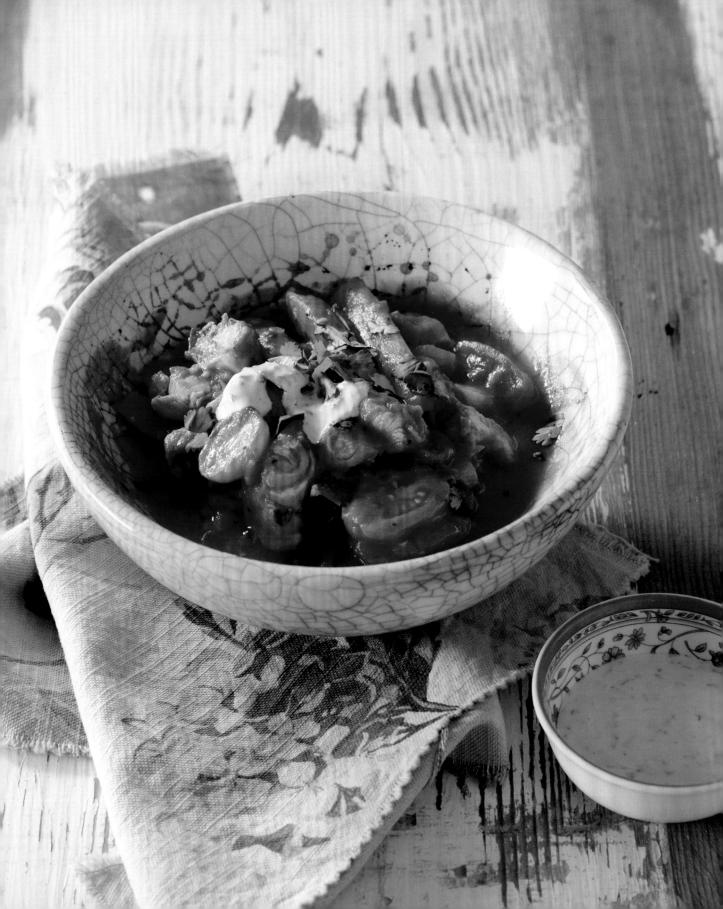

1 SERVE =
2 units protein
1 unit vegetables
½ unit fats

Seared tuna with Asian greens and soy

SERVES 4   PREP 10 mins   COOK 6 mins

4 × 200 g tuna steaks
2 teaspoons peanut oil
2 bunches baby bok choy (pak choi),
   leaves separated and washed
4 spring onions (scallions),
   finely slivered
½ cup coriander (cilantro) leaves
½ cup mint leaves
lime wedges

DRESSING

2 tablespoons light soy sauce
2 teaspoons lime juice
1 teaspoon grated ginger

1 In a cup, mix all dressing ingredients.

2 Heat a heavy-based frying pan over medium heat. Brush tuna steaks with oil. Add to pan and cook for 3 minutes each side.

3 Meanwhile, bring a little water to a simmer in a wok. Put bok choy into a bamboo steamer and place steamer in wok. Cover wok and steam bok choy for 2–3 minutes.

4 Divide bok choy between serving plates and arrange tuna steaks on top. Sprinkle with spring onion, coriander and mint and drizzle the dressing over. Offer lime wedges.

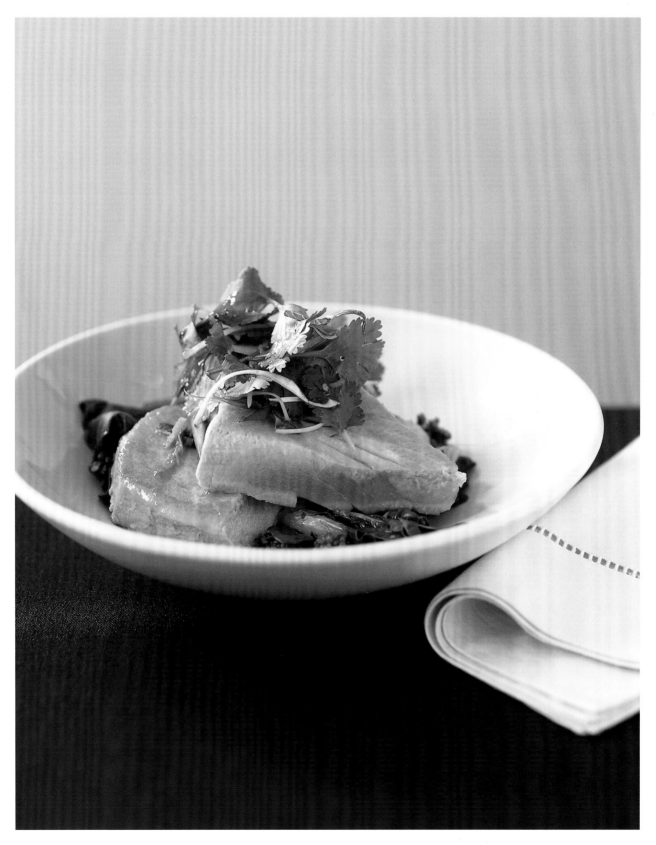

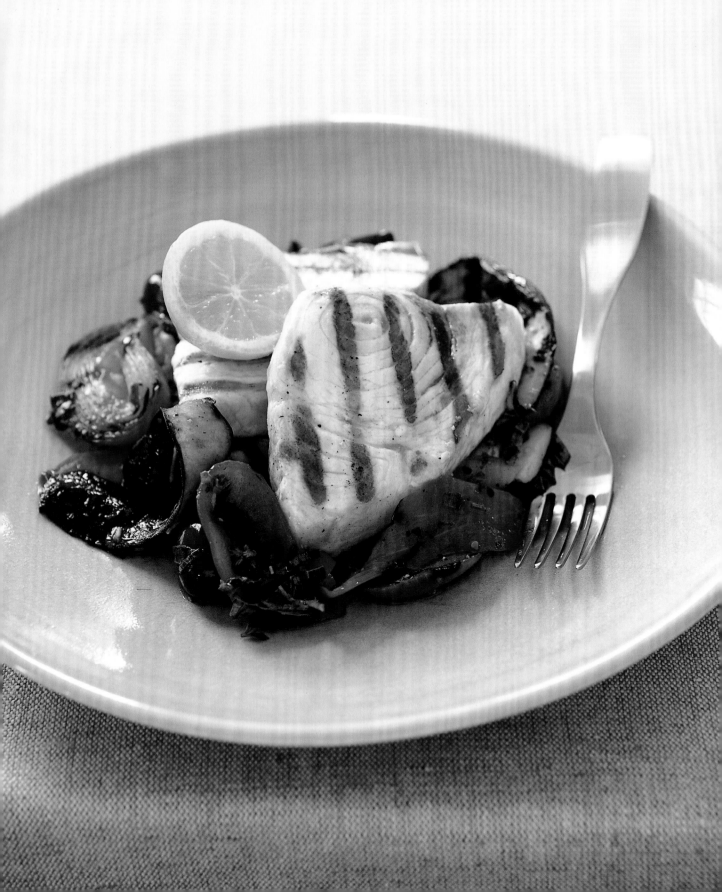

1 SERVE =
2 unit protein
1 unit vegetables
2 units fats

Barbecued swordfish with charred Mediterranean vegetables and olives

SERVES 4　PREP 15 mins　COOK 10 mins

1 red capsicum (pepper),
　seeded and thickly sliced
1 yellow capsicum (pepper),
　seeded and thickly sliced
2 zucchini (courgette),
　sliced lengthways
1 red (Spanish) onion,
　thickly sliced
2 tablespoons olive oil
2 cloves garlic, chopped
8 kalamata olives
2 teaspoons balsamic vinegar
1 tablespoon chopped flat-leaf
　(Italian) parsley
¼ cup torn basil
juice of ½ lemon
olive oil spray
4 × 200 g swordfish steaks
lemon wedges

1　Preheat a grill plate or barbecue grill to high.

2　Place capsicum, zucchini and onion in a bowl with half the oil and lightly season. Toss to coat thoroughly. Transfer to grill plate and cook, turning occasionally, for 3–5 minutes, or until charred and slightly wilted. Return vegetables to bowl. Add garlic, olives, balsamic vinegar, parsley, basil, lemon juice and remaining oil and toss lightly. Cover with plastic wrap and allow flavours to infuse while cooking the fish.

3　Lightly spray swordfish steaks with oil spray and lightly season. Char-grill for 2 minutes each side, or until cooked. Divide vegetables between serving plates and top with fish. Serve with lemon wedges.

Steamed bream with lemon and capers

SERVES 4   PREP 15 mins   COOK 10 mins

1 small red (Spanish) onion,
    finely diced
1 tablespoon capers, chopped
2 tablespoons flat-leaf
    (Italian) parsley
2 tablespoons olive oil
juice and finely grated zest
    of 2 lemons
4 × 200 g bream fillets
300 g baby squash
150 g baby spinach

1 Preheat oven to 200°C.

2 In a small bowl, combine onion, capers, parsley, 1 tablespoon of the oil and half the lemon juice and zest.

3 Tear off 4 large pieces of foil. Place a fish fillet in the centre of each and spoon over lemon and caper mixture. Bring together the long sides of each foil parcel and fold the edge over several times. Now fold in the short ends of the foil several times to ensure the parcel is well sealed. Transfer parcels to a baking tray and cook for 10 minutes, or until fish is cooked through. (The exact cooking time will depend on the thickness of the fillets.)

4 Meanwhile, steam squash for 5 minutes, or until cooked. Drain and slice thickly while still hot. Transfer to a large bowl and add spinach leaves. Toss to combine, and drizzle with remaining lemon juice and zest. Season lightly and serve alongside the steamed bream.

Fish kebabs with spiced corn and tomato

SERVES 4   **PREP** 20 mins + marinating time   **COOK** 25 mins

200 g reduced-fat natural yoghurt
2 teaspoons curry powder
4 cloves garlic, crushed
3 teaspoons finely grated ginger
800 g thick white fish fillets,
   skin and bones removed,
   cut into large cubes
¼ cup coriander (cilantro) leaves
lemon wedges, to serve

SPICED CORN AND TOMATO
1 tablespoon olive oil
1 teaspoon cumin seeds
1 teaspoon ground turmeric
¼ teaspoon chilli powder
3 tomatoes, diced
1 × 350 g tin corn kernels,
   drained

This is a great summer meal. The spiced corn and tomato would also make a lovely accompaniment to barbecued meats or chicken.

1   In a large bowl, combine the yoghurt, curry powder, garlic and ginger. Add the fish and toss gently to coat with spice mixture. Cover and marinate for 15 minutes.

2   To prepare the spiced corn and tomato, heat the olive oil in a medium saucepan over medium heat and cook the spices for 1 minute or until fragrant. Add the tomato and cook for 3–4 minutes or until softened. Add the corn and ½ cup (125 ml) water and bring to the boil, then reduce the heat and simmer for 5 minutes or until thickened.

3   Preheat the oven grill to medium–high. Thread the fish onto eight skewers. Place on an oiled tray or grill plate and grill for 5 minutes each side, or until cooked through (the cooking time will depend on the thickness of the fish).

4   Sprinkle the kebabs with coriander leaves and serve with the spiced corn and tomato, lemon wedges and steamed rice from your daily bread allowance.

> **TIP** If you are using wooden skewers, soak them in water for about 20 minutes so they don't scorch during cooking. You could also make the kebabs with chicken.

Parmesan fish fingers with homemade wedges

SERVES 4   PREP 25 mins   COOK 40 mins

6 medium potatoes, cut into wedges
2 tablespoons olive oil
2 teaspoons Cajun spice mix (optional)
50 g grated parmesan
½ cup (85 g) polenta
2 eggs
700 g thin fish fillets, skin and bones removed, cut into 5 cm fingers
olive oil spray
lemon wedges, to serve
reduced-fat tartare sauce, to serve

The parmesan and polenta coating gives the fish fingers a wonderful crunch, and the potato wedges are equally delicious with or without the Cajun spices.

1   Preheat the oven to 200°C and line two baking trays with baking paper.

2   Toss the potato wedges with the olive oil and spice mix (if using) and place on one of the trays in a single layer. Bake for 35–40 minutes, turning once or twice, until golden and crisp.

3   Meanwhile, combine the parmesan and polenta in a bowl. Place the eggs in a separate bowl and lightly beat them. Dip the fish pieces in the egg and then in the polenta mixture, shaking off any excess. Place on the other baking tray, spray with olive oil and bake for 20 minutes or until crisp.

4   Serve the fish fingers and potato wedges with lemon wedges, tartare sauce and a salad to the side.

> **TIP** For best results, use a thin white fish such as flathead, whiting or snapper to make the fish fingers.

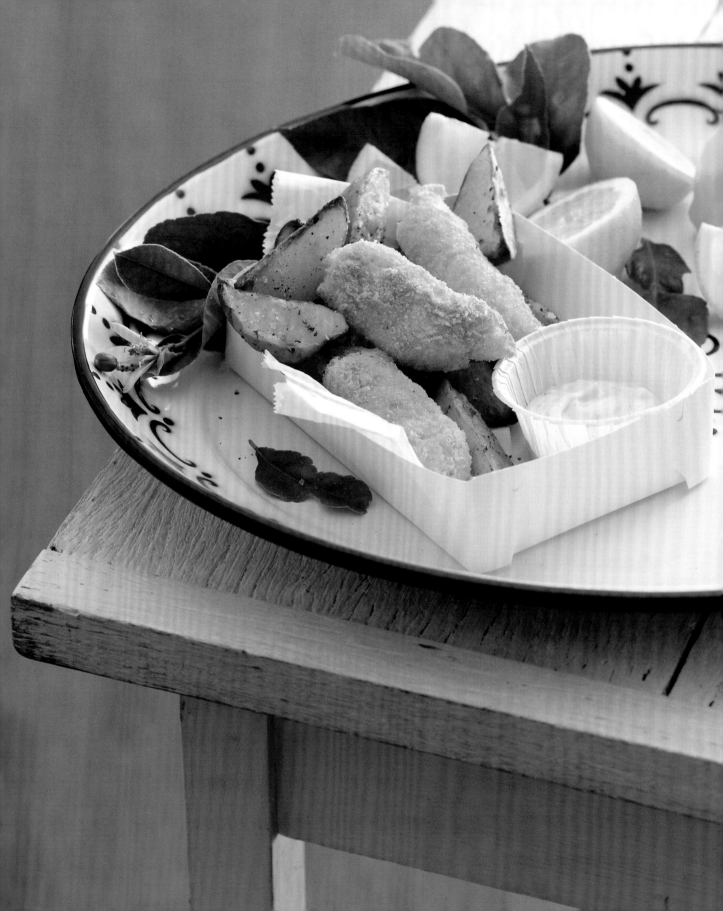

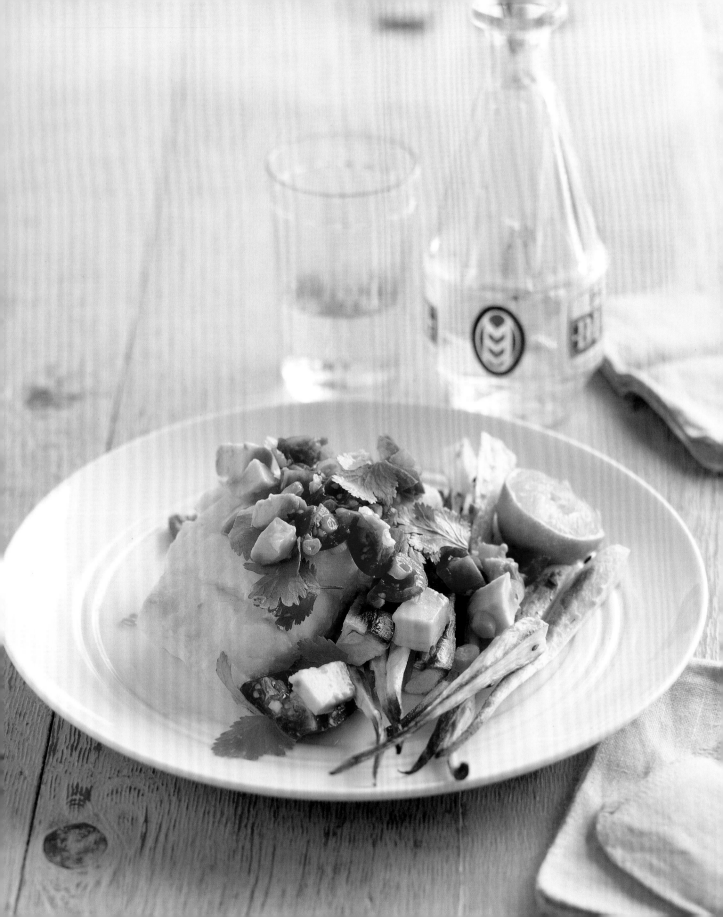

Steamed fish with chunky guacamole and cumin-roasted parsnip

SERVES 4   PREP 15 mins   **COOK** 30 mins

1 tablespoon vegetable oil
500 g small parsnips, peeled
   and quartered lengthways
1 teaspoon cumin seeds
4 × 200 g snapper or other white
   fish fillets, skin removed and
   pin-boned
lime halves (optional), to serve

CHUNKY GUACAMOLE

1 avocado (about 250 g), peeled,
   seeded and cut into cubes
1 small red (Spanish) onion,
   finely chopped
250 g cherry tomatoes, quartered
handful coriander (cilantro) or
   flat-leaf (Italian) parsley leaves,
   coarsely chopped
¼ cup (60 ml) lime juice
1 red chilli, or to taste, finely chopped

This unusual combination of flavours works beautifully and will impress at a dinner party. Serve this refreshing dish with a green salad to increase your vegetable units for the day.

1 For the chunky guacamole, place all the ingredients in a bowl and toss gently to combine well.

2 Preheat the oven to 180°C. Place the oil and parsnip in a roasting tin and toss to combine well. Roast for 20 minutes, then sprinkle over the cumin seeds. Roast for another 10 minutes or until the parsnip is very tender, then season with salt and pepper.

3 Meanwhile, pour water into the base of a steamer or a wok fitted with a steamer basket and bring to the boil. Place the fish on a plate which will fit into the steamer, cover and steam for 8 minutes or until just cooked through.

4 Serve the fish immediately with the guacamole, roast parsnip and lime halves (if using).

Seafood platter

SERVES 8 **PREP** 25 mins + marinating time **COOK** 3 mins

1 tablespoon olive oil

2 tablespoons lemon juice

2 cloves garlic, crushed

2 tablespoons chopped
   flat-leaf (Italian) parsley

250 g uncooked prawns, peeled
   and deveined, or 200 g squid
   hoods, cut into rings or pieces

8 scallops

300 g clams or mussels, scrubbed
   and debearded

150 g white fish fillets, skin and
   bones removed, cut into strips

12 oysters

CREAMY TOMATO SAUCE

¼ cup (75 g) reduced-fat mayonnaise

1 tablespoon tomato ketchup

1 teaspoon Worcestershire sauce

2 teaspoons lemon juice

VINAIGRETTE

2 golden shallots, finely chopped

2 tablespoons extra virgin olive oil

1 tablespoon white wine vinegar

1 tablespoon lemon or lime juice

1 teaspoon brown sugar

What better way to enjoy the company of friends than over a platter of freshly grilled seafood? The dipping sauces enhance the wonderful flavours.

1 Combine the olive oil, lemon juice, garlic and parsley and brush over the prawns or squid, scallops, clams or mussels and fish. Cover and marinate in the refrigerator for 30 minutes.

2 To make the tomato sauce, combine all the ingredients in a small bowl, then transfer to a dipping bowl and set aside until ready to serve.

3 To make the vinaigrette, combine all the ingredients in a small bowl, then transfer to a dipping bowl and set aside until ready to serve.

4 Heat a chargrill or barbecue to medium. Add the marinated seafood and grill, turning, for 2–3 minutes or until just cooked. Arrange on a platter with the oysters and serve with the sauce and vinaigrette to the side.

TIP To save time on the day of the barbecue, you can make the marinade, sauce and vinaigrette in advance and store them in the refrigerator until ready to use.

Cajun fish fillets

SERVES 4   PREP 15 mins   **COOK** 15 mins

60 g skim-milk powder
1 cup (250 ml) water
1 tablespoon paprika
2 teaspoons ground cumin
1 teaspoon turmeric
1 teaspoon chilli powder
800 g white fish fillets (whiting,
    snapper, flathead, etc)
2 tablespoons olive oil
400 g reduced-fat natural yoghurt
1 small cucumber, finely diced

1 Preheat oven to 200°C. Line a baking tray with baking paper.

2 Mix milk powder and water in a small bowl. In a separate bowl, mix ground spices.

3 Dip fish fillets into the milk, then roll in the mixed spices.

4 Heat oil in a frying pan over high heat. Rapidly fry the fish, in batches, for 2 minutes each side, or until golden. Be careful not to overcrowd the pan, as the fish will stew. Place all fillets on prepared baking tray and bake for 5 minutes.

5 Mix yoghurt and cucumber and lightly season. Serve fish with lemon wedges and Yoghurt Sauce (see page 536) and with salad or vegetables.

1 SERVE =
1 unit protein
2 units bread
1 unit vegetables
1 unit fats

Thai fish burgers

SERVES 4   PREP 20 mins   COOK 10 mins

400 g boneless white fish fillets,
    coarsely chopped
2 spring onions, trimmed and
    finely chopped
1 small red chilli, finely chopped
1 stalk lemongrass, trimmed
    and finely chopped
1 tablespoon fish sauce
small handful coriander (cilantro)
    leaves, finely chopped (optional)
vegetable oil spray
4 × 70 g wholegrain buns or
    bread rolls, split in half
1 Lebanese (small) cucumber,
    thinly sliced
small handful Asian salad mix
1 avocado, halved, seeded and sliced
½ small red (Spanish) onion,
    thinly sliced
2 tablespoons sweet chilli sauce

These are perfect to serve for lunch when you've got some mates coming over to watch the footy. If you're short of time, substitute the chilli, lemongrass, fish sauce and coriander in the patties with 2 tablespoons of bought Thai red curry paste.

1 Place the fish in a food processor, then process until a coarse paste forms. Transfer to a bowl, then add the spring onion, chilli, lemongrass, fish sauce and coriander (if using) and stir to mix well. Season to taste, then divide into four even-sized portions.

2 Spray a non-stick frying pan with vegetable oil and heat over medium heat. Add the fish cakes and cook for 5 minutes on each side or until golden and cooked through.

3 Meanwhile, toast the buns or rolls on both sides and place the bases on four plates. Top each with one-quarter of the cucumber and salad mix. Place a fish cake on top, then add the avocado and onion and drizzle over the chilli sauce. Place the lids on top and serve.

TIP Asian salad mix is available from most supermarkets and can include shiso leaves, mizuna and cress.

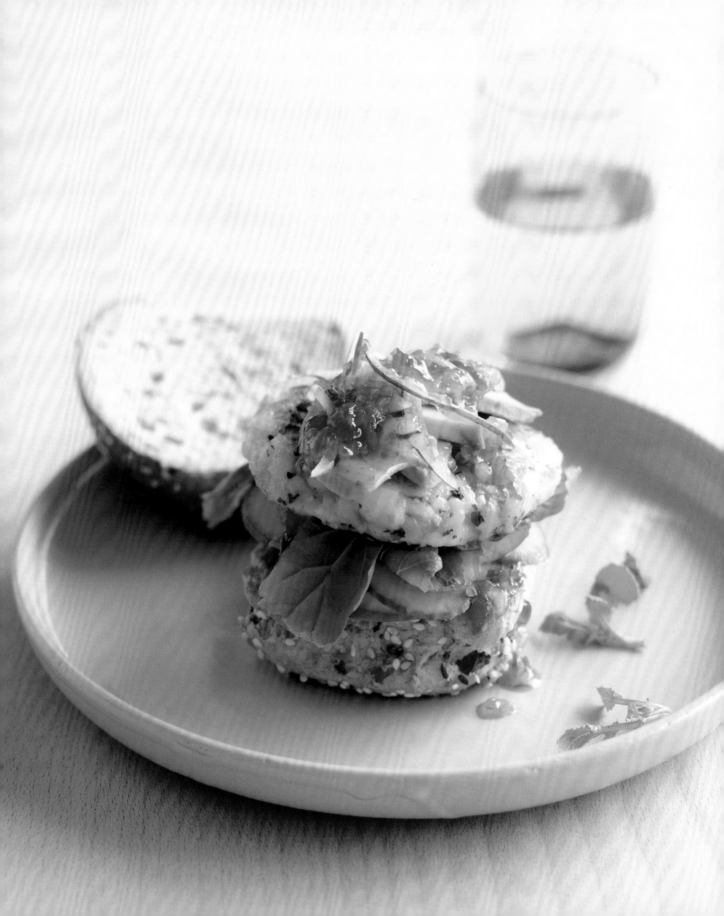

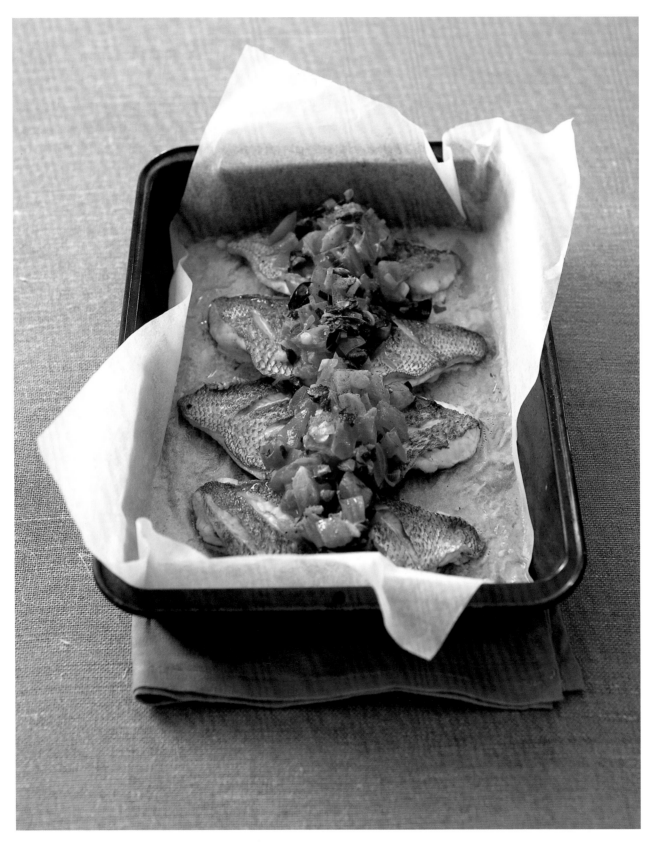

1 SERVE =
2 units protein
½ unit vegetables
2 units fats

Baked snapper with basil, capers and tomato

SERVES 4   PREP 10 mins   COOK 20 mins

2 tablespoons olive oil
1 clove garlic, crushed
½ red chilli, finely chopped
3 spring onions (scallions),
   finely sliced
¼ cup roughly chopped basil
1 tablespoon dried oregano
2 tablespoons capers
¼ cup (60 ml) white wine
4 tomatoes, seeded and
   roughly chopped
4 × 200 g snapper fillets

1   Heat half the oil in a small saucepan over medium heat. Add garlic, chilli and spring onion and cook, stirring, for 2 minutes, or until garlic is golden. Reduce heat to medium–low, then add herbs, capers and wine and cook, stirring occasionally, for 5 minutes. Remove from heat and stir through chopped tomato.

2   Heat a large non-stick frying pan over high heat. Brush fish with remaining oil and sear each side for 2 minutes. Transfer to an ovenproof baking dish and spoon sauce over fish. Bake for 6–8 minutes, or until cooked – when cooked, the flesh will flake away easily when pressed with a fork.

3   Serve with a green salad.

VARIATION

Experiment with different ingredients in the baking dish. For example, top 800 g whiting or flathead with onion slices, chopped parsley, lemon zest and fresh thyme. Pour over white wine, or lemon juice mixed with crushed garlic, and a drizzle of oil.

1 SERVE =
1 unit protein
1 unit dairy
1 unit vegetables
2 units fats

Tomatoes stuffed with tuna, basil and spinach

SERVES 4   PREP 15 mins   COOK 20 mins

8 medium-sized ripe tomatoes
400 g tinned tuna in spring water,
    drained and flaked
½ red (Spanish) onion, finely diced
¹/₃ cup shredded basil
1 × 250 g packet frozen spinach,
    defrosted
1 tablespoon finely grated
    lemon zest
200 g reduced-fat ricotta
freshly ground black pepper
2 tablespoons olive oil

1 Preheat oven to 170°C.

2 Slice tops off tomatoes and carefully remove flesh with a teaspoon, reserving lids and flesh for later. Place tomato shells upside down on paper towels to drain.

3 Place tuna, onion, basil, spinach, lemon zest, ricotta and tomato flesh in a bowl, season well with pepper and combine thoroughly. Spoon tuna mixture into tomato shells and replace tops. Transfer tomatoes to an ovenproof dish and drizzle with olive oil. Bake for 20 minutes, or until heated through. Serve with roasted zucchini or rocket salad.

1 SERVE =
2 units protein
1 unit dairy
1½ units vegetables

Fish pie

SERVES 4   PREP 25 mins   COOK 1 hour 15 mins

300 g pumpkin (squash), peeled,
    seeded and chopped
400 g swede, peeled and chopped
25 g grated parmesan cheese
800 g barramundi fillets, skin
    removed, pin-boned and cut
    into 2.5 cm pieces
3 cups (750 ml) reduced-fat milk
1 fresh bay leaf
finely grated zest of 1 lemon
¼ cup (35 g) cornflour
2½ tablespoons chopped chives

**Fish pie is always a popular choice for dinner. Use any firm
white fish for this, such as snapper, blue eye or ling.**

1 Cook the pumpkin and swede in a large saucepan of boiling water
   for 15 minutes or until tender. Drain well, then mash, stir through
   the cheese and set aside, keeping warm.

2 Preheat the oven to 180°C. Line the base of a 2.5 litre capacity baking
   dish with the fish pieces.

3 Place 600 ml of the milk, the bay leaf and lemon zest in a saucepan
   and bring to simmering point. Meanwhile, in a small bowl, mix the
   cornflour with the remaining milk until a smooth paste forms. Stirring
   constantly, add the paste to the simmering milk mixture in a steady
   stream, then cook, stirring, for 2–3 minutes or until thickened. Remove
   the bay leaf, then pour the mixture over the fish in the baking dish.

4 Spoon over the mash, spreading it as evenly as you can without
   pushing it into the sauce. Bake for 45–50 minutes or until the sauce
   is bubbling and the fish is cooked through. Serve immediately.

Sesame ocean trout with mixed mushrooms

SERVES 4   **PREP** 15 mins   **COOK** 10 mins

3 limes, quartered
1 tablespoon black sesame seeds
2 teaspoons white sesame seeds
4 × 200 g ocean trout fillets,
  skin removed
1 tablespoon canola oil
1 clove garlic, crushed
1 × 2 cm piece fresh ginger,
  finely sliced
3 spring onions (scallions),
  finely sliced
400 g mixed mushrooms
  (oyster, shiitake, Swiss brown),
  large ones sliced
6 baby bok choy (pak choi), halved
2 tablespoons oyster sauce
2 tablespoons water
¹⁄₃ cup roughly chopped coriander
  (cilantro)

1   Preheat oven 200°C. Squeeze enough lime quarters to yield 2 tablespoons lime juice, and reserve the others.

2   In a small bowl, combine the sesame seeds. Sprinkle seeds over fish, then transfer fillets to a baking tray. Bake for 10 minutes, or until cooked – when cooked, the flesh will flake away easily when pressed with a fork.

3   Meanwhile, heat oil in large frying pan or wok over high heat. Add garlic, ginger and spring onions and cook for 2 minutes, or until onions are soft. Add mushrooms and bok choy and toss together. Add lime juice, oyster sauce and water and stir-fry for 2–3 minutes. Finally, toss through coriander. Place stir-fried mushrooms on plates and top with ocean trout. Serve the remaining lime wedges on the side.

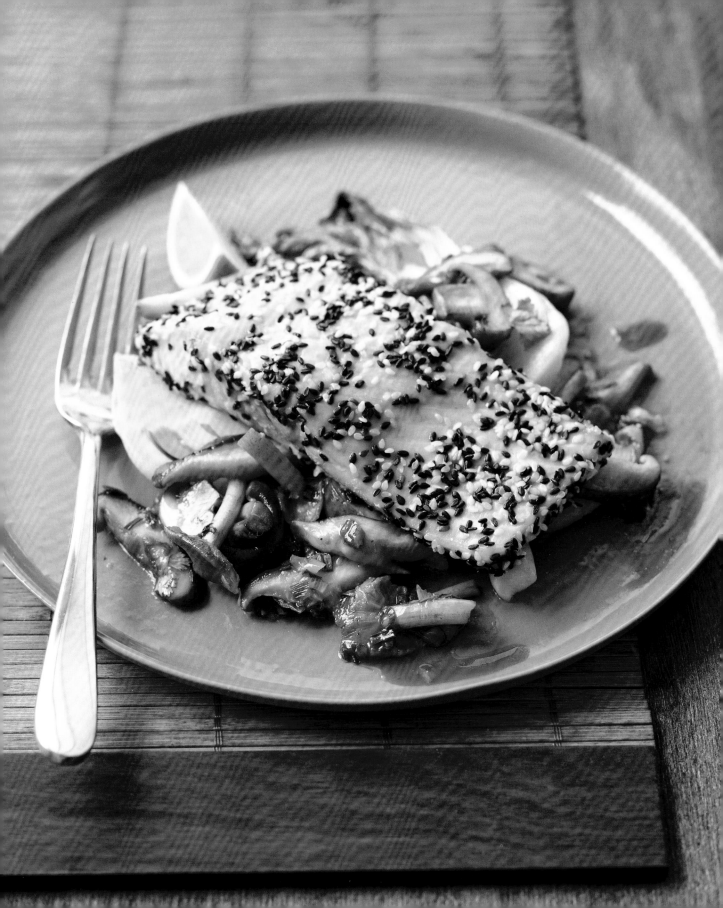

1 SERVE =
2 units protein
1½ units vegetables
1½ units fat

Salt and pepper calamari with mango and watercress salad

SERVES 4   PREP 20 mins   COOK 5 mins

800 g squid hoods, cleaned
1 teaspoon salt flakes
1 teaspoon coarsely ground
   black peppercorns
1 tablespoon vegetable oil
2 spring onions, sliced
1 red chilli, sliced (optional)

MANGO AND WATERCRESS SALAD
1 mango, peeled, seed removed
   and sliced
1 cucumber, peeled, halved
   lengthways and sliced
1 bunch (350 g) watercress,
   stalks discarded
½ red (Spanish) onion, peeled,
   halved and thinly sliced
1 tablespoon lime juice
2 teaspoons soy sauce
1 teaspoon sesame oil
1 teaspoon vegetable oil
pinch of sugar

This dish is popular in restaurants and cafes, and now you can make it at home whenever the mood takes you. It's perfect for enjoying on a sunny day by the water.

1   To prepare the salad, combine the mango, cucumber, watercress and onion in a large bowl. Mix together the remaining ingredients to make a dressing and pour over the salad. Gently toss to combine.

2   Cut the squid hoods into 5 cm squares then, using a sharp knife, score the inside in a criss-cross pattern.

3   Combine the salt and pepper in a bowl. Add the calamari and stir to coat.

4   Heat the oil in a wok or large frying pan over high heat. Add the squid in two batches and stir-fry for about 2 minutes or until just cooked and coloured. Add the spring onion and chilli (if using) for the last 30 seconds of cooking. Serve immediately with the mango and watercress salad.

TIP Watercress is a delicious alternative to rocket or other salad leaves. It has a peppery, mustardy flavour that works well in salads, sandwiches and soups. Look for dark green leaves with no yellowing.

1 SERVE =
2 units protein
1½ units vegetables
1 unit fats

Grilled salmon with warm Mexican vegetable salsa

SERVES 4 PREP 15 mins COOK 17 mins

1 tablespoon olive oil

2 onions, coarsely chopped

1 red capsicum (pepper), trimmed, seeded and coarsely chopped

1 cinnamon stick

1 teaspoon cumin seeds

½ teaspoon dried chilli flakes (optional)

3 roma (plum) tomatoes, coarsely chopped

small handful coriander (cilantro) leaves (optional), chopped

1 teaspoon finely grated lime zest

2 tablespoons lime juice, or to taste

olive oil spray

4 × 200 g salmon fillets, skin removed

The zesty flavours of this easy-to-make salsa go beautifully with salmon, but work just as well with poached or grilled chicken. Serve with steamed greens on the side if you like to increase your vegetable intake.

1 Heat the oil in a large saucepan over medium heat, then add the onion, capsicum and cinnamon stick and cook, stirring, for 5–6 minutes or until the vegetables have softened. Add the cumin seeds, chilli flakes (if using) and tomato, then cook, stirring, for 3–4 minutes or until the tomato has softened a little. Remove from the heat, discard the cinnamon stick and stir in the coriander (if using), lime zest and juice. Transfer the salsa to a bowl, season with salt and pepper and set aside.

2 Wipe out the pan and place over medium heat. Once hot, spray with olive oil, then add the salmon and cook for 4–5 minutes. Turn it over and cook for another 1–2 minutes or until cooked but still a little pink in the middle. Serve immediately with the salsa alongside.

TIP You could add some chopped avocado from your daily fat allowance to the salsa: just stir it gently through the salsa when it comes off the heat.

1 SERVE =
2 units protein
1½ units vegetables
1 unit fats

Spanish-style fish stew

SERVES 4 **PREP** 10 mins **COOK** 35 mins

1 tablespoon olive oil
1 onion, finely chopped
3 cloves garlic, crushed
2 sticks celery, finely sliced
1 bulb fennel, finely sliced
½ teaspoon chilli flakes
2 teaspoons mild Spanish paprika
1 litre salt-reduced fish or
  chicken stock
2 × 400 g tins chopped tomatoes
2 bay leaves
1 teaspoon sugar
800 g mixed seafood, such as white
  fish fillets, prawns, mussels,
  scallops and calamari
1 tablespoon lemon juice
3 tablespoons chopped flat-leaf
  (Italian) parsley, plus extra
  leaves to garnish
lemon wedges, to serve (optional)

This stew has quite a light texture, which allows the seafood to be the star. Pay a visit to your fishmonger and use whatever looks fresh on the day.

1 Heat the olive oil in a large saucepan over medium heat and saute the onion, garlic, celery and fennel until soft but not coloured. Stir in the chilli and paprika, and saute for a further minute.

2 Add the stock, tomato, bay leaves and sugar. Bring to the boil, then reduce the heat and simmer, uncovered, for 25 minutes. You can cool the fish stew base at this stage and freeze until required. Otherwise, carry on with the recipe.

3 Add the seafood to the pan and gently submerge it in the liquid. Cover and simmer for 5 minutes until the fish is just cooked. Gently stir in the lemon juice and parsley, and season to taste. Garnish with extra parsley leaves and serve with lemon wedges, if liked.

VARIATIONS

Pan-fried or grilled white fish fillets or prawns may be served on top of the stew with the parsley and lemon wedges, instead of adding seafood to the stew at step 3. Carry out steps 2 and 3 to make the stew base ahead of time. Refrigerate or freeze, depending on when you wish to use it. Instead of cooking the seafood in the saucepan at step 3, you could place your seafood in a large ovenproof dish, pour over the prepared stew base, then cover and bake in a preheated 180°C oven for 20–30 minutes or until the seafood is just cooked.

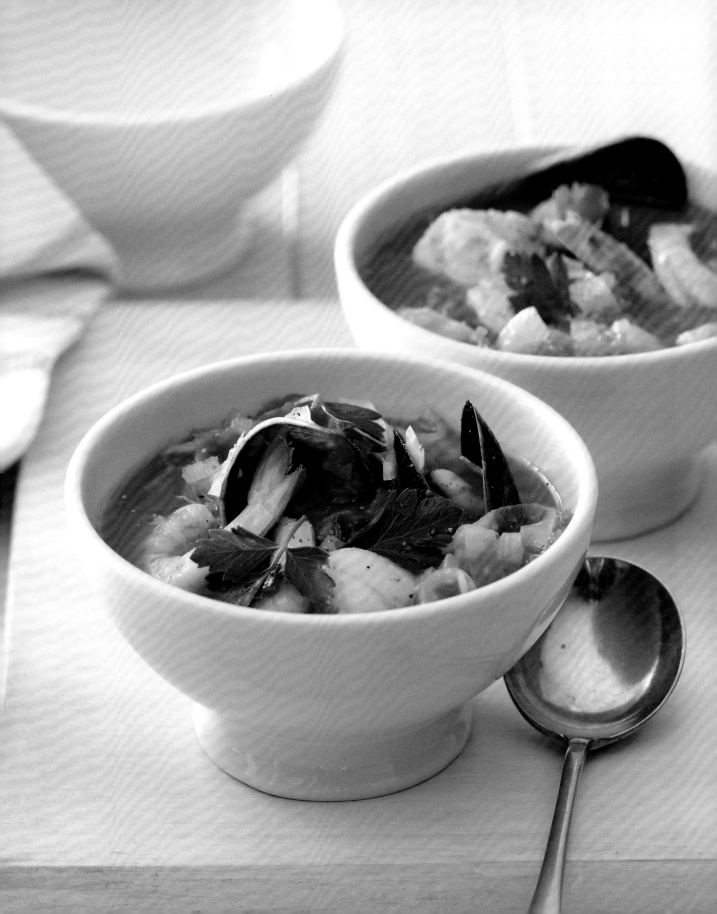

Baked whole fish with Chinese flavours and stir-fried snowpeas

SERVES 4   PREP 25 mins   COOK 20 mins

4 × 400 g whole white fish (such as
   snapper or barramundi), scaled
   and cleaned
3 cloves garlic, thinly sliced
1 × 3 cm piece ginger, peeled
   and cut into fine matchsticks
2½ tablespoons salt-reduced
   soy sauce
2½ tablespoons Chinese shaohsing
   rice wine or dry sherry
2 teaspoons sesame oil
1–2 handfuls coriander leaves
   (optional)
lemon wedges (optional), to serve

STIR-FRIED SNOWPEAS

2 teaspoons vegetable oil
200 g snowpeas (mange-tout),
   cut into fine matchsticks
1 leek, trimmed and white part
   cut into fine matchsticks
2 carrots, cut into fine matchsticks
110 g snowpea shoots

If you haven't cooked whole fish before, then this is an easy recipe to get you started. The aromatic flavours of the sauce complement the fish perfectly.

1 Preheat the oven to 200°C.

2 Using a large sharp knife, make 3 or 4 diagonal slashes in each side of the fish, taking care not to cut all the way through (this helps the fish to cook evenly). Place the fish in a large roasting tin. Scatter the garlic and ginger over the fish, then sprinkle over the soy sauce, rice wine and sesame oil. Cover the dish with foil, then bake for 15–20 minutes or until cooked through.

3 To make the stir-fried snowpeas, heat the oil in a wok over medium–high heat. Add the snowpeas, leek, carrot and snowpea shoots, then stir-fry for 5–6 minutes or until the vegetables are just tender.

4 Serve the fish with the vegetables piled on top and scattered with coriander, with lemon wedges on the side (if using).

TIP Instead of using whole fish, you could use four 200 g white fish fillets and reduce the cooking time accordingly.

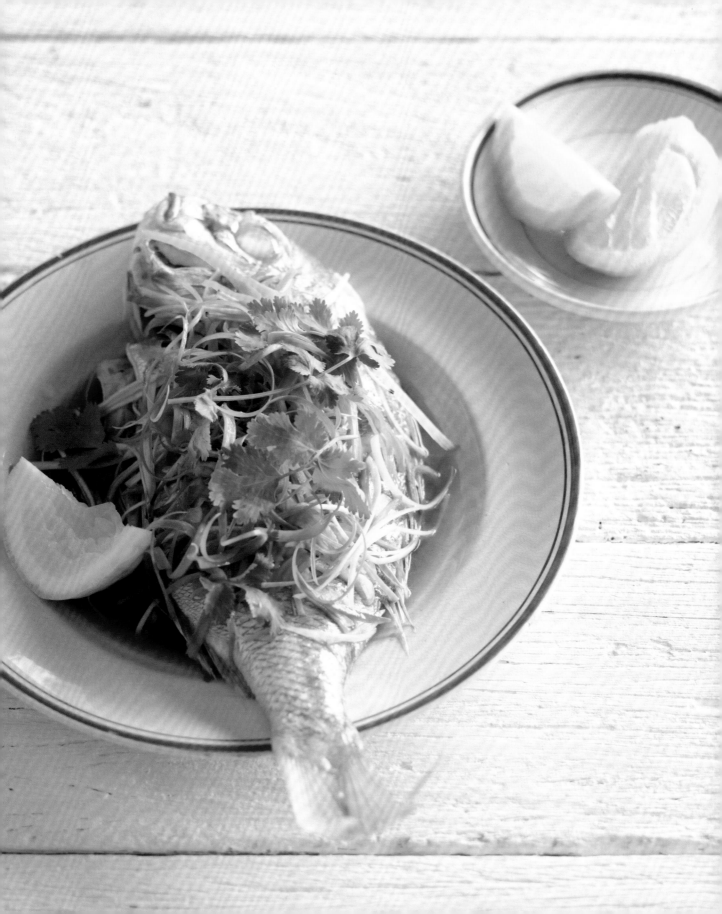

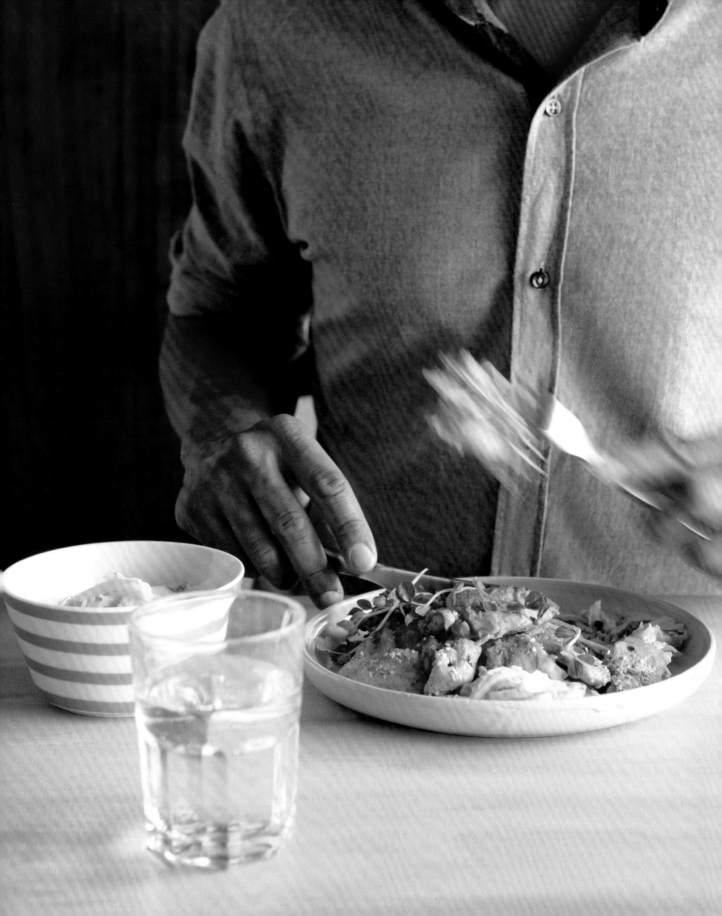

chicken and pork

Mediterranean chicken salad

SERVES 4   PREP 20 mins   COOK 35 mins

2 red capsicums (peppers), trimmed,
  seeded and cut into 5 cm pieces
8 small truss tomatoes, halved
4 Japanese eggplants (aubergines),
  trimmed and halved lengthways
3 zucchini (courgettes), trimmed and
  thickly sliced on the diagonal
1 tablespoon olive oil
1½ teaspoons smoked paprika
olive oil spray
800 g skinless chicken thigh fillets,
  trimmed of fat
2–3 tablespoons balsamic vinegar,
  or to taste
small handful basil leaves (optional)
1 head radicchio, tough outer leaves
  discarded, torn

**This is a more substantial salad that you could easily enjoy for
dinner. The happy marriage of flavours will suit everyone.**

1 Preheat the oven to 180°C.

2 Place the capsicum, tomato, eggplant, zucchini, olive oil and paprika
   in a large roasting tin and toss to combine well. Spray another large
   roasting tin with olive oil, add the chicken and toss to coat. Roast the
   vegetables and the chicken for 35 minutes or until cooked through.
   Transfer the vegetables to a bowl.

3 Transfer the chicken to a board, reserving the cooking juices. When
   cool enough to handle, cut the chicken into 1 cm thick slices and
   add to the vegetables in the bowl along with the balsamic vinegar,
   reserved cooking juices, basil (if using) and radicchio (if using).

4 Season to taste and toss to combine well, then divide among plates
   and serve immediately.

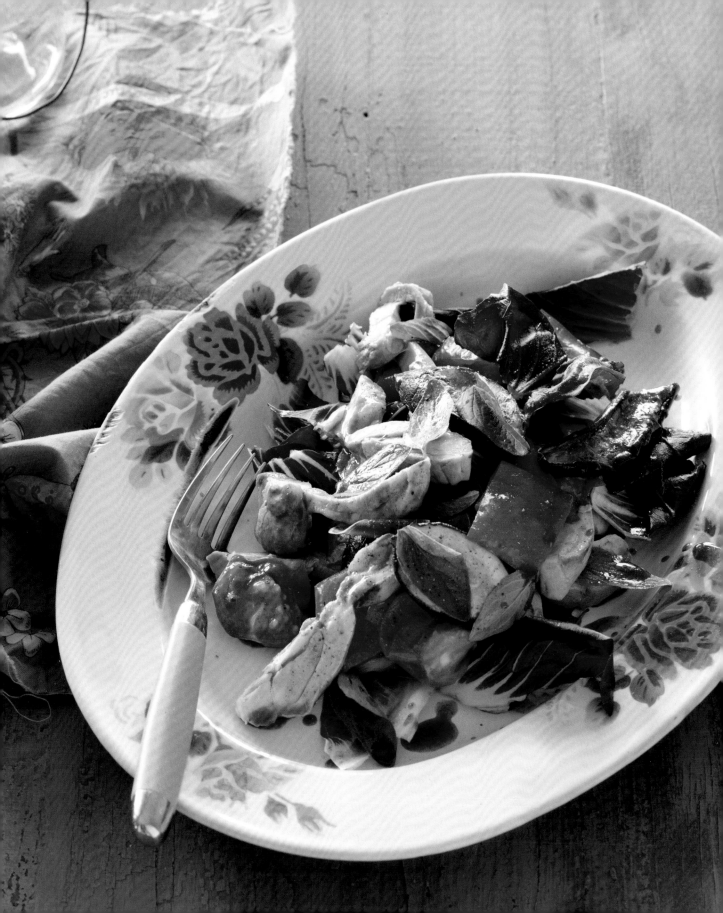

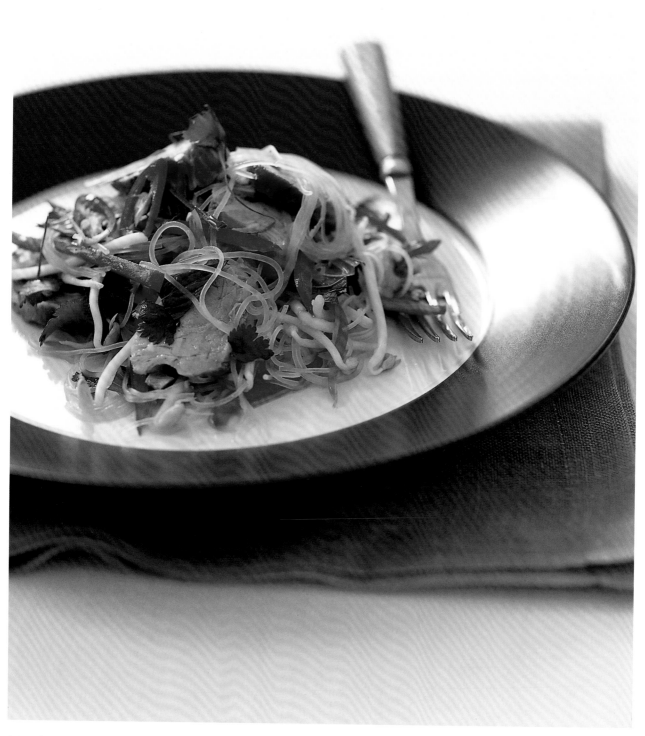

1 SERVE =
1 unit protein
1 unit bread
½ unit vegetables
½ unit fats

Thai pork and noodle salad

SERVES 4   PREP 10 mins + resting time   **COOK** 15 mins

1 × 400 g lean pork fillet
2 teaspoons peanut oil
2 tablespoons fish sauce
⅓ cup (80 ml) lime juice
1 teaspoon sugar
2 teaspoons chopped garlic
2 teaspoons chopped ginger
1 red chilli, sliced
3 kaffir lime leaves,
   finely shredded
1 cup (80 g) bean sprouts
½ red capsicum (pepper),
   seeded and finely sliced
1⅓ cups cooked vermicelli
   (glass) noodles
1 bunch mint leaves
1 bunch coriander (cilantro) leaves

1 Heat a frying pan over medium heat. Coat pork fillet with oil and cook for 12 minutes, turning to brown entire surface. Set aside for 10 minutes to rest.

2 Meanwhile, mix fish sauce with lime juice and sugar in a small bowl.

3 Thinly slice meat and place in a serving bowl with garlic, ginger, chilli, lime leaves, bean sprouts, capsicum, noodles and mint and coriander leaves. Pour dressing over salad and toss well.

Warm chicken salad

SERVES 4   PREP 10 mins + marinating and resting time   COOK 15 mins

1 tablespoon herb mustard
1 clove garlic, crushed
juice of 1 lime
800 g chicken tenderloins
50 g snowpeas (mange-tout)
100 g rocket (arugula) leaves
12 cherry tomatoes, halved
1 small avocado, sliced
$^1/_3$ cup basil, roughly chopped
½ red (Spanish) onion, finely sliced
1 tablespoon olive oil
2 teaspoons balsamic vinegar

1 Mix mustard, garlic and lime juice in a bowl. Add chicken, turning to coat thoroughly. Cover and chill for 30 minutes.

2 Bring a small saucepan of lightly salted water to a boil. Blanch snowpeas for 3 minutes. Drain and cool under cold running water.

3 Preheat griller or a grill plate to hot. Cook chicken for 5 minutes each side. Remove from heat and set aside for 5 minutes to rest.

4 Place snowpeas, rocket, tomatoes, avocado, basil and onion in a large salad bowl. Add oil and balsamic vinegar and gently toss. Arrange salad on serving plates, then top with chicken and serve immediately.

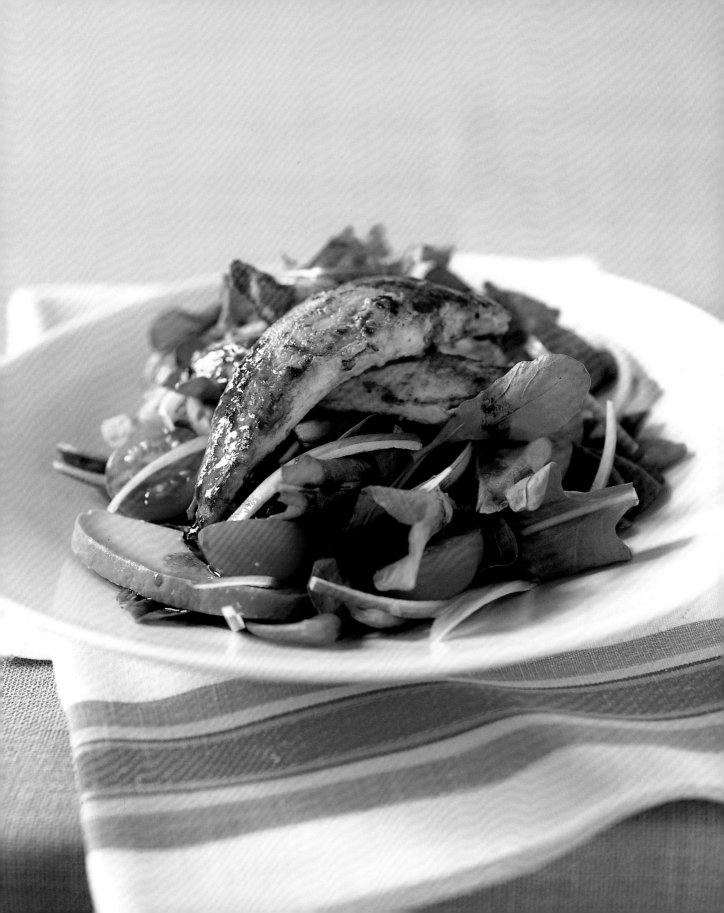

1 SERVE =
2 units protein
1½ units vegetables
1 unit fats

Chicken stir-fry with broccoli and capsicum

SERVES 4   PREP 15 mins   COOK 20 mins

1 head broccoli, broken into florets
2 tablespoons water
2 teaspoons dry sherry
   (or Chinese shaohsing rice wine)
1 tablespoon soy sauce
2 teaspoons cornflour (cornstarch)
1 teaspoon sesame oil
1 tablespoon peanut oil
1 tablespoon freshly grated ginger
½ clove garlic, crushed
800 g skinless chicken breast,
   cut into small pieces
1 onion, quartered
1 red capsicum (pepper),
   seeded and sliced

1 Bring a small saucepan of lightly salted water to a boil. Blanch broccoli for 2 minutes. Drain and cool under cold running water.

2 In a cup, mix water, sherry, soy sauce and cornflour, and set aside.

3 Heat a wok or large frying pan over medium heat. Add oils and, when smoking, add ginger and garlic. Cook for a few seconds, stirring constantly, then add chicken and stir-fry for 6–8 minutes, or until chicken is cooked. Remove from wok and set aside.

4 Add onion and capsicum to wok and stir-fry for 5 minutes, or until vegetables begin to soften. Add broccoli and toss to combine. Stir cornflour mixture, then pour into wok and stir over high heat until sauce has thickened. Return chicken to wok and toss to combine and heat through.

5 Serve with rice from your daily bread allowance, if desired.

1 SERVE =
2 units protein
½ unit bread
1 unit fats

Chicken and tarragon meatloaf

SERVES 5   PREP 20 mins   COOK 1 hour 10 mins

1½ tablespoons olive oil
1 small Granny Smith apple,
  peeled and diced
1 onion, finely chopped
1 clove garlic, finely chopped
1 tablespoon tarragon,
  finely chopped
2 slices bread, crumbled
  into breadcrumbs
1 egg, lightly beaten
3 spring onions (scallions),
  finely sliced
1 small zucchini (courgette), grated
1 tablespoon fruit chutney
1 kg lean minced (ground) chicken

1 Preheat oven to 150°C. Lightly grease a loaf tin.

2 Heat oil in a large frying pan over medium heat. Add apple, onion and garlic and cook for 8 minutes, or until soft and golden.

3 In a large bowl, combine onion mixture, tarragon, breadcrumbs, egg, spring onion, zucchini, chutney and chicken. Lightly season. Spoon into prepared loaf tin and bake for 1 hour. Allow to cool in the tin, then turn out onto your work surface and cut into 5 thick slices.

4 Serve with salad.

1 SERVE =
1 unit protein
2 units bread
1 unit vegetables
2 units fats

Portuguese chicken salad with charred lemons

SERVES 4   PREP 10 mins + marinating time   COOK 30 mins

400 g skinless chicken breast fillets
2 lemons, halved

MARINADE
juice and finely grated zest
   of 1 lemon
2 cloves garlic, crushed
2 tablespoons olive oil
1 teaspoon chilli flakes

SALAD
12 spears asparagus, blanched
500 g baby potatoes, steamed
   and halved
100 g mixed salad leaves
2 tablespoons oil-free
   balsamic dressing

1 Mix all marinade ingredients in a large ceramic bowl. Add chicken and toss to coat thoroughly. Cover bowl and refrigerate for 30 minutes.

2 Preheat a grill plate or barbecue grill to high and cook chicken for 5 minutes each side, or until cooked through. Remove chicken and set aside. Cook lemons, flesh-side down, for 3 minutes.

3 Meanwhile, toss together all salad ingredients and divide among four plates. Slice chicken and arrange on top of the salad, and serve with a charred lemon half on the side of each plate.

TIP For a tasty alternative, try chickpeas in this recipe in place of the potato.

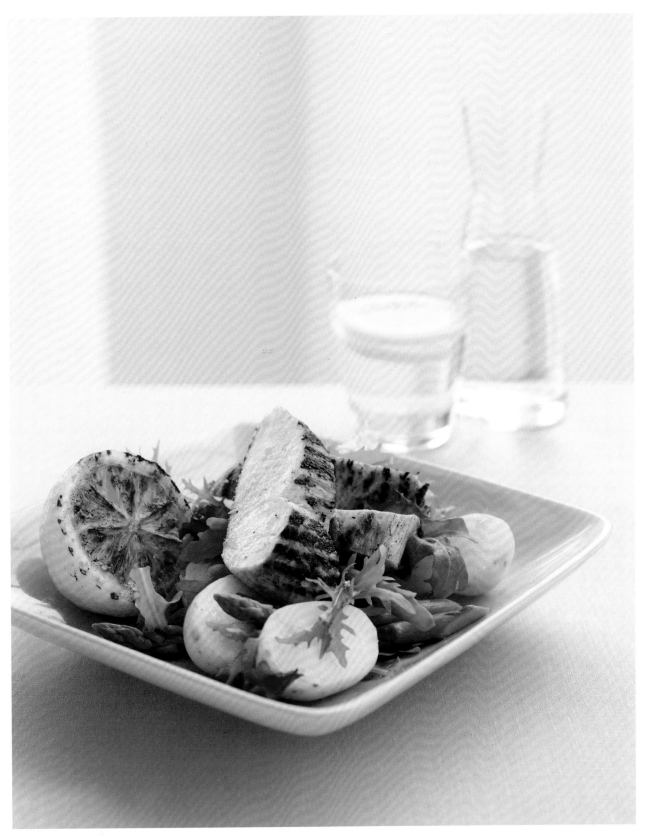

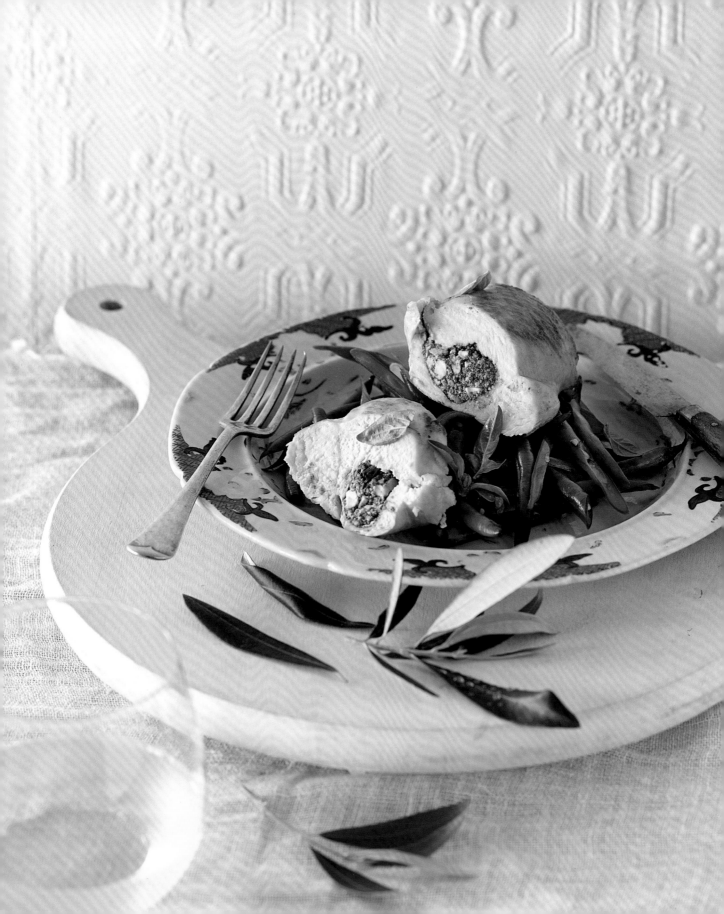

1 SERVE =
2 units protein
½ unit dairy
½ unit vegetables*
* or 1½ units with serving suggestion

Chicken breasts stuffed with feta and olive tapenade

SERVES 4   PREP 15 mins   COOK 10 mins

4 × 200 g chicken breast fillets
100 g reduced-fat feta, crumbled
1 clove garlic, crushed
2 tablespoons olive tapenade
4 large basil leaves,
   plus extra to serve
olive oil spray
200 g green beans, trimmed
1 tablespoon balsamic vinegar

These chicken breasts taste as good as they look, and are perfect for an informal dinner with friends. Prepare them in advance, then pan-fry them when you're ready to eat.

1 Cut a deep pocket into the thickest side of the chicken breasts to create a pocket.

2 Combine the feta, tapenade and garlic in a bowl. Place a basil leaf in each pocket, then divide the feta mix among the pockets. Secure with a skewer, then lightly spray the chicken pieces with olive oil.

3 Heat a non-stick frying pan over medium heat and pan-fry the chicken for 5 minutes each side or until cooked through (the time can vary, depending on the thickness of the breasts).

4 Meanwhile, blanch the beans in boiling water for 1–2 minutes (or cook them in a microwave). Drain and toss with the balsamic vinegar.

5 Garnish the chicken with extra basil leaves and serve with the green beans and a green salad.

TIP To make your own olive tapenade, process 1 cup (150 g) pitted Kalamata olives, 2 chopped anchovy fillets, ½ small clove garlic, chopped, 2 tablespoons rinsed capers and 1 tablespoon olive oil to a coarse puree. Stir in 2 teaspoons sherry vinegar, to taste. Season with freshly ground black pepper. Serve any leftovers as a dip or sandwich spread.

Baked yoghurt chicken with tomato, mint and cucumber salad

SERVES 4 **PREP** 15 mins + marinating time **COOK** 15 mins

½ teaspoon Chinese five-spice
  powder
1 teaspoon chilli powder
2 teaspoons soy sauce
1 clove garlic, crushed
1 tablespoon olive oil
200 g reduced-fat natural yoghurt
4 × 200 g skinless chicken breasts

SALAD
2 Lebanese (small) cucumbers, sliced
4 Roma (plum) tomatoes, sliced
½ red (Spanish) onion, finely sliced
¼ cup mint leaves
1 tablespoon olive oil
1 teaspoon lemon juice

1 In a bowl, gently fold five-spice powder, chilli powder, soy sauce, garlic and oil through yoghurt. Coat chicken with mixture and allow to stand at least 4 hours.

2 Preheat oven to 180°C. Line a baking dish with baking paper.

3 Heat a non-stick frying pan over medium heat. Add chicken and cook for 2 minutes each side. Transfer to prepared baking dish and bake for 6–8 minutes, or until cooked through. Remove and allow chicken to rest for 5 minutes. Carve into thick slices.

4 To make the salad gently toss all ingredients. Divide between four serving plates, then add chicken and serve.

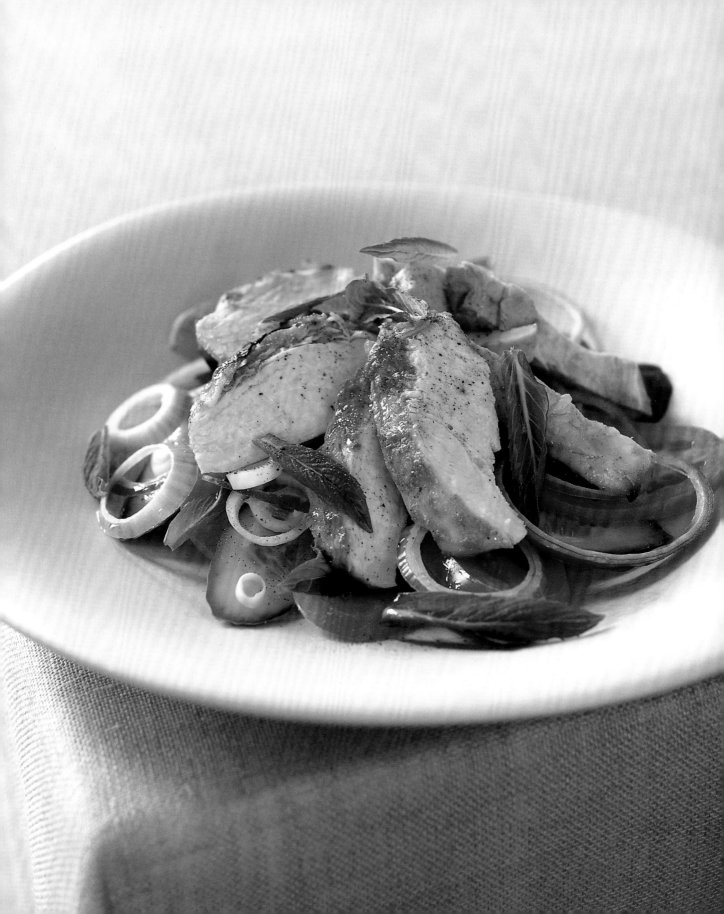

1 SERVE =
2 units protein
½ unit fruit
2 units vegetables
1 unit fats

Brussels sprout, swede, apple and rocket salad with pork

SERVES 4   PREP 20 mins   COOK 45 mins

400 g brussels sprouts, tough
    outer leaves removed,
    halved lengthways
300 g swedes, peeled and
    cut into 1 cm pieces
2 pink lady apples, halved, cored
    and each half cut into 5 wedges
olive oil spray
2 × 400 g pieces pork fillet,
    trimmed of fat
large handful baby rocket leaves
2 teaspoons poppy seeds (optional)

DRESSING
2½ tablespoons horseradish cream
1 tablespoon lemon juice
1 tablespoon olive oil

A substantial salad to serve for dinner. Instead of the pork fillets, you could serve this salad with grilled lean pork chops.

1 Preheat the oven to 180°C.

2 Place the sprouts, swede and apple in a single layer in a large roasting tin, then spray with olive oil. Cover the tin tightly with foil and bake for 25 minutes. Remove the foil, then cook for another 20 minutes or until the vegetables and apple are tender and light golden. Remove from the oven and set aside to cool to room temperature, then transfer to a large bowl.

3 Meanwhile, heat a non-stick ovenproof frying pan over medium–high heat, then spray the pan with olive oil and add the pork. Cook, turning often, for 3–4 minutes or until golden all over. Transfer the pan to the oven and cook for 7–8 minutes or until the pork is cooked through but still a little pink in the middle. Remove from the oven and leave to cool to room temperature, then slice.

4 For the dressing, combine the ingredients in a bowl with 2½ tablespoons water and whisk to combine well.

5 Add the rocket to the bowl with the sprout mixture, then pour over the dressing and, using your hands, toss to combine well. Divide among plates, then sprinkle over the poppy seeds (if using). Place slices of pork on top and serve immediately.

TIP This salad also tastes great with cold leftover roast pork.

1 SERVE =
2 units protein
1 unit fruit
1½ units vegetables
1½ units fats

3–4 tablespoons vindaloo paste
3 cloves garlic, crushed
1 × 3 cm piece ginger, peeled
   and finely chopped
100 ml white vinegar
800 g pork steaks, trimmed of fat,
   cut into 1 cm wide strips
1 tablespoon vegetable oil
2 large onions, thinly sliced
1½ cups (375 ml) salt-reduced
   chicken stock
400 g cherry tomatoes,
   roughly chopped

MANGO AND CUCUMBER SALAD
1 large mango, peeled and stone
   removed, flesh thinly sliced
2 Lebanese (small) cucumbers,
   thinly sliced
6 radishes, trimmed and thinly sliced
small handful baby rocket leaves
small handful coriander (cilantro)
   leaves (optional)
2 tablespoons lemon juice

Spicy pork vindaloo with mango and cucumber salad

SERVES 4   PREP 25 mins   COOK 15 mins

This is super-quick to make and will really impress your dinner guests – the light and refreshing salad is a great contrast to the spicy pork. You could use chicken breast in place of the pork if you prefer.

1 Place the paste, garlic, ginger and vinegar in a shallow dish and combine. Add the pork and toss to coat with the marinade. Cover with plastic wrap and set aside for 30 minutes, then drain, reserving the marinade (squeeze the pork to remove as much liquid as possible).

2 Heat half the oil in a large saucepan over medium heat, then add the onion and cook, stirring, for 4–5 minutes or until softened. Meanwhile, heat the remaining oil in a large, non-stick frying pan over medium heat, add the pork and cook, stirring, for 4–5 minutes or until the pork has changed colour, then remove from the heat.

3 Add the pork, stock, tomato and reserved marinade to the pan with the onion and bring to simmering point. Cook, stirring occasionally, over medium heat for 4–5 minutes or until the pork is cooked through.

4 To make the salad, place all the ingredients in a large bowl and toss to combine well.

5 Divide the pork vindaloo among four plates and serve with the salad alongside.

TIP Vindaloo paste is available in jars from most supermarkets.

Pork rissoles with red grapefruit and watercress salad

SERVES 4   PREP 25 mins + refrigerating time   COOK 20 mins

400 g lean minced pork
1 small onion, grated
1 egg, lightly beaten
1 clove garlic, crushed
1 small zucchini (courgette),
   finely grated
2 tablespoons chopped flat-leaf
   (Italian) parsley
1 tablespoon tomato paste (puree)
2 teaspoons Worcestershire sauce
½ teaspoon curry powder
olive oil spray

RED GRAPEFRUIT AND
WATERCRESS SALAD

1 Lebanese (small) cucumber,
   halved and cut into 1 cm slices
½ bunch (175 g) watercress,
   trimmed, washed and dried
2 red grapefruit, segmented
   (reserve any excess juice)
½ red (Spanish) onion, thinly sliced
2 teaspoons extra virgin olive oil

The pork rissoles are enhanced by the vibrant colours and flavours in this stunning salad.

1   Preheat the oven to 200°C. Line a baking tray with baking paper.

2   Combine the pork, onion, egg, garlic, zucchini, parsley, tomato paste, Worcestershire sauce and curry powder in a large bowl. Form the mixture into 12 balls, then place on the prepared tray and flatten slightly. Refrigerate for at least 30 minutes.

3   Spray the rissoles with olive oil and bake for 20 minutes or until golden and cooked through.

4   Meanwhile, to prepare the salad, combine the cucumber, watercress, grapefruit and onion in a bowl. Drizzle with the olive oil and reserved grapefruit juice and toss gently. Serve with the rissoles.

TIP You will find the easiest way to combine the rissole ingredients is by using your hands. Just make sure you have cleaned them thoroughly beforehand. Leftovers are great for lunch the next day – you could even make a double batch for work or school lunches.

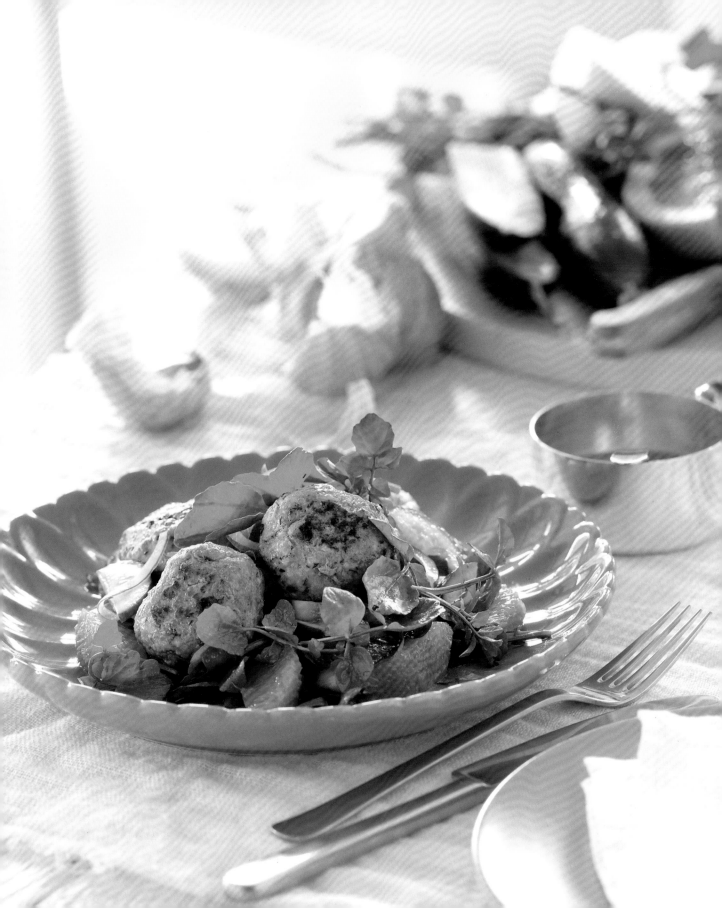

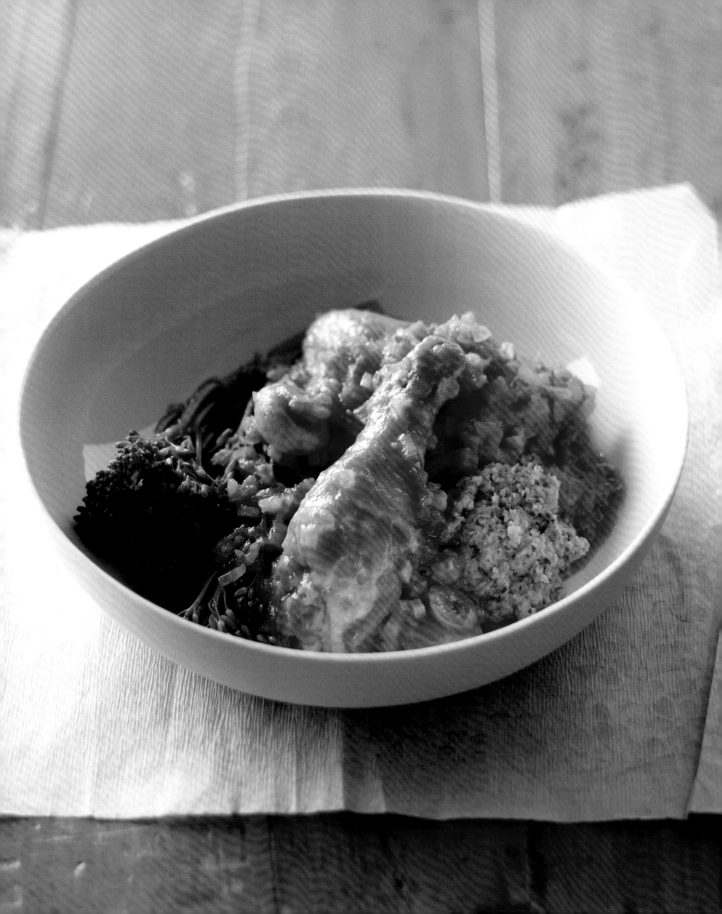

Chicken cacciatore with roasted cauliflower puree

SERVES 4   PREP 20 mins   COOK 55 mins

1 tablespoon olive oil
1 large onion, finely chopped
2 cloves garlic, crushed
2 sticks celery, finely chopped
2 carrots, thinly sliced
300 g button mushrooms, trimmed
4 skinless chicken thighs
4 skinless chicken drumsticks
2 × 400 g tins chopped tomato
200 ml white wine
2 sprigs rosemary
steamed broccolini, to serve

ROASTED CAULIFLOWER PUREE
1 head cauliflower, trimmed
   and cut into small florets
olive oil spray
½ cup (125 ml) salt-reduced
   chicken stock

A classic dinner-party dish, with the roasted cauliflower puree adding a new twist on mashed potato.

1 To make the cauliflower puree, preheat the oven to 180°C. Place the cauliflower in a large roasting tin, then spray with olive oil. Roast for 45 minutes or until golden and tender.

2 Heat the chicken stock in a small saucepan, then transfer to a food processor or blender along with the roasted cauliflower and process to a smooth puree. Set aside.

3 Meanwhile, heat the olive oil in a large saucepan over medium heat. Add the onion, garlic, celery and carrot and cook, stirring, for 5 minutes or until the vegetables start to soften. Add the mushrooms and cook, stirring, for 2–3 minutes or until they start to soften.

4 Add the chicken, tomato and wine to the pan, topping up with a little water if necessary to just cover the chicken. Add the rosemary, then bring the mixture to simmering point. Cook over low–medium heat for 45 minutes or until the chicken is just cooked through. Using a slotted spoon, transfer the chicken to a warmed platter, cover and keep warm.

5 Increase the heat to high, then simmer the sauce for 5–6 minutes or until reduced and thickened. Meanwhile, place the cauliflower puree in a small saucepan, cover and warm through over low heat for 3–4 minutes.

6 Serve the chicken with the sauce spooned over and the cauliflower puree and steamed broccolini to the side.

Chicken tikka with cherry tomato and cucumber salad

SERVES 4   PREP 15 mins   COOK 10 mins

2 tablespoons curry paste (use whatever you have to hand)
400 g reduced-fat natural yoghurt
800 g chicken breast fillets, trimmed of fat and cut into strips
4 wholemeal flatbreads
lime wedges, to serve

CHERRY TOMATO AND CUCUMBER SALAD

250 g cherry tomatoes, quartered
2 Lebanese (small) cucumbers, peeled and diced
1 red (Spanish) onion, finely diced
3 tablespoons coriander (cilantro) leaves
2 tablespoons lemon juice

A tikka masala curry paste works very well in this recipe. It is deliciously aromatic, with a rich, slightly smoky flavour.

1 Combine the curry paste and half the yoghurt in a large bowl. Add the chicken and mix to coat.

2 Preheat a chargrill or barbecue to medium. Grill the chicken, turning, for about 5–10 minutes or until browned and cooked through.

3 Meanwhile, combine all the salad ingredients in a medium bowl and toss gently to combine.

4 Place a quarter of the chicken strips on each flatbread and serve with the cherry tomato and cucumber salad, an extra dollop of yoghurt and lime wedges.

TIP For greater depth of flavour, coat the chicken in the yoghurt mixture the night before and leave it to marinate in the fridge overnight.

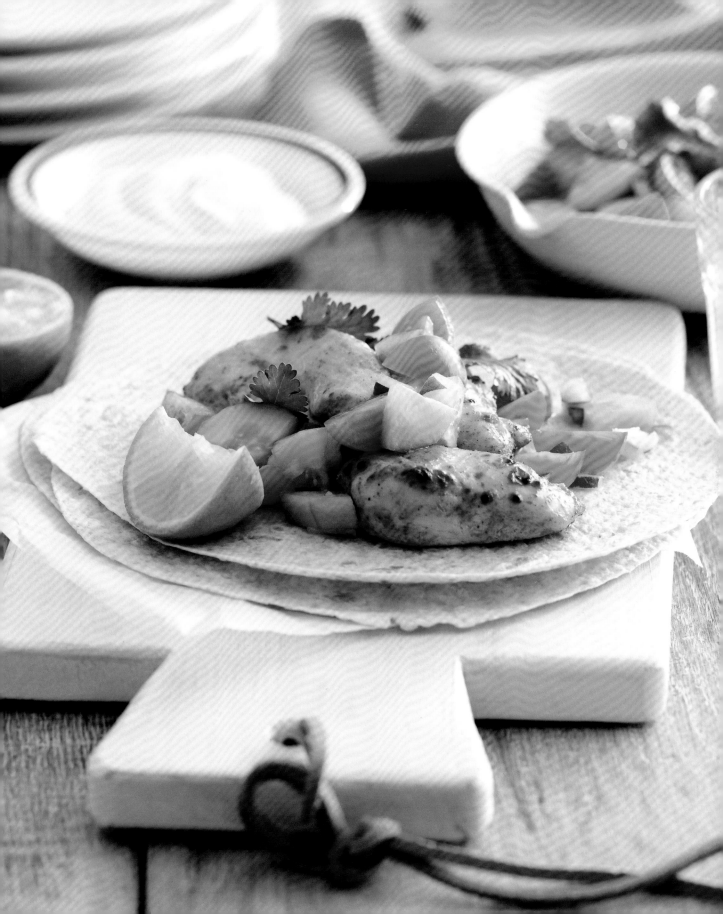

Teriyaki pork with steamed ginger bok choy

SERVES 4   PREP 15 mins + marinating time   COOK 12 mins

3 tablespoons teriyaki sauce
2 cloves garlic, crushed
1 tablespoon honey
2 teaspoons salt-reduced soy sauce
2 × 400 g lean pork fillets,
   trimmed of fat
vegetable oil spray

STEAMED GINGER BOK CHOY
8 baby bok choy, halved lengthways
1 × 3 cm piece ginger, cut into
   fine matchsticks

In this recipe, the pork is quickly pan-fried before being transferred to the oven to finish cooking. This ensures that the meat cooks evenly all the way through, and prevents it burning on the outside due to the honey in the marinade.

1   Place the teriyaki sauce, garlic, honey and soy sauce in a bowl and stir to combine well. Add the pork fillets, turning to coat, then cover with plastic wrap and refrigerate for at least 2 hours. Drain well, reserving the marinade.

2   Preheat the oven to 180°C. Heat a non-stick ovenproof frying pan over medium heat. Once hot, spray the pan with vegetable oil and add the pork. Cook, turning, for 4–5 minutes or until light golden, then transfer the pan to the oven. Cook for 8 minutes or until the pork is cooked through but still a little pink in the middle. Transfer the pork to a plate and set aside, keeping warm.

3   Add the reserved marinade to the pan, place on the stove and bring to simmering point. Cover and keep warm over low heat.

4   Meanwhile, steam the bok choy and ginger for 7–8 minutes or until the bok choy is tender.

5   Cut the pork into 1 cm thick slices. Divide the bok choy and pork among plates, then spoon the reserved marinade over and serve.

TIP If you have time, throw the marinade together the night before and marinate the pork overnight for a more intense flavour.

1 SERVE =
2 units protein
½ unit bread
1½ units vegetables
1 unit fats

Chicken and carrot meatballs

SERVES 4   PREP 30 mins   COOK 25 mins

800 g lean minced chicken
2 large carrots, finely grated
1 egg
70 g fresh breadcrumbs
½ teaspoon ground nutmeg
olive oil spray
1 tablespoon olive oil
2 onions, thinly sliced
2 cloves garlic, crushed
1 tablespoon tomato paste (puree)
½ cup (125 ml) red wine or
    salt-reduced chicken stock
2 × 400 g tins chopped tomato
2 tablespoons chopped oregano
    (optional)

These make a refreshing change from regular beef-based meatballs.

1   Preheat the oven to 180°C. Place the mince, carrot, egg, breadcrumbs and nutmeg in a large bowl, season to taste, then, using clean hands, mix well. Form the mixture into balls about the size of a large walnut.

2   Spray a large roasting tin with olive oil, then add the meatballs and roast, turning them occasionally, for 25 minutes or until cooked through.

3   Meanwhile, heat the tablespoon of oil in a large heavy-based saucepan over medium heat, then add the onion and garlic and cook, stirring, for 5–6 minutes or until softened. Add the tomato paste and cook, stirring, for 1–2 minutes, then add the wine or stock and the tomato. Reduce the heat to low and cook, stirring occasionally, for 15 minutes. Add the oregano (if using) and season to taste.

4   Divide the meatballs among warmed bowls, then pour over the sauce and serve.

1 SERVE =
1½ units protein
1½ units bread
1 unit fats
* 1 unit vegetables with serving
suggestion

Chicken nuggets with potato wedges

SERVES 4   PREP 20 mins   COOK 35 mins

4 medium potatoes,
   cut into wedges
olive oil spray
lemon wedges, to serve

NUGGETS
500 g chicken breast fillets,
   trimmed of fat and cut
   into bite-sized pieces
2 eggs, lightly beaten
½ cup (75 g) cornflake crumbs
olive oil spray

This is bound to be a favourite with the kids. They'll enjoy helping you prepare them too, particularly smashing the cornflakes!

1 Preheat the oven to 200°C.

2 Spray the potato wedges with olive oil and place in a single layer on a baking tray. Bake for 30–35 minutes or until crisp and golden, turning from time to time.

3 Meanwhile, line a baking tray with baking paper and prepare the chicken. Dip the chicken pieces into the egg and then into the cornflake crumbs to coat. Place in a single layer on the baking tray, spray with olive oil and bake for 15–20 minutes or until golden and crisp.

4 Serve the wedges and nuggets with lemon wedges and your favourite salad or steamed vegetables.

TIP If you prefer, the cornflake crumbs may be replaced with breadcrumbs. Make your own breadcrumbs by pulsing day-old slices of wholemeal bread in a food processor until fine crumbs are formed.

VARIATION

Use sweet potato instead of the potato and flavour with a little Cajun spice mix before baking.

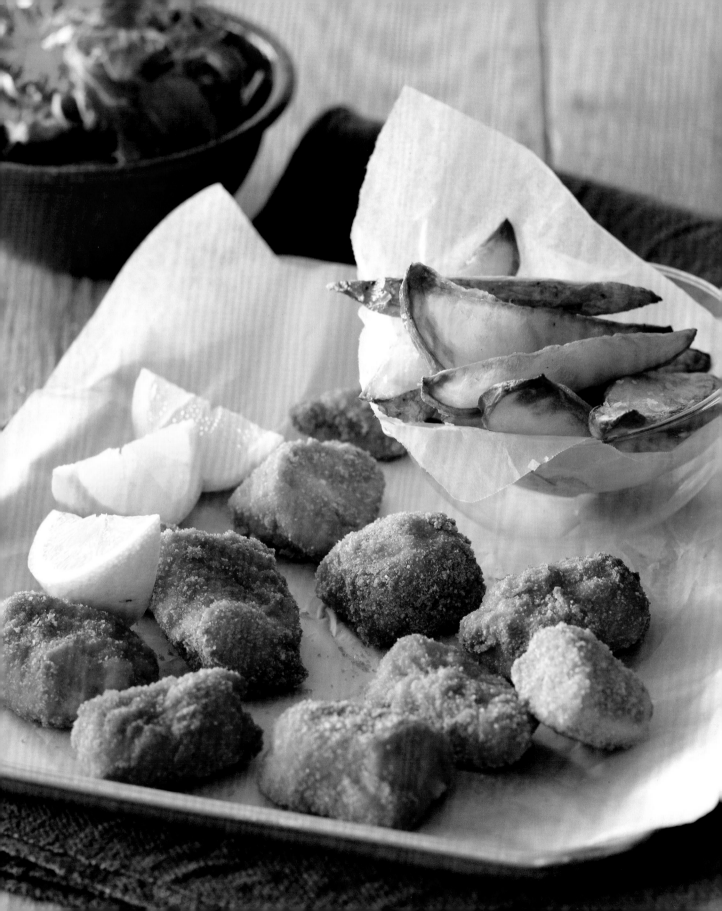

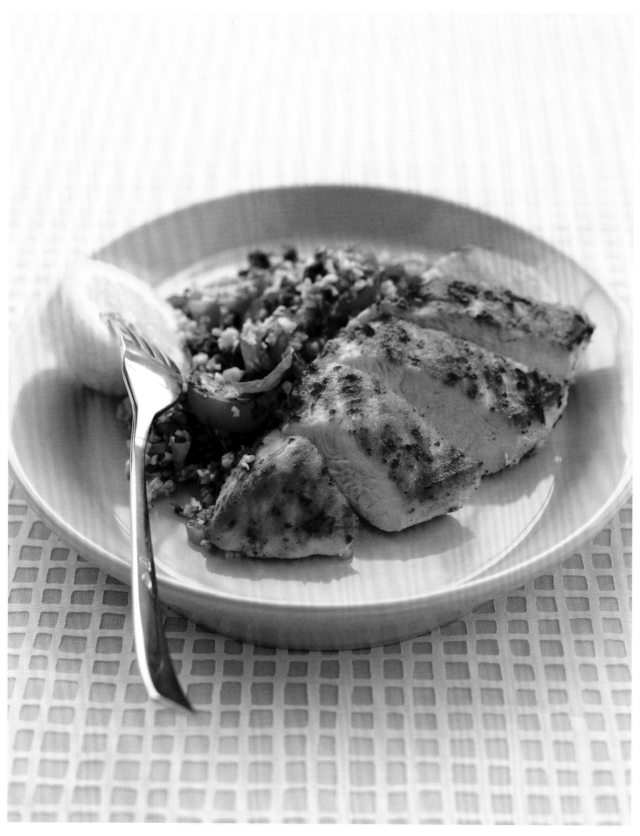

1 SERVE =
2 units protein
2 units bread
½ unit vegetables
3 units fats

Chargrilled pesto chicken with tabouleh

SERVES 4 PREP 20 mins COOK 15 mins

4 × 200 g skinless chicken
   breast fillets
1 lemon, cut into wedges

PESTO (or use bought pesto)
 1 cup loosely packed basil leaves
1 clove garlic, crushed
1 tablespoon lemon juice
1 tablespoon olive oil
1 tablespoon pine nuts

TABOULEH
1 cup (160 g) burghul (cracked wheat)
2 cups (500 ml) boiling water
4 spring onions (scallions),
   finely sliced
12 cherry tomatoes, halved
2 tablespoons chopped mint
juice of 1 lemon
2 tablespoons olive oil
½ cup roughly chopped flat-leaf
   (Italian) parsley

1 Place pesto ingredients in a food processor and blend to a coarse paste. Rub pesto into chicken. Preheat a grill plate or barbecue grill to high. Cook chicken for 6 minutes each side, or until cooked through.

2 Meanwhile, place burghul in a heatproof bowl, pour boiling water over and leave for 15 minutes. Fluff with a fork, then add remaining tabouleh ingredients and stir to combine.

3 Slice chicken and serve with tabouleh and lemon wedges and a side salad.

1 SERVE =
2 units protein
1 unit vegetables
1 unit fats

Chicken satay with peanut sauce

SERVES 4   PREP 25 mins + marinating time   COOK 10 mins

800 g chicken breast fillets,
   cut into 1 cm thick pieces
2 tablespoons soy sauce
2 tablespoons lime juice
2 cloves garlic, crushed
1 tablespoon vegetable oil
2 teaspoons mild curry powder
small handful of coriander (cilantro)
   leaves, to serve (optional)

PEANUT SAUCE
1 tablespoon oyster sauce
1 tablespoon peanut butter
2 tablespoons sweet chilli sauce
1 tablespoon lime juice

CUCUMBER SALAD
1 Lebanese (small) cucumber,
   seeded and cut into thin strips
100 g bean sprouts
2 spring onions, thinly sliced
1 red capsicum (pepper),
   thinly sliced
1 tablespoon lime juice
1 teaspoon light soy sauce

The peanut sauce is only mildly spicy, so the whole family can tuck into this popular dish with confidence. Any leftover satay sticks would make a great lunchbox addition.

1 Place the chicken, soy sauce, lime juice, garlic, oil and curry powder in a bowl and mix well. Cover and marinate in the refrigerator for at least 1 hour.

2 To make the peanut sauce, combine all the ingredients in a bowl. If you want to heat the sauce to serve, warm gently in a microwave.

3 To prepare the salad, toss all the ingredients together.

4 Heat a barbecue or chargrill to medium. Thread the chicken onto skewers and cook for 3–4 minutes each side or until cooked through. Garnish with coriander leaves (if using) and serve with the peanut sauce and cucumber salad.

TIP Many kids love peanut sauce, but for those who have a peanut allergy, the skewers are just as delicious served with sweet chilli sauce instead. If you're using bamboo skewers, soak them in water for 20 minutes or so before use to prevent scorching while grilling. You'll need 16 skewers for this recipe. If you feel like a change, swap the chicken for diced beef or pork.

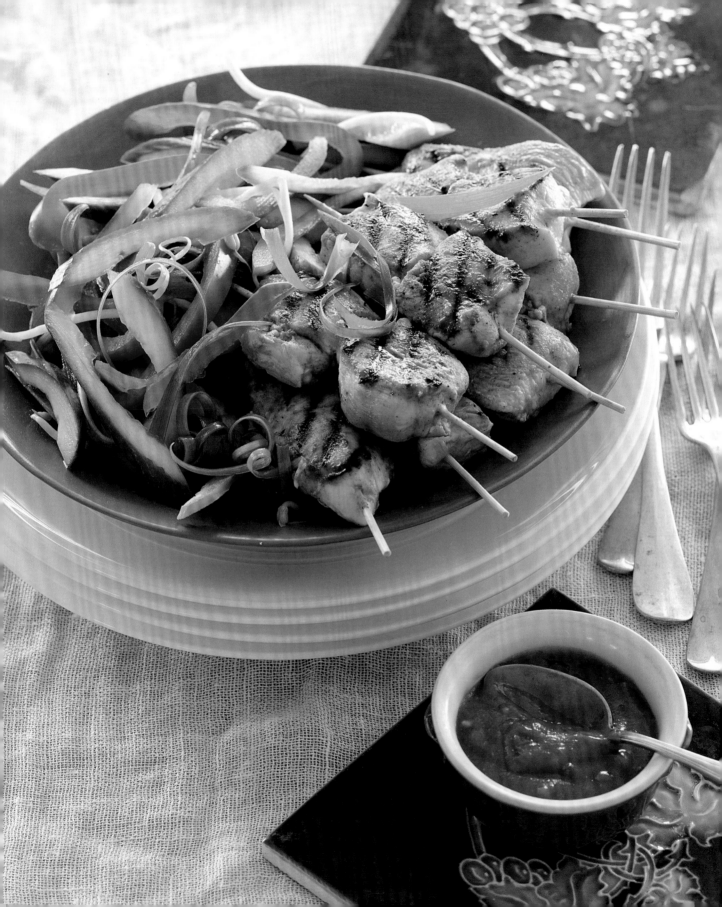

Korean chicken with speedy kimchi

SERVES 4   PREP 30 mins + standing time   COOK 20 mins

800 g chicken breast fillets,
   cut into thin strips
1½ tablespoons salt-reduced
   soy sauce
2 teaspoons sesame oil
1 clove garlic, crushed
1½ tablespoons honey
1 tablespoon mirin
2 teaspoons vegetable oil
large handful snowpea shoots
   (optional)
2 teaspoons toasted sesame seeds

SPEEDY KIMCHI
½ Chinese cabbage, trimmed
   and cut into 5 cm pieces
3 spring onions, trimmed
   and cut into 2 cm pieces
4 cloves garlic, crushed
1 tablespoon finely chopped ginger
1 tablespoon white vinegar
1 teaspoon dried chilli flakes

Kimchi, Korean pickled vegetables, are a delicious crunchy addition to this dinner inspired by Korean flavours.

1 To make the kimchi, place the cabbage in a saucepan with ½ cup (125 ml) water, then cover the pan and place over medium–high heat for 4–5 minutes or until the cabbage has wilted. Drain well. Transfer the cabbage to a large bowl, then add the spring onion. Place the remaining ingredients in a food processor and process until smooth. Pour over the cabbage, then toss to combine well. Cover the bowl tightly with plastic wrap and set aside for 30 minutes or until cool.

2 Meanwhile, place the chicken in a large bowl with the soy sauce, sesame oil, garlic, honey and mirin and toss to coat the chicken. Cover the bowl with plastic wrap, then leave to marinate for 1 hour.

3 Drain the chicken well, reserving the marinade. Heat the oil in a large wok over medium–high heat, then add the chicken, in two batches, and stir-fry for 5–6 minutes or until cooked through. Return all the chicken to the pan, add the reserved marinade and simmer for 2–3 minutes or until reduced and thickened slightly.

4 Serve the chicken and kimchi with snowpea shoots (if using) and sesame seeds scattered on top.

TIP The chicken can be marinated up to 24 hours in advance.

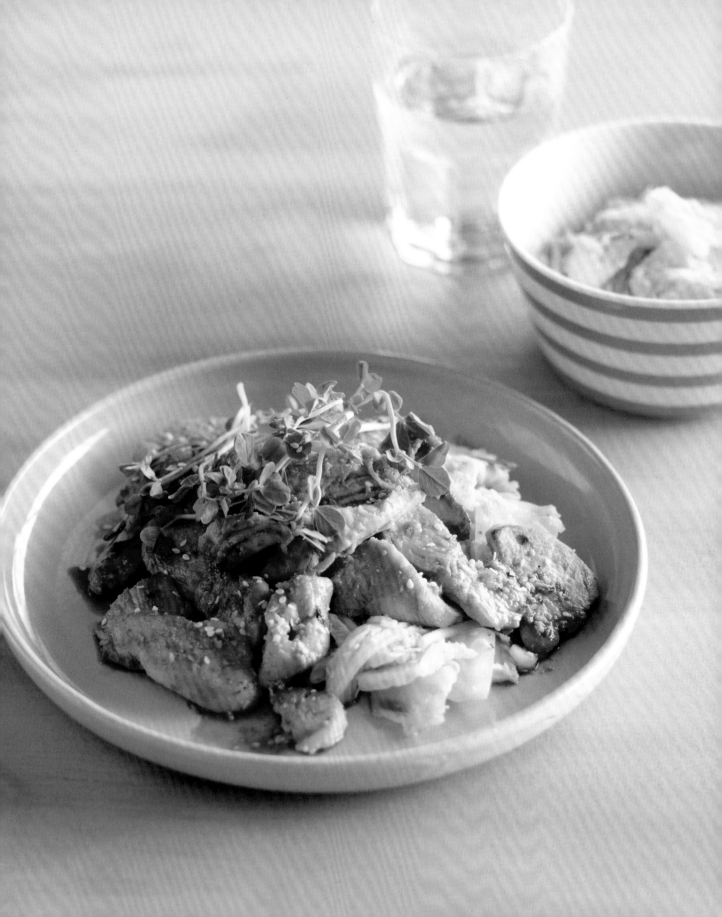

1 SERVE =
2 units protein
1½ units vegetables
2 units fats

Roasted chicken with thyme, red onions and butternut pumpkin

SERVES 4   PREP 20 mins   COOK 1 hour

finely grated zest and juice of 1 lemon
1 clove garlic, roughly chopped
1 tablespoon picked lemon
   thyme leaves
¼ cup chopped flat-leaf
   (Italian) parsley
2 tablespoons olive oil
1.5 kg skinless chicken drumsticks
   and thighs on the bone, trimmed
   of fat
4 red (Spanish) onions,
   peeled and halved
600 g butternut pumpkin, peeled
   and cut into 4 cm pieces

1 Preheat oven to 180°C.

2 Place lemon zest, lemon juice, garlic, thyme, parsley and half the oil in a food processor and blend until smooth. Grease a large ovenproof baking dish with the remaining oil, arrange chicken pieces in the dish and spoon on herb mixture. Rub mixture into chicken pieces and season lightly. Add onions and pumpkin to dish and cover with foil. Roast for 20 minutes. Remove foil, baste chicken with cooking juices, and bake for a further 40 minutes.

3 Serve with steamed greens or a salad.

Coq au vin

SERVES 4   PREP 15 mins   COOK 1 hour 10 mins

2 tablespoons olive oil

100 g lean bacon, sliced

350 g small brown onions, peeled

1 clove garlic, crushed

900 g skinless chicken drumsticks
   and thighs on the bone, trimmed
   of fat

2 cups (500 ml) red wine

1 cup (250 ml) chicken stock

3 Roma (plum) tomatoes, diced

2 bay leaves

1 tablespoon cornflour
   (cornstarch) mixed with
   2 tablespoons cold water

250 g button mushrooms

200 g green beans, trimmed

2 tablespoons chopped flat-leaf
   (Italian) parsley

1   Heat half the oil in a large heavy-based saucepan over high heat. Add bacon, onion and garlic and cook for 5 minutes, or until onion is soft. Remove from pan and set aside. Return pan to heat, add remaining oil and cook chicken in batches for 5 minutes, or until golden. Return all chicken and bacon mixture to pan, add wine, stock, tomatoes and bay leaves and bring to a boil. Reduce heat and simmer, covered, for 45 minutes, or until chicken is tender. Remove lid, stir in cornflour mixture and mushrooms and simmer, uncovered, for a further 10 minutes.

2   Meanwhile, steam beans in a steamer for 5 minutes. Serve coq au vin sprinkled with parsley and with beans on the side.

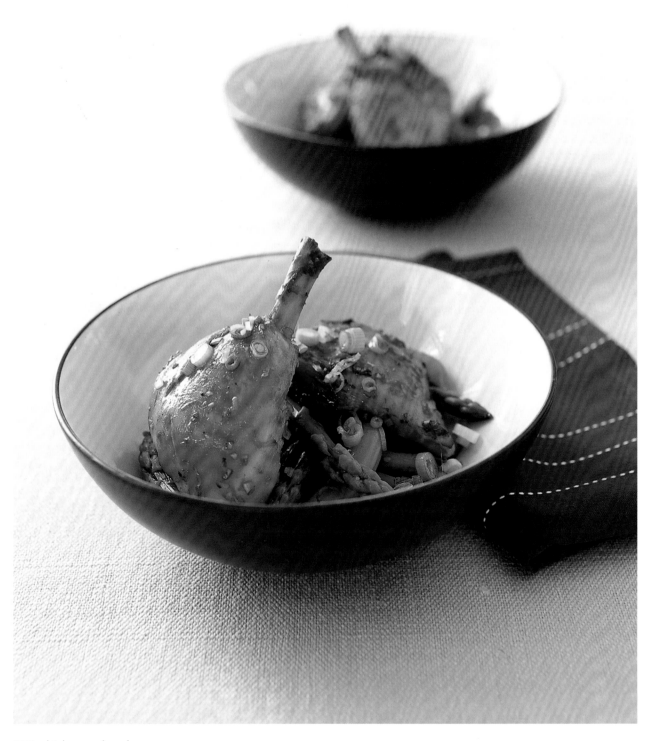

1 SERVE =
2 units protein
1 unit vegetables
½ unit fats

Lemongrass and soy chicken with sugar snap peas and asparagus

SERVES 4   PREP 10 mins + marinating time   COOK 30 mins

800 g skinless chicken pieces on
   the bone, excess fat removed
150 g sugar snap peas
16 spears asparagus
½ cup finely sliced spring
   onion (scallion)
lime wedges

MARINADE

1 stalk lemongrass,
   finely chopped
2 cloves garlic, crushed
2 teaspoons grated ginger
½ cup (125 ml) light soy sauce
½ cup (125 ml) chicken stock
2 teaspoons olive oil
2½ tablespoons dry sherry
   (or Chinese shaohsing rice wine)

1   Mix all marinade ingredients in a bowl. Add chicken and toss to
    coat thoroughly. Cover with plastic wrap and refrigerate, turning
    occasionally, for anywhere from 2 hours to overnight – the longer
    you leave it, the better the result.

2   Preheat oven to 180°C.

3   Tip chicken and marinade into a baking dish, then bake for 30 minutes,
    basting occasionally.

4   Meanwhile, bring a small saucepan of lightly salted water to
    a boil. Blanch vegetables for 2–3 minutes. Drain and divide between
    4 serving plates. Arrange chicken on top of vegetables and brush with
    pan juices. Sprinkle with spring onion and serve with lime wedges.

Baked piri piri chicken with roasted capsicum, fennel and tomato salad

SERVES 4 **PREP** 20 mins **COOK** 1 hour

2 teaspoons olive oil
2 cloves garlic, coarsely chopped
1 teaspoon dried chilli flakes,
   or to taste
1½ teaspoons finely grated lemon zest
2 tablespoons white wine vinegar
olive oil spray
1 × 1.2 kg chicken, butterflied (ask
   your butcher to do this for you)
1 lemon, cut into wedges
2 red capsicums (peppers), trimmed,
   seeded and cut into 2 cm pieces
1 bulb fennel, trimmed and cut
   into thin wedges
400 g grape tomatoes, halved
small handful coarsely chopped
   coriander (cilantro) or flat-leaf
   (Italian) parsley leaves (optional)

Spice up dinnertime with this piri piri paste – it's so easy to make and adds a zesty bite to all kinds of meat and fish. This is a much healthier homemade version of a takeaway staple.

1 Preheat the oven to 180°C.

2 Place the oil, garlic, chilli, lemon zest, vinegar and ½ teaspoon finely ground black pepper in a bowl and stir to combine.

3 Spray the base and sides of a large roasting tin with olive oil. Using your fingers, carefully lift the skin around the opening to the chicken breast where the wishbone is, pushing your fingers between the skin and the flesh to create a cavity. Carefully work your fingers all the way down to the thighs and leg to loosen the thigh and leg skin. Push the chilli mixture under the skin to cover the chicken flesh as evenly as possible, then place the chicken and lemon wedges in the prepared tin, along with the capsicum and fennel.

4 Roast the chicken and vegetables for 40 minutes or until the vegetables are tender and lightly charred, then transfer the capsicum and fennel to a large bowl. Add the tomato to the roasting tin, then continue to roast for another 20 minutes or until the chicken is cooked through and the tomato is tender. Transfer the tomato to the bowl of vegetables, then scatter over the coriander or parsley (if using) and toss to combine.

5 Pour off the pan juices from the roasting tin into a small bowl and skim off any fat that rises to the top. Add the pan juices to the bowl of vegetables and toss lightly to coat. Divide the vegetable mixture among warmed plates. Cut the chicken into four pieces, then divide among the plates and serve.

1 SERVE =
2 units protein
1 unit dairy
3 units fats

Baked chicken breast stuffed with parsley, lemon and pine nuts

SERVES 4   **PREP** 15 mins + refrigerating time   **COOK** 20 mins

2 spring onions (scallions),
   finely sliced
200 g reduced-fat ricotta
finely grated zest of 1 lemon
¼ cup chopped flat-leaf
   (Italian) parsley
1 tablespoon lemon juice
¼ cup pine nuts, lightly toasted
4 × 180 g skinless chicken breast fillets
8 thin slices prosciutto
1 tablespoon olive oil

1 In a small bowl, combine the spring onions, ricotta, lemon zest and juice, parsley and pine nuts. Season lightly, then cover and refrigerate for 10 minutes.

2 Meanwhile, with a sharp knife, make a long incision along the side and into the centre of each chicken breast, being careful not to cut through to the other side.

3 Spoon a quarter of the ricotta mixture into each breast. Place 2 slices of prosciutto on your work surface, overlapping them slightly. Place a stuffed chicken breast across the prosciutto, then roll up and secure with toothpicks. Repeat with remaining chicken and prosciutto.

4 Preheat oven to 180°C.

5 Heat oil in a frying pan over high heat. Add chicken and cook for 4 minutes each side, then transfer to a baking tray. Bake for 10 minutes, or until cooked through.

6 Serve chicken with mixed steamed vegetables.

1 SERVE =
1 unit protein
1 unit bread
¼ unit dairy
1 unit vegetables
1 unit fats

Chicken laksa

SERVES 4   **PREP** 10 mins   **COOK** 15 mins

60 g rice vermicelli noodles

1 tablespoon vegetable oil

2 tablespoons laksa paste or
   red curry paste (or more to taste)

2½ cups (625 ml) salt-reduced
   chicken stock

400 g chicken breast fillet,
   thinly sliced

100 g shiitake mushrooms,
   sliced if large

1 cup (250 ml) reduced-fat coconut-
   flavoured evaporated milk

100 g Chinese greens, sliced
   (such as pak choy or bok choy)

100 g shiitake mushrooms
   (or other mushrooms)

2 kaffir lime leaves,
   shredded (optional)

½ cup (15 g) roughly torn
   coriander (cilantro)

50 g bean sprouts

sliced cucumber, red chilli,
   lime wedges and fish sauce,
   to serve (optional)

Laksa is traditionally made with full-fat coconut milk, which has made it off-limits for those watching their weight; this light version puts it firmly back on the menu.

1 Prepare the noodles according to the packet instructions.

2 Heat the oil in a large saucepan over medium heat. Add the paste and cook, stirring, for 2–3 minutes or until fragrant.

3 Pour in the stock and bring to the boil, then reduce the heat and simmer for 5 minutes. Add the chicken, mushrooms and milk and simmer for 5 minutes or until the chicken is just cooked. Add the Chinese greens, mushrooms, lime leaves and noodles.

4 Divide the laksa, coriander and bean sprouts among four bowls and finish with cucumber, chilli, lime juice and fish sauce, to taste.

TIP You can use Thai green curry paste (see page 541) in place of laksa paste, if preferred. Curry pastes vary in heat from brand to brand so you may have to adjust the quantity. Coconut-flavoured evaporated milk is available from your local supermarket in the long-life milk section.

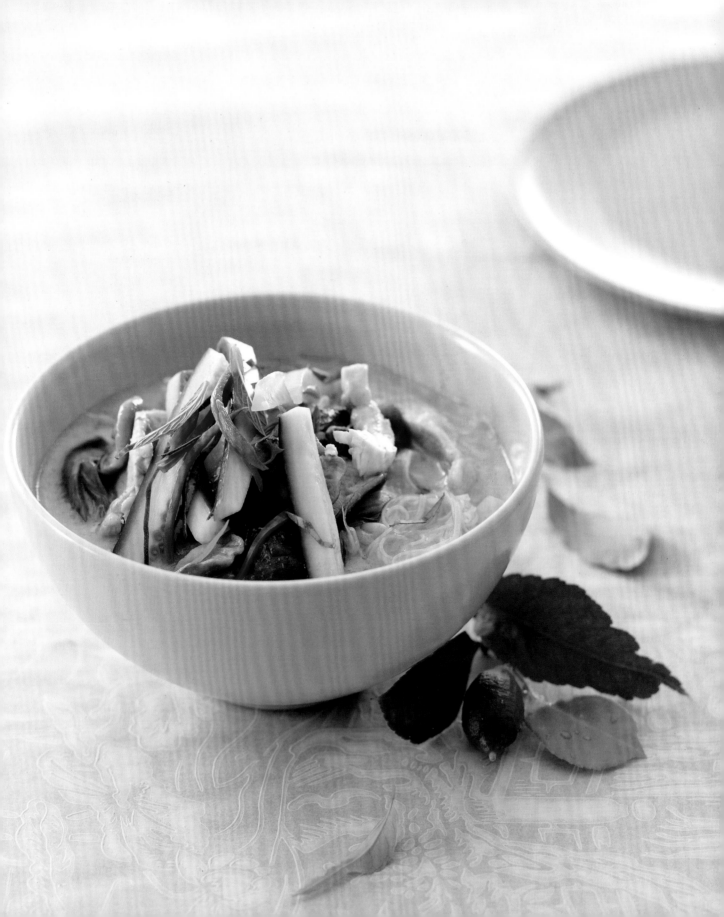

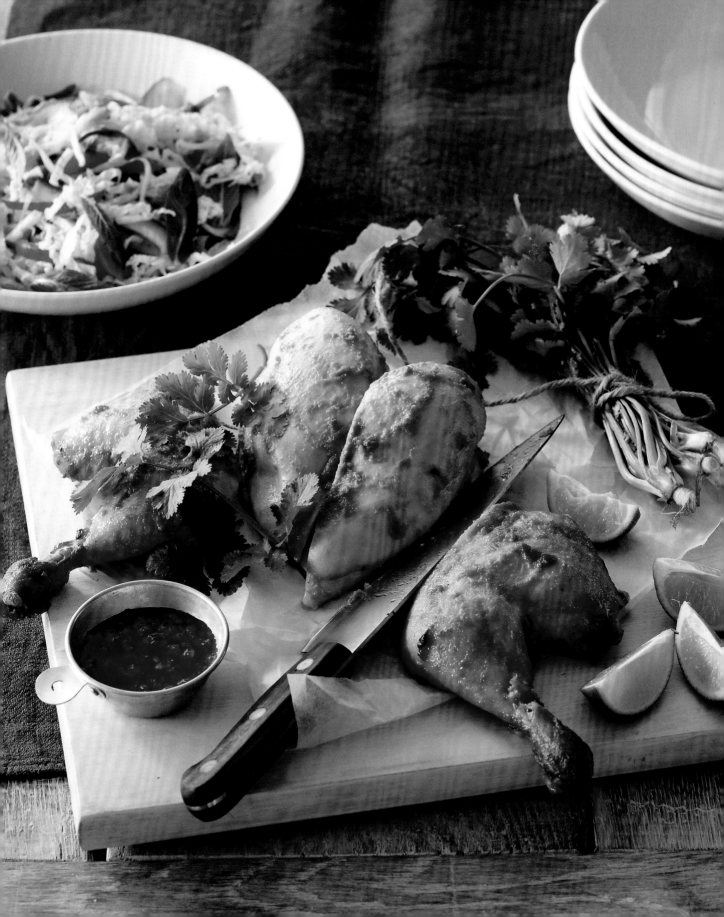

Green roast chicken curry with a fresh cabbage and cucumber salad

SERVES 4   PREP 25 mins   COOK 40 mins

1.5 kg whole chicken
2 tablespoons Thai Green Curry Paste
   (see page 541)
100 ml reduced-fat coconut milk
2 tablespoons fish sauce
1 clove garlic, crushed
1 tablespoon brown sugar
   or palm sugar
¼ teaspoon white pepper
roughly chopped mint
   or coriander (cilantro),
   to serve
lime wedges, to serve
sweet chilli sauce, to serve

CABBAGE AND CUCUMBER SALAD

100 g Chinese cabbage,
   finely shredded
1 Lebanese (small) cucumber,
   cut into ribbons
large handful of bean sprouts
1 red capsicum (pepper),
   thinly sliced
2 spring onions, finely sliced
2 tablespoons mint leaves
1 tablespoon lime juice
2 teaspoons fish sauce
½ teaspoon sugar or powdered
   sweetener

This unusual recipe brings together the comforting familiarity of roast chicken and the unique flavours of Thailand.

1 Preheat the oven to 190°C.

2 Remove the backbone from the chicken, then open out the chicken and flatten gently with your hands. Remove the skin and wings, and then place the chicken in a large roasting tin.

3 Combine the curry paste, coconut milk, fish sauce, garlic, brown sugar and white pepper. Pour the curry mixture evenly over the chicken and bake for about 40 minutes or until golden and cooked through.

4 Meanwhile, prepare the salad. Combine the cabbage, cucumber, sprouts, capsicum, spring onion and mint in a large bowl. Whisk together the lime juice, fish sauce and sugar and toss through the vegetables.

5 Sprinkle the chicken with mint or coriander leaves and serve with the salad, lime wedges and sweet chilli sauce.

TIP Any leftover chicken can be served for lunch the following day with salad or in a sandwich or wrap.

Chicken, tomato and rosemary hotpot

SERVES 4   PREP 15 mins   COOK 1 hour 10 mins

2 tablespoons olive oil
800 g skinless chicken thigh fillets,
   cut into 4 cm cubes
2 leeks, sliced and washed
2 carrots, finely chopped
2 sticks celery, chopped
2 cloves garlic, crushed
1 cup (250 ml) chicken stock
½ cup (125 ml) white wine
1 × 400 g tin chopped tomatoes
1 tablespoon chopped rosemary
2 tablespoons roughly chopped
   flat-leaf (Italian) parsley

1 Heat oil in a large saucepan over high heat. Add chicken in batches and cook, stirring occasionally, for 5 minutes, or until browned. Remove from pan and set aside.

2 Reduce heat to medium, then add leek and cook for 8 minutes, or until soft. Add carrot, celery and garlic and cook for 10–12 minutes, or until vegetables are soft. Add stock, wine and tomato and bring to a boil. Reduce heat to low, then return chicken to pan and simmer gently for 35 minutes.

3 Add herbs and season to taste. Serve with a mixed green salad.

Chicken breast with roast tomato and mozzarella

SERVES 4   PREP 10 mins   COOK 25 mins

4 Roma (plum) tomatoes
1 tablespoon olive oil
1 small onion, sliced
¼ cup basil
4 × 200 g skinless chicken breasts
80 g mozzarella, thinly sliced

1 Preheat oven to 180°C. Line a baking tray with baking paper.

2 Cut tomatoes in half lengthways. Place, cut-side up, on prepared tray and lightly season. Bake for 15–20 minutes. Remove from oven and allow to cool slightly before chopping each half into 3 pieces.

3 Meanwhile, heat oil in a frying pan over medium heat. Add onion and basil and cook for 5 minutes, or until onion is soft. Strain off and reserve oil, and remove onion and basil to a plate.

4 Return pan to heat and add reserved oil. Add chicken and cook for 6 minutes each side, or until cooked through and lightly browned on both sides.

5 Heat grill to medium. Divide chicken between 4 serving plates and cover meat with a layer of tomato and onion mixture. Top with mozzarella slices and place under the griller until cheese has melted and is golden.

6 Serve with salad or vegetables.

Vietnamese-style prawn and chicken salad

SERVES 4   **PREP** 20 mins + standing time   **COOK** 17 mins

vegetable oil spray
4 × 200 g skinless chicken breast
   fillets, trimmed of fat
400 g peeled cooked prawns
about ½ cabbage, thinly sliced
   (you'll need 6 cups sliced cabbage)
2 carrots, cut into very fine matchsticks
3 spring onions, trimmed and
   thinly sliced
large handful mint leaves
   (optional)
handful coriander (cilantro)
   leaves (optional)
1 or 2 red chillies (optional),
   chopped

DRESSING

2½ tablespoons rice wine vinegar
¼ cup (60 ml) lime juice
¼ cup (60 ml) fish sauce
1 clove garlic, crushed
1 teaspoon finely grated lemon zest
1 tablespoon shaved palm sugar
   or powdered sweetener

This satisfying salad is just perfect for dinner on a warm summer's night. If you want to serve this for lunch though, just halve the amount of prawns and chicken, and accompany with some rice from your bread allowance. Use white, red or savoy cabbage – or a mixture, for added colour and texture.

1 Preheat the oven to 200°C.

2 Heat a non-stick ovenproof frying pan over medium–high heat. Once hot, spray with vegetable oil, add the chicken breasts and cook for 1 minute. Turn the chicken breasts over, add ½ cup (125 ml) water to the pan, then cover tightly with foil and transfer to the oven to cook for 15 minutes. Remove from the oven and leave to stand, covered, for 30 minutes or until the chicken has cooled to room temperature.

3 For the dressing, place all the ingredients in a bowl, stir to combine well and set aside.

4 Cut the chicken into thin slices on the diagonal, then place in a large bowl. Add the prawns, vegetables, herbs (if using) and chilli (if using), and toss to combine well. Pour over the dressing, toss again, then divide among bowls and serve.

TIP Omit the prawns and double the amount of chicken if you prefer.

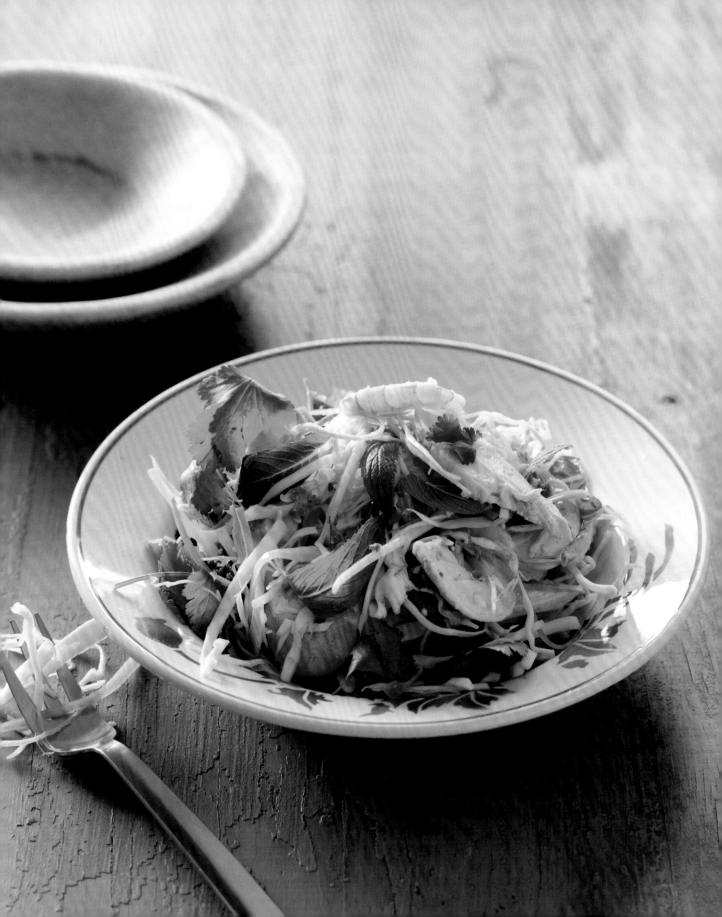

Roast pork stuffed with prunes and sage

SERVES 4   PREP 30 mins   COOK 1 hour

1 onion, finely chopped
120 g pitted prunes, halved
1½ tablespoons chopped sage leaves
1 rolled pork loin, trimmed of fat
olive oil spray

BEAN AND ROCKET SALAD
400 g green or yellow beans, trimmed
1 tablespoon extra virgin olive oil
2 teaspoons mustard seeds
1 clove garlic, crushed
1 tablespoon hot English mustard
2 tablespoons white wine vinegar
large handful rocket leaves

The flavours of this stuffing will permeate the meat as it cooks, resulting in sweet and succulent meat. Take care to trim all the fat off the loin, including the top layer of skin that is traditionally cooked as crackling.

1 Preheat the oven to 200°C.

2 Combine the onion, prunes and sage in a small bowl, then season to taste with salt and pepper and stir to combine well. Remove the kitchen twine from the pork, then unroll on a chopping board. Place the prune mixture down the thinner end of the pork, then roll the pork up around the stuffing to enclose. Using kitchen twine, tie the pork firmly at 2.5 cm intervals to form a neat shape.

3 Spray the base and sides of a large roasting tin with olive oil, then place the pork in the dish. Roast the pork for 15 minutes, then reduce the oven temperature to 180°C. Roast for 50 minutes or until the pork is cooked through but still a little pink in the middle, or until cooked to your liking. Transfer the pork to a warmed plate, then cover and set aside to rest for 15 minutes. Pour the roasting juices into a small bowl and set aside, skimming off any fat that settles on top.

4 To make the salad, bring a saucepan of water to the boil. Add the beans, then cook over high heat for 3–4 minutes or until tender. Drain well, then set aside. Heat the olive oil in a small frying pan over medium heat, then add the mustard seeds and cook, swirling the pan, for 2 minutes or until the seeds start to pop. Add the garlic and cook for another 30 seconds, then remove from the heat. Add the mustard and vinegar to the pan, then pour the mixture into a large bowl. Add the reserved roasting juices, beans and rocket to the bowl and toss to combine well, then divide among warmed plates.

5 Cut the pork into 1 cm thick slices, then divide among plates and serve.

TIP Mustard seeds can be found in the spice section of most supermarkets.

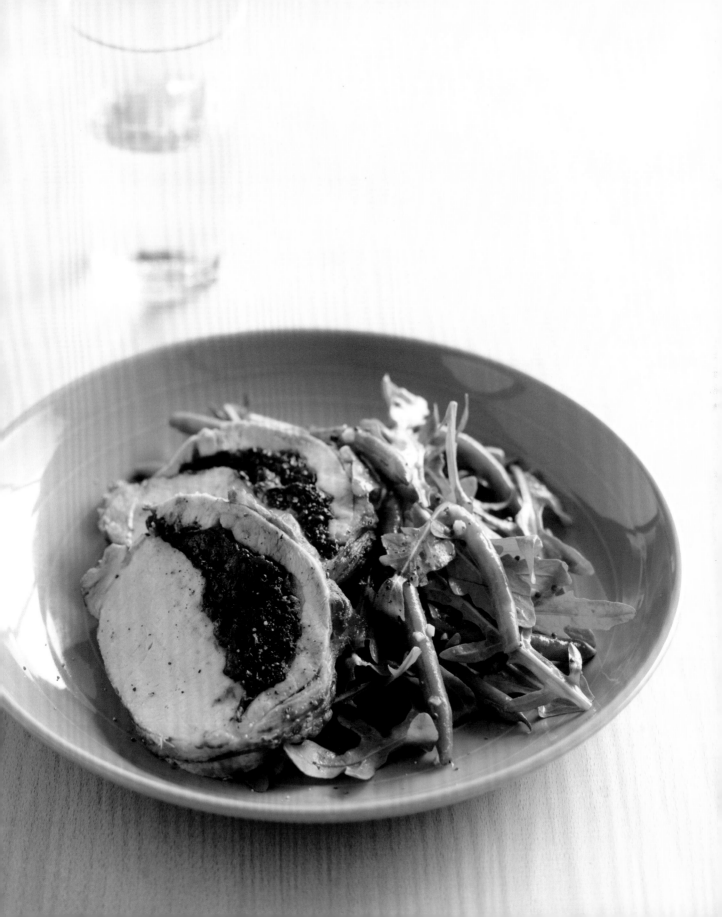

1 SERVE =
2 units protein
¼ unit dairy
1 unit fruit
1 unit vegetables

Pork fillet with roasted pears and creamed greens

SERVES 4   PREP 30 mins   COOK 35 mins

olive oil spray
4 small pears (about 400 g),
    halved and cored
1 tablespoon balsamic vinegar
800 g pork fillets, trimmed of fat

CREAMED GREENS
200 g baby spinach leaves
1 bunch watercress, washed
    and trimmed, leaves coarsely
    chopped
large handful rocket, coarsely chopped
²/₃ cup (160 ml) reduced-fat
    evaporated milk
3 teaspoons cornflour (cornstarch)

Use any lean cut of pork you like for this – cutlets or leg steaks would work well. Take care not to overcook pork; lean pork is much tastier and juicier if left just a little pink in the middle.

1 Preheat the oven to 180°C.

2 Spray the base of a small roasting tin with olive oil. Add the pears, cut-side down, then roast for 35 minutes or until tender.

3 Meanwhile, spray a large ovenproof frying pan with olive oil, then heat over medium–high heat. Add the pork fillets and cook, turning often, for 3–4 minutes or until browned all over. Transfer the pan to the oven, then roast for 15 minutes or until cooked through but still a little pink in the middle.

4 To make the creamed greens, place the spinach, watercress and rocket in a large saucepan with 2 tablespoons water. Cover the pan, then cook over medium–high heat for 4–5 minutes or until the spinach has wilted. Add the milk and bring to the boil. Combine the cornflour with 1 tablespoon water in a small bowl to form a smooth paste. Stirring constantly, add the paste to the pan and cook until the liquid boils and thickens. Season to taste with salt and pepper.

5 Cut the pork into thick slices, then serve with the roasted pears and creamed greens.

TIP Use packham pears if they are in season.

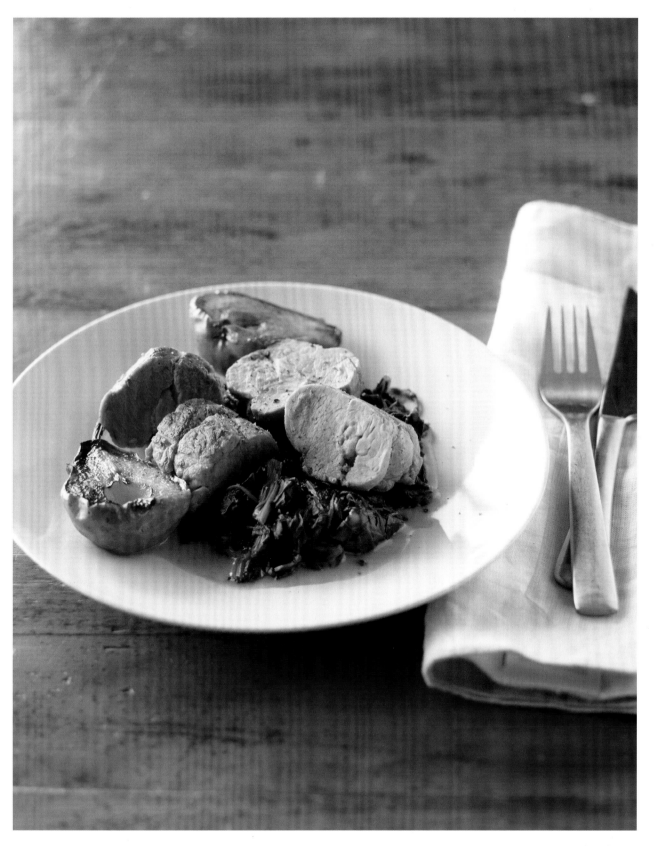

1 SERVE =
2 units protein
1 unit vegetables
1 unit fats

Marinated chicken with steamed greens

SERVES 4   **PREP** 15 mins + marinating and resting time   **COOK** 35 mins

2 cloves garlic, crushed
2 teaspoons freshly grated ginger
2 spring onions (scallions), sliced
1 tablespoon chopped coriander
   (cilantro) stalks
¼ cup (60 ml) light coconut milk
2 tablespoons fish sauce
2 teaspoons dry sherry
   (or Chinese rice wine)
1 tablespoon dark soy sauce
2 teaspoons sesame oil
1 large red chilli, finely sliced
800 g skinless chicken thigh fillets,
   trimmed of fat
4 baby bok choy (pak choi)
handful roughly chopped coriander
   (cilantro) leaves

1   Place garlic, ginger, spring onions, coriander stalks and coconut milk in a food processor and blend to form a paste. Transfer paste to a large bowl and add fish sauce, sherry, soy sauce, sesame oil and chilli, stirring to combine. Add chicken and toss to coat thoroughly. Cover and refrigerate for 1 hour.

2   Preheat oven to 200°C.

3   Transfer chicken pieces to a rack placed in a baking dish and bake for 35 minutes. Remove chicken from oven, cover with foil and set aside to rest for 5 minutes.

4   Meanwhile, steam bok choy and divide among serving plates. Add chicken, sprinkle with extra coriander and serve with extra steamed greens, such as choy sum, and rice or noodles from your daily bread allowance, if desired.

1 SERVE =
1 unit protein
½ unit fats

1 SERVE =
2 units protein

Chargrilled balsamic chicken

SERVES 4   **PREP** 10 mins + marinating time   **COOK** 6 mins

This recipe is a great example of how effective a few well-chosen ingredients can be – in this case, a clever combination of balsamic vinegar, garlic, olive oil and chicken.

$^1/_3$ cup (80 ml) balsamic vinegar
3 cloves garlic, crushed
1 tablespoon olive oil
800 g chicken thigh fillets,
   trimmed of fat and halved
lime wedges, to serve

1 Combine the vinegar, garlic and olive oil in a bowl. Add the chicken and toss to coat, then cover and marinate in the refrigerator for at least 30 minutes or overnight.

2 Heat a chargrill or barbecue to medium. Add the chicken pieces and cook for 3 minutes each side or until cooked through. Serve with lime wedges tand a salad.

Chicken with dijon mustard and white wine

SERVES 4   **PREP** 10 mins   **COOK** 45 mins

4 × 200 g skinless chicken breasts
2 ripe tomatoes, diced
zest and juice from 1 lemon
1 clove garlic, crushed
¼ cup tarragon leaves, torn
1 tablespoon Dijon mustard
¼ cup (60 ml) white wine
½ cup (125 ml) chicken stock

1 Preheat oven to 180°C.

2 Place chicken in an ovenproof baking dish and sprinkle tomato over.

3 In a bowl, mix remaining ingredients. Pour mixture over chicken and cover dish with a lid or piece of foil. Bake for 45 minutes.

4 Serve with vegetables or salad.

1 SERVE =
2 units protein
½ unit fruit
2 units vegetables

Chicken sausages with parsnip mash and apple slaw

SERVES 4   PREP 25 mins   COOK 20 mins

800 g parsnips, peeled and chopped
pinch ground nutmeg
olive oil spray
800 g (about 12) chicken or
    other reduced-fat sausages

APPLE SLAW
about ½ cabbage, very finely
    shredded (you'll need 6 cups
    shredded cabbage)
2 sticks celery, very thinly sliced,
    leaves reserved
2 apples, halved, cored
    and thinly sliced
¼ cup (60 ml) lemon juice
small handful flat-leaf (Italian)
    parsley leaves (optional)

Everybody loves sausages for dinner, and chicken sausages are much lower in fat than ones made from beef or pork. Serve with some mustard on the side if you like.

1   Cook the parsnips in a large saucepan of boiling water for 20 minutes or until very tender. Drain well, then mash to a coarse puree and season with nutmeg, salt and pepper.

2   Meanwhile, spray a large non-stick frying pan with olive oil and heat over low–medium heat. Add the sausages and cook, turning often, for 20 minutes or until golden and cooked through.

3   For the apple slaw, place all the ingredients in a bowl and toss to combine well. Season with salt and pepper.

4   Divide the sausages, parsnip mash and apple slaw among four plates and serve immediately.

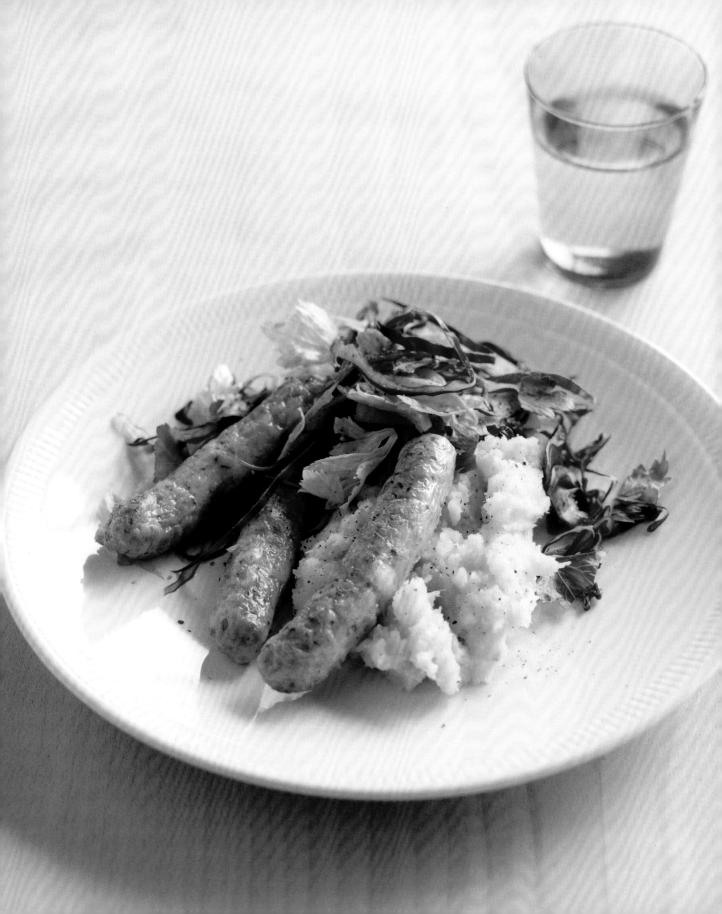

1 SERVE =
2 units protein
½ unit fruit
1 unit vegetables
1½ units fats

Fennel roasted pork with mustard cabbage

SERVES 4   PREP 15 mins   **COOK** 2 hours

3 teaspoons ground fennel
3 cloves garlic, crushed
1 tablespoon extra virgin olive oil
800 g piece pork neck,
    trimmed of fat
½ cup (125 ml) salt-reduced
    chicken stock
2 apples, peeled, quartered
    and cored

MUSTARD CABBAGE
2 teaspoons extra virgin olive oil
1 small onion, thinly sliced
1 clove garlic, crushed
½ savoy cabbage, core removed
    and thinly sliced
1 tablespoon seeded mustard

Pork and apple is a classic combination, enhanced here by the aniseed flavour of the fennel.

1 Preheat the oven to 130°C.

2 Combine the fennel, garlic and olive oil to make a paste. Place the pork in a roasting tin and rub all over with the fennel paste. Season with salt and pepper. Pour in the stock, then cover tightly with foil and roast for 1½ hours.

3 Increase the oven temperature to 220°C. Remove the foil and add the apples to the roasting tin. Return to the oven for 20 minutes, then remove the pork and apples from the tin, cover them loosely with foil and set aside. Drain the juices from the roasting tin into a small saucepan.

4 To prepare the cabbage, heat the olive oil in a heavy-based frying pan, add the onion and stir until it just starts to colour. Add the garlic and cabbage and cook, stirring, for 10 minutes or until just tender. Stir in the mustard and season to taste.

5 Simmer the meat juices until reduced and slightly thickened, then serve with the sliced pork, apples and cabbage.

TIP Take the pork out of the refrigerator and bring it to room temperature before cooking – this will ensure even cooking. Resting time after cooking is important as it allows the juices to settle, making the meat more tender and easier to slice. Leftover pork can be used for sandwiches the next day – it's delicious with mustard and salad.

1 SERVE =
2 units protein
½ unit bread
1½ units vegetables*
1 unit fats
* or 2½ units with serving suggestion

Chicken meatballs

SERVES 4   PREP 25 mins   COOK 35 mins

Children often enjoy lending a helping hand to roll these meatballs and are delighted with the finished dish, knowing they helped prepare it.

olive oil spray
2 slices wholemeal bread,
    crusts removed
¹/₃ cup (60 ml) reduced-fat milk
800 g lean minced chicken
1 onion, finely chopped
2 cloves garlic, crushed
3 tablespoons chopped coriander
    (cilantro)
3 tablespoons chopped flat-leaf
    (Italian) parsley
2 teaspoons ground cumin
2 teaspoons finely grated
    lemon zest

TOMATO SAUCE

1 tablespoon extra virgin olive oil
1 onion, finely chopped
2 cloves garlic, crushed
2 teaspoons ground cumin
2 teaspoons paprika
2 × 400 g tins chopped tomatoes
2 tablespoons chopped coriander
    (cilantro)
2 tablespoons chopped flat-leaf
    (Italian) parsley
1 tablespoon lemon juice
    (or to taste)

1   Preheat the oven to 200°C. Spray a large baking tin with olive oil.

2   Place the bread slices in a bowl, pour over the milk and set aside to soak for a few minutes.

3   Place the minced chicken, onion, garlic, herbs, cumin and lemon zest in a large mixing bowl. Squeeze the excess milk from the soaked bread and add the bread to the bowl. Using your hands, mix all the ingredients until well combined. Roll tablespoons of the mixture into balls, then place them in the baking tin. Bake for 15 minutes or until the meatballs are cooked through and lightly golden.

4   Meanwhile, to prepare the tomato sauce, heat the olive oil in a large frying pan over medium heat and fry the onion for 4–5 minutes or until softened. Add the garlic and spices and cook for a further 30 seconds. Stir in the tomatoes and 1 cup (250 ml) water and bring to the boil, then reduce the heat and simmer for 10 minutes.

5   Add the baked meatballs to the sauce and simmer for an extra 10–15 minutes or until the sauce has thickened. Stir in the coriander, parsley and lemon juice and season to taste. Serve with rice, couscous or pasta from your daily allowance, with a crisp salad to the side.

TIP Use a jar of salt-reduced ready-made pasta sauce as a short cut if you don't have time to make your own. Having wet hands while rolling the meatballs will make the task a lot easier. The meatballs can be frozen either before or after baking.

1 SERVE =
2 units protein
½ unit bread
1 unit vegetables
1½ units fats

Whole poached chicken and vegetables with parsley-almond sprinkle

SERVES 4   PREP 20 mins   COOK 1 hour 10 mins

2 litres salt-reduced chicken stock
    or water, plus extra if needed
1 × 1.2 kg chicken, trimmed of fat
3 sprigs thyme
1 bay leaf
1 bunch yellow or orange Dutch
    (baby) carrots (about 350 g),
    trimmed
8 salad onions, white part only,
    trimmed and halved lengthways
4 chat potatoes, halved
4 small turnips, trimmed,
    peeled and halved

PARSLEY-ALMOND SPRINKLE
large handful flat-leaf (Italian)
    parsley leaves
2 tablespoons lemon juice
1 tablespoon olive oil
2 tablespoons blanched almonds

The parsley-almond sprinkle provides a delightfully crunchy contrast to the moist, tender chicken in this delicious dinner. Save the leftover cooking liquid and freeze it in an airtight container. It will keep for up to 3 months, and you can use it as you would chicken stock. Enjoy the leftover cooked chicken for lunch the next day.

1   Place the stock, chicken, thyme, bay leaf, carrots, salad onions, potatoes and turnips in a large saucepan or stockpot, adding a little extra stock or water to cover the chicken as necessary. Bring to simmering point, then cover and cook over low heat for 1 hour 10 minutes (do not allow the liquid to boil at any time or the chicken will be tough). Without lifting the lid, remove the saucepan from the heat and leave to stand while you prepare the sprinkle.

2   For the parsley-almond sprinkle, preheat the oven to 180°C. Place the almonds on a baking tray and roast for 7–8 minutes or until golden, then leave to cool slightly and coarsely chop. Combine the nuts with the rest of the ingredients in a food processor, then process until very finely chopped.

3   Remove the chicken and vegetables from the pan, reserving the cooking liquid. Break the chicken into large pieces, discarding the skin, then divide among bowls along with the vegetables. Skim the fat from the surface of the reserved cooking liquid and spoon a little into the bowls. Scatter with the parsley-almond mixture and serve immediately.

TIP You could use hazelnuts or walnuts instead of the almonds.

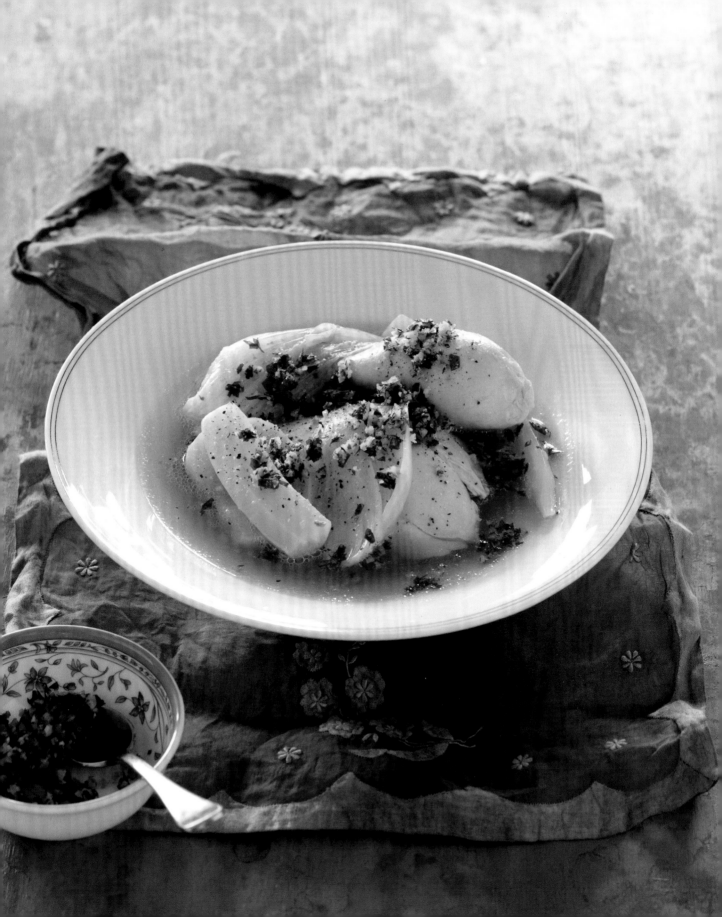

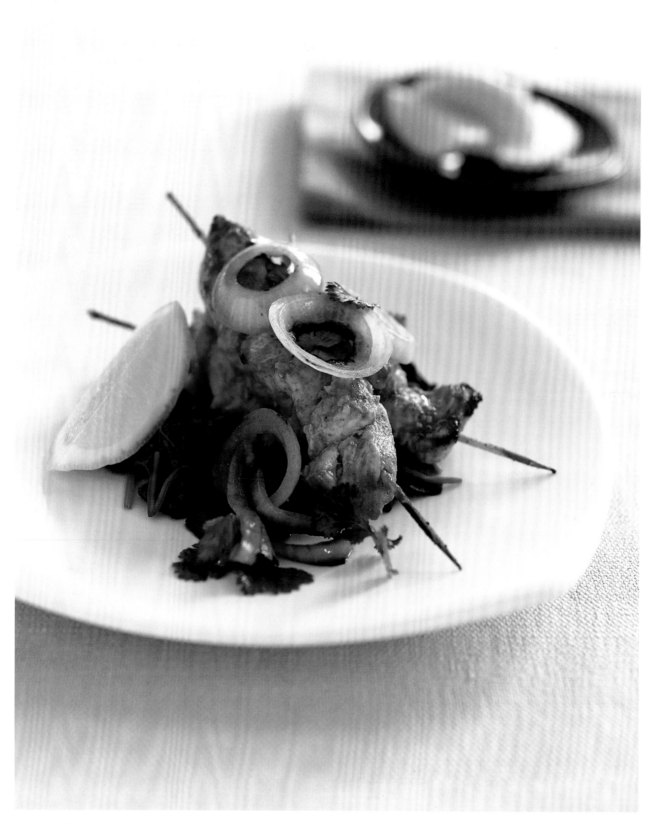

1 SERVE =
2 units protein
½ unit dairy
1 unit vegetables
1 unit fats

Tandoori chicken with garlic spinach

SERVES 4   **PREP** 20 mins + marinating time   **COOK** 15 mins

⅓ cup (100 g) tandoori paste
1 teaspoon ground cumin
1 tablespoon lemon juice
400 g reduced-fat natural yoghurt
1½ cloves garlic, crushed
800 g skinless chicken thigh fillets,
    cut into 2 cm cubes
2 teaspoons olive oil
3 small onions, thickly sliced
¼ cup (60 ml) water
300 g baby spinach leaves
1 cup coriander (cilantro) leaves
lemon wedges
mango chutney

1 In a plastic container, mix tandoori paste, cumin, lemon juice, two-thirds of the yoghurt and two-thirds of the garlic. Add chicken, coat thoroughly and refrigerate for 3 hours at least.

2 Soak 8 bamboo skewers in warm water for 30 minutes.

3 Preheat oven to 180°C. Line 2 baking trays with baking paper. Thread chicken pieces onto skewers.

4 Heat oil in a non-stick frying pan over medium heat and saute onion until soft. Transfer to a prepared baking tray.

5 Increase heat to high. Add chicken skewers and cook for 2 minutes one side and 1 minute other side. Transfer to second baking tray. Bake for 6–8 minutes. Slip baking tray with onion into oven for final 2 minutes of cooking time.

6 Meanwhile, bring water to a simmer in a large saucepan. Add spinach and cook, stirring gently, until limp. Add remaining garlic and stir gently to combine.

7 Toss coriander and warm onion to combine.

8 Serve wilted spinach topped with onion mixture and chicken skewers and offer lemon wedges, chutney and remaining yoghurt.

Pork loin with tomato and sage

SERVES 4   PREP 15 mins   COOK 20 mins

1 × 800 g pork loin
16 sage leaves
1 tablespoon olive oil
2 tablespoons lemon juice
3 large ripe tomatoes,
   cut into 1 cm dice
½ cup (125 ml) white wine
200 g broccolini
200 g carrots
2 tablespoons flat-leaf (Italian)
   parsley leaves

1   Cut pork loin into 8 steaks. Place steaks, cut-side up, on a chopping board and cover with plastic wrap. Using a rolling pin, lightly flatten to 5 mm thickness. Remove plastic wrap and place 4 sage leaves on half of the steaks, then top with the remaining steaks. Secure with a toothpick at either end.

2   Heat oil in a heavy-based frying pan over medium heat. Add pork and cook for 5 minutes each side, or until browned. Remove from pan, cover lightly with foil and set aside to rest.

3   Return pan to heat, add lemon juice, tomatoes and wine and bring to a boil. Reduce heat and simmer for 2 minutes. Return pork to pan and continue to simmer for 8 minutes.

4   Meanwhile, steam broccolini and carrots. Divide vegetables among serving plates and arrange pork alongside. Sprinkle pork with parsley and serve immediately.

1 SERVE =
2 units protein
½ unit bread
1 unit vegetables
2 units fats

Chicken and vegetable country stew

SERVES 4   PREP 15 mins   COOK 40 mins

2 tablespoons olive oil
800 g chicken thigh fillets,
   trimmed of fat and cut
   into 2 cm pieces
1 large onion, finely chopped
2 cloves garlic, crushed
2 sticks celery, sliced
2 carrots, finely diced
1 tablespoon tomato paste (puree)
2 medium potatoes, peeled
   and finely diced
2 cups (500 ml) salt-reduced
   chicken stock
1 teaspoon dried oregano
1 tablespoon Worcestershire sauce
1 zucchini (courgette),
   cut into 1 cm dice
½ cup (60 g) frozen peas
½ cup (80 g) frozen corn
1½ tablespoons cornflour (cornstarch)
roughly chopped flat-leaf (Italian)
   parsley, to serve

Worcestershire sauce is the secret ingredient in this tasty and easy-to-prepare stew, which is delicious on a winter's night.

1 Heat the olive oil in a large heavy-based saucepan over medium–high heat. Add the chicken in batches and cook for 2–3 minutes or until golden. Remove and set aside. Add the onion, garlic, celery and carrot to the pan and cook for 5 minutes or until the onion has softened.

2 Stir in the tomato paste, then add the potato, stock, oregano and Worcestershire sauce and return the chicken to the pan. Bring to the boil, then reduce the heat and simmer, covered, for 15 minutes.

3 Add the zucchini, peas and corn and cook for a further 10 minutes or until all the vegetables are tender and cooked through.

4 Mix the cornflour with 3 tablespoons water and add to the pan, stirring until the sauce has thickened. Season to taste, then garnish with parsley and serve.

TIP There will be leftovers, so freeze these in individual containers for a quick lunch to grab in a rush.

Spanish pork

SERVES 4   PREP 20 mins + standing time   COOK 25 mins

large pinch saffron threads (optional)
1 tablespoon olive oil
1 onion, finely chopped
2 cloves garlic, thinly sliced
2 carrots, thinly sliced
1 large yellow capsicum (pepper),
    trimmed, seeded and cut
    into 2 cm pieces
1 large red capsicum (pepper),
    trimmed, seeded and cut
    into 2 cm pieces
2 teaspoons smoked paprika
3 sprigs thyme
150 ml medium–dry sherry
150 ml salt-reduced chicken stock
olive oil spray
8 small pork cutlets (about 1.25 kg
    total weight), trimmed of fat

Saffron is an expensive ingredient, but lovely to include in a special dinner like this, and a little bit goes a long way.

1   Combine the saffron and ⅓ cup (80 ml) hot water in a small bowl, then stand for 1 hour to infuse.

2   Heat the olive oil in a large heavy-based saucepan over medium heat. Add the onion, garlic, carrot and capsicum and cook, stirring, for 5–6 minutes or until the onion has softened. Add the paprika and thyme and cook, stirring, for 1–2 minutes, then add the sherry, stock and saffron (if using). Bring to simmering point, then cook over low heat for 20 minutes or until the capsicum has softened.

3   Meanwhile, heat a large non-stick frying pan over medium heat and, when hot, spray with olive oil. Working in batches, cook the cutlets, turning once, for 8 minutes or until cooked through, keeping the cooked cutlets warm while you cook the remainder.

4   Divide the vegetables and juices among warmed bowls or plates, then place the cutlets on top and serve.

TIP Smoked paprika and saffron can be found in the spice section of most supermarkets.

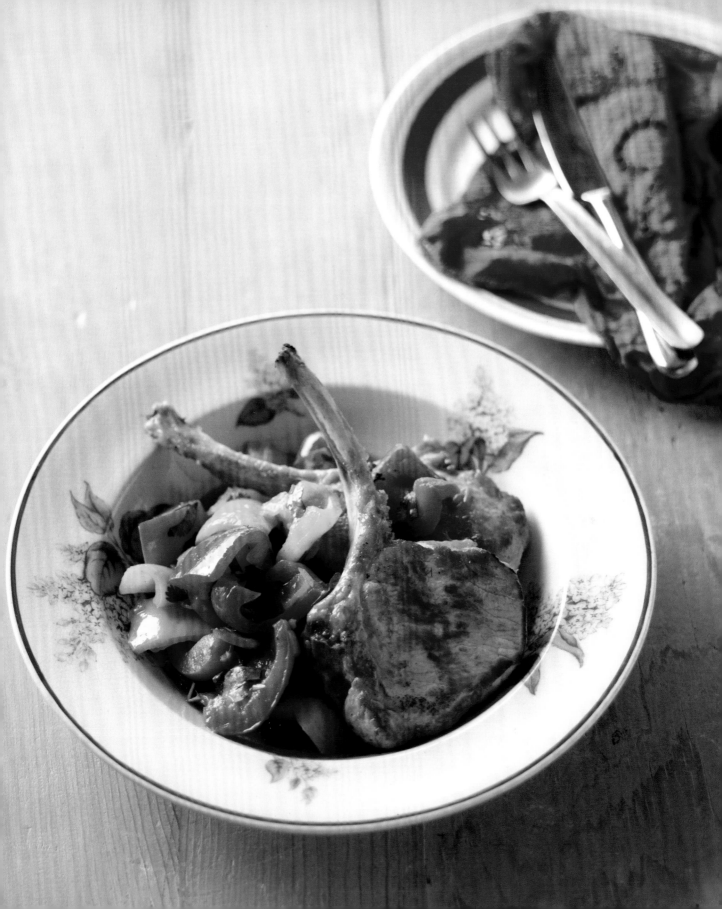

1 SERVE =
2 units protein
½ unit dairy
½ unit fruit
1½ units vegetables

Thai-spiced chicken with cucumber and pineapple salad

SERVES 4   **PREP** 40 mins + marinating time   **COOK** 35 mins

1½ teaspoons ground turmeric

2 stalks lemongrass, trimmed
and finely chopped

3 cloves garlic, crushed

2 tablespoons fish sauce

2 small red chillis, or to taste,
coarsely chopped

175 ml reduced-fat coconut-
flavoured evaporated milk

1 kg skinless chicken pieces,
trimmed of fat

vegetable oil spray

CUCUMBER AND PINEAPPLE SALAD

½ large cucumber, thinly sliced

300 g pineapple, peeled, cored
and very thinly sliced

large handful coriander (cilantro)
sprigs, leaves picked (optional)

2½ tablespoons lime juice

TOMATO JAM

4 ripe tomatoes (about 500 g),
coarsely chopped

½ red capsicum (pepper),
trimmed, seeded and
coarsely chopped

1 red chilli, or to taste,
finely chopped

2 tablespoons fish sauce

1 tablespoon caster sugar
or powdered sweetener

This dish is so simple to make, yet is bound to impress your dinner guests – the aromatic baked chicken is accompanied by a zesty salad and homemade tomato jam.

1 Combine the turmeric, lemongrass, garlic, fish sauce and chilli in a food processor and process to a coarse paste. Add the evaporated milk and process to combine well. Transfer the mixture to a bowl, add the chicken pieces and toss to coat. Cover with plastic wrap and refrigerate for 4 hours, or overnight if you have time.

2 Preheat the oven to 180°C and spray a large baking dish with vegetable oil. Drain the chicken pieces, then place them in the dish in a single layer. Roast for 35–40 minutes or until cooked through and golden.

3 Meanwhile, for the tomato jam, combine the tomato and capsicum in a food processor and process until smooth. Place in a small saucepan with the remaining ingredients and bring to simmering point. Cook over low–medium heat for 25 minutes or until reduced and very thick, then set aside until needed.

4 Place the cucumber, pineapple, coriander and lime juice in a bowl and toss to combine well.

5 Serve the chicken pieces with the salad and a spoonful of tomato jam.

TIP The tomato jam can be made a day in advance and kept in an airtight container in the fridge. If you have any leftover you could serve it with the Thai Fish Burgers on page 220.

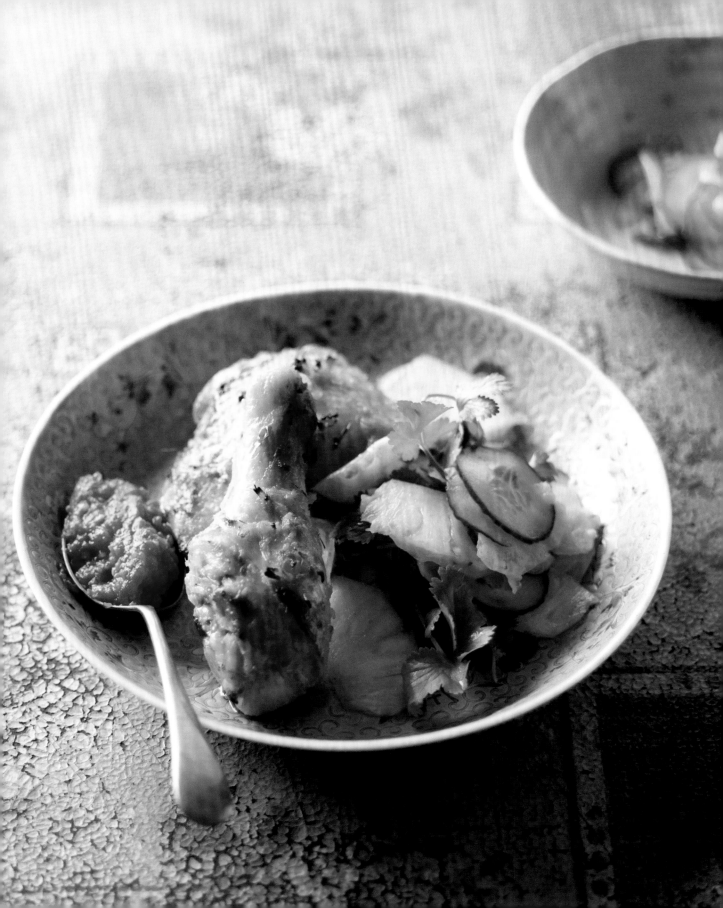

Mediterranean-style chicken with olives and capers

SERVES 4   PREP 15 mins   COOK 35 mins

1 tablespoon olive oil

800 g chicken thigh fillets,
   trimmed of fat and halved

1 cup (250 ml) red wine vinegar

1 cup (250 ml) salt-reduced
   chicken stock

1 × 400 g tin chopped tomatoes

½ cup (15 g) chopped flat-leaf
   (Italian) parsley

12 black olives, pitted and chopped

2 teaspoons capers, rinsed
   and drained

175 g broccolini

100 g green beans, trimmed

The classic combination of tomatoes, capers and olives has always been a winner. Here it works beautifully with pan-fried chicken and steamed greens.

1 Heat the olive oil in a large saucepan over medium heat. Add the chicken in batches and cook until browned.

2 Return all the chicken to the pan and add the vinegar. Bring to the boil and cook for about 5 minutes until the vinegar has reduced by half. Add the stock and tomatoes and simmer for 15 minutes or until the chicken is cooked through. Stir in the parsley, olives and capers.

3 Meanwhile, steam the broccolini and beans for 10 minutes or until tender. Serve with the chicken.

1 SERVE =
2 units protein
½ unit fruit
1 unit vegetables
1 unit fats

Cajun turkey skewers with orange and red onion salad

SERVES 4   PREP 20 mins   COOK 6 mins

800 g turkey tenderloins,
   trimmed of fat and cut
   into strips
1 tablespoon olive oil
2 tablespoons Cajun spice mix

ORANGE AND RED ONION SALAD
100 g mixed salad leaves
2 oranges, peeled and sliced
2 tomatoes, sliced
1 red (Spanish) onion, sliced
2 teaspoons olive oil
2 teaspoons sherry or
   red wine vinegar

These spicy skewers would also work well with chicken or pork. If you are using wooden skewers, soak them in water for about 20 minutes before use to prevent scorching during cooking.

1 In a large bowl, combine the turkey, olive oil and spice mix until the meat is well coated. Divide the meat into eight portions, then thread each portion onto a skewer to make eight kebabs.

2 To make the salad, combine the salad leaves, orange, tomato and onion in a large bowl. Sprinkle the olive oil and vinegar over the top and gently toss to coat.

3 Heat a chargrill or large frying pan over medium heat and cook the turkey skewers for 2–3 minutes each side or until cooked through. Serve with the salad.

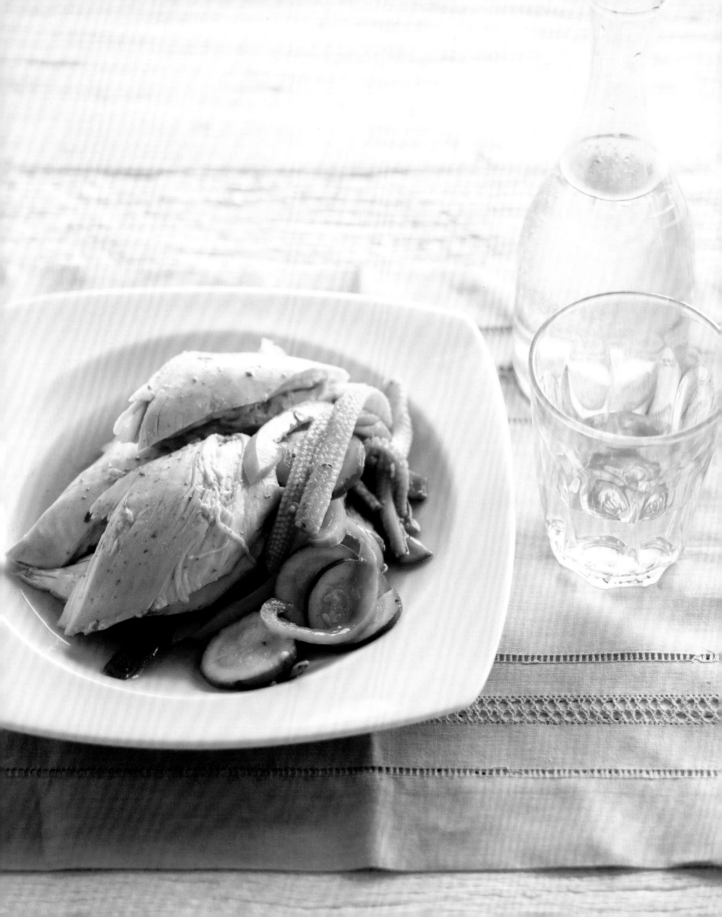

Master-stock chicken with stir-fried vegetables

SERVES 4 **PREP** 25 mins **COOK** 1 hour 30 mins

2 star anise

1 × 4 cm piece ginger,
   peeled and sliced

1 cinnamon stick

4 cloves garlic, 2 bruised with the
   flat part of a knife, 2 crushed

1 cup (250 ml) salt-reduced
   light soy sauce

1 cup (250 ml) medium–dry sherry

$^1/_3$ cup (75 g) firmly packed
   brown sugar

1 × 1.2 kg chicken

1 tablespoon vegetable oil

1 yellow capsicum (pepper),
   trimmed, seeded and
   finely sliced

250 g baby corn,
   halved lengthways

4 zucchini (courgettes),
   trimmed and sliced

1 × 3 cm piece ginger,
   peeled and finely chopped

Cooking chicken in master stock, a lightly spiced poaching liquid, is a great way to add flavour and colour without adding fat. You can use the same batch of stock over and over; in fact, its flavour only improves with time. Let it cool and store it in the freezer, then when you come to use it again, thaw it in the fridge and strain it (you may need to top it up with a little water) before simmering. You'll need a very large, deep saucepan or a stockpot for this recipe, as the chicken is cooked whole in the stock.

1 Combine the star anise, ginger, cinnamon, bruised garlic, soy sauce, sherry, sugar and 1 cup (250 ml) water in a large deep saucepan or stockpot. Bring to simmering point, then add the chicken, carefully pushing it into the hot liquid as far as it will go. Bring back to simmering point, then reduce the heat to low, cover and gently simmer for 30 minutes (do not let it simmer rapidly as this will make the chicken tough). Carefully turn the chicken over, then cover and cook over low heat for another 30 minutes. Remove the pan from the heat and leave to stand, covered, for 30 minutes to finish cooking the chicken.

2 Carefully remove the chicken and drain over a large bowl. Strain and reserve the master stock for another use. Using your hands, break the chicken into large chunks, removing the skin and bones, then divide among plates.

3 Meanwhile, heat the oil in a wok over medium–high heat. Add the capsicum, corn and zucchini and stir-fry for 3 minutes or until the vegetables have softened. Add the crushed garlic and ginger and cook for another minute or so, then serve immediately with the chicken.

TIP Star anise is a star-shaped spice commonly used in Chinese cooking. It lends a sweet aniseed flavour to dishes, and is available from delis and Asian grocers.

1 SERVE =
2 units protein
1½ units fruit
2½ units vegetables
1 unit fats

Chicken with cranberry-braised red cabbage

SERVES 4   PREP 30 mins   COOK 30 mins

1 tablespoon olive oil
about ²/₃ red cabbage,
    finely shredded (you'll need
    8 cups shredded cabbage)
120 g dried cranberries
1½ cups (375 ml) cranberry juice
1 sprig rosemary
olive oil spray
4 × 200 g skinless chicken breast
    fillets, butterflied (ask your
    butcher to do this for you)
1 quantity Parsnip, Carrot and
    Orange Mash (see page 485)

A great combination of flavours. Use turkey instead of chicken here and you could serve this for Christmas dinner!

1 Heat the oil in a large saucepan over low–medium heat. Add the cabbage, then cover and cook, stirring often, for 10 minutes or until wilted. Add the cranberries, cranberry juice and rosemary and cook, stirring often, for 20 minutes or until the cabbage is tender and the liquid has reduced. Discard the rosemary.

2 Meanwhile, preheat the oven to 200°C. Spray a baking dish with olive oil, place the chicken in and cover the dish tightly with foil. Bake for 8 minutes, then remove from the oven and leave to stand, covered, for 5 minutes; the chicken should be cooked through. Season to taste with salt and pepper and cut into thick slices. Divide the cabbage, chicken and mash among plates and serve.

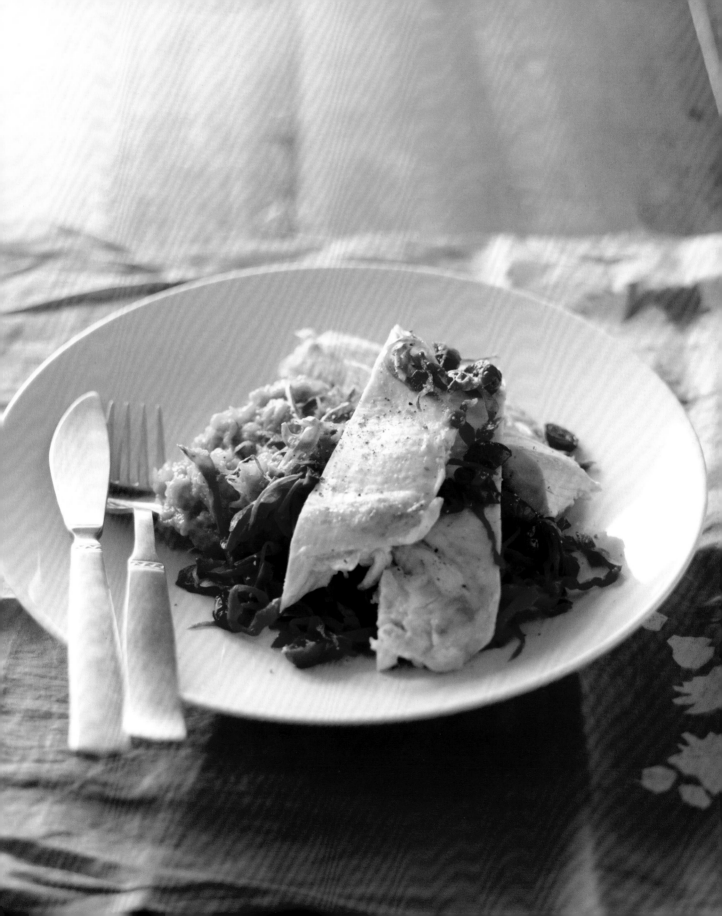

1 SERVE =
2 units protein
½ unit fruit
1½ units vegetables
2 units fats

Fennel-crusted pork fillet with parsnip and baked apple

SERVES 4   PREP 15 mins + refrigerating time   COOK 30 mins

1 × 800 g lean pork fillet
2 tablespoons ground fennel
2 tablespoons olive oil
2 apples, quartered and cored
2 teaspoons brown sugar
2 tablespoons water
4 parsnips, peeled and
    cut into chunks
4 sprigs rosemary
200 g green beans

1 Preheat oven 180°C.

2 Remove all sinew from pork. Season well, then roll in fennel. Wrap in plastic wrap and refrigerate for 10–15 minutes.

3 Heat a large frying pan over high heat. Coat pork with half the oil and cook each side for 3 minutes, or until golden. Set aside, covered.

4 Place apples in an ovenproof dish, sprinkle with brown sugar and water and cover with foil. Set aside. Place parsnip, rosemary and remaining oil in a baking dish and toss to coat. Bake for 10 minutes.

5 Transfer apples in their dish to oven. At the same time, add pork to the parsnip dish. After a further 10 minutes cooking, the parsnip should be golden, the pork cooked and the apples soft.

6 Meanwhile, bring a small saucepan of lightly salted water to a boil. Add beans and cook for 5–6 minutes, then drain.

7 Turn off the oven, transfer pork to a plate and allow to rest, covered, for 5 minutes. Slice pork thickly and serve with parsnip, apple and green beans.

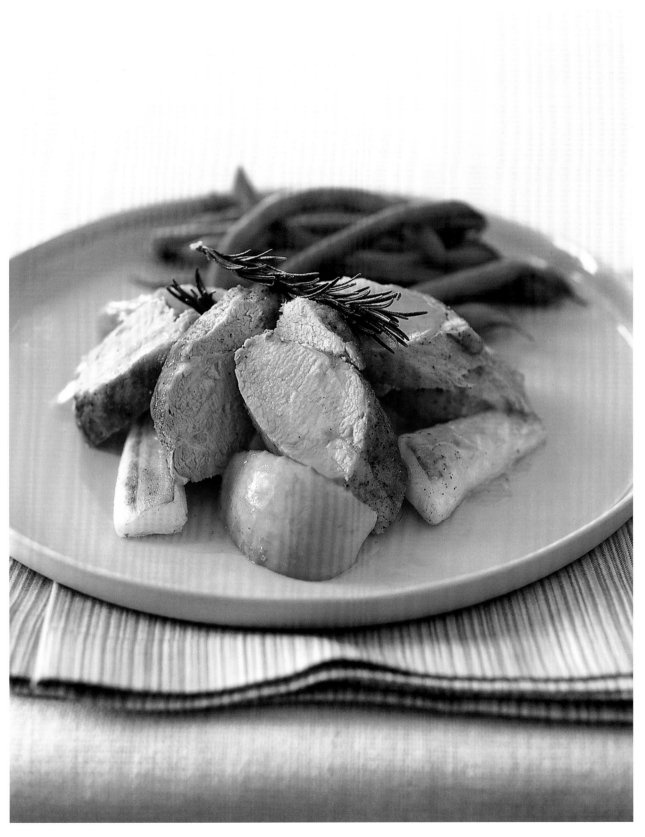

Chicken gumbo

SERVES 4   PREP 20 mins   COOK 40 mins

2 teaspoons ground cumin
2 teaspoons smoked paprika
1 teaspoon chilli powder
1 teaspoon garlic powder
1 teaspoon onion powder
1 teaspoon dried oregano
800 g chicken thighs, trimmed
    and cut into quarters
1 tablespoon extra virgin olive oil
1 onion, chopped
2 cloves garlic, crushed
2 sticks celery, diced
1 green capsicum (pepper),
    seeded and diced
1 × 400 g tin chopped tomatoes
1 cup (250 ml) salt-reduced
    chicken stock
roughly chopped flat-leaf
    (Italian) parsley, to serve
Tabasco sauce, to serve

A jewel in the crown of Cajun cuisine, a gumbo is a cross between a soup and a stew. Whatever you call it, this recipe promises a warming meal that is bursting with flavour.

1   Combine the cumin, paprika, chilli powder, garlic powder, onion powder and oregano in a large bowl. Add the chicken pieces and toss to coat well in the spice mix.

2   Heat the olive oil in a medium saucepan over medium heat. Add the chicken and cook, stirring regularly, until browned. Remove and set aside.

3   Add the onion to the pan and cook for 5 minutes or until softened, then stir in the garlic, celery and capsicum and cook for 1 minute. Add the chopped tomatoes and stock and simmer for 15 minutes. Return the chicken to the pan, then cover and simmer for 15 minutes or until the chicken is cooked through.

4   Sprinkle with parsley and a few drops of Tabasco sauce, and serve with rice from your daily bread allowance and a salad or vegetables to the side.

TIP If the spices start to burn when you remove the chicken from the saucepan, add a little water. You could replace some of the chicken with sliced lean sausages.

Poached chicken breast with soy, ginger and spring onion

SERVES 4   PREP 10 mins + resting time   COOK 15 mins

2 tablespoons light soy sauce
1 tablespoon dry sherry
   (or rice wine)
1 × 2 cm piece ginger, sliced
¼ cup coriander (cilantro) leaves,
   plus extra for garnish
5 spring onions (scallions),
   finely sliced
1 litre chicken stock
4 × 200 g skinless chicken breasts

1   In a large saucepan or deep frying pan, bring soy sauce, sherry, ginger, ¼ cup coriander, two-thirds of the spring onion and chicken stock to a boil.

2   Add chicken, then reduce heat and simmer for 12 minutes. Remove from heat but allow chicken to rest in liquid for 5 minutes. Slice chicken thickly and place on serving plate. Pour over a little poaching liquid and top chicken with extra coriander and remaining spring onion.

3   Serve with your favourite steamed green and rice from your daily bread allowance.

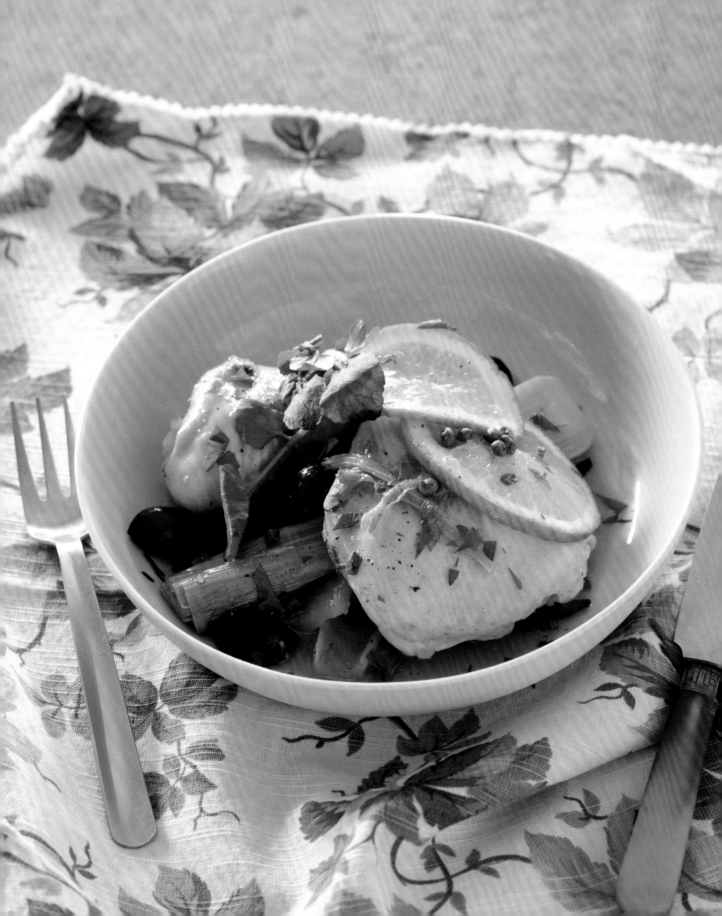

1 SERVE =
2 units protein
1 unit fruit
1½ units vegetables

Oven-steamed chicken with celery, leeks, capers, garlic and orange

SERVES 4   PREP 20 mins   COOK 1 hour

2 cloves garlic, thinly sliced
4 sticks celery, cut into 10 cm lengths
4 leeks, trimmed, washed and
  quartered lengthways
2½ tablespoons drained capers
½ cup (60 g) pitted black olives
300 ml orange juice
1 kg skinless chicken pieces,
  trimmed of fat
1 orange, thinly sliced
small handful watercress sprigs, torn

Steaming is such a healthy way to cook food, and you don't even need a steamer basket for this recipe. The chicken pieces are steamed in a small amount of liquid in a roasting tin in the oven, tightly covered with foil to seal. Serve this with a fresh green salad on the side if you like.

1   Preheat the oven to 180°C.

2   Place the garlic, celery, leek, capers, olives and orange juice in a large roasting tin. Season with salt and pepper, then cover tightly with foil. Bake for 25 minutes or until the vegetables have started to soften.

3   Remove the foil and add the chicken in a single layer, then scatter the orange slices evenly on top to cover the chicken. Replace the foil and bake for 35–40 minutes or until the vegetables are very soft and the chicken is cooked through.

4   Divide the chicken and vegetable mixture among warmed plates, then pour over the pan juices. Serve immediately scattered with watercress.

TIP Chicken, or any meat or fish for that matter, tends to taste better when cooked on the bone, and the weight specified here includes the bones. You could use 800 g skinless chicken thigh fillets if you prefer – just cook them for a little less time (about 20 minutes should suffice).

Honey-mustard pork with warm cabbage salad

SERVES 4   PREP 15 mins   COOK 15 mins

800 g pork fillet, trimmed of fat
   and cut into 4 cm slices
olive oil spray
¼ cup (60 ml) salt-reduced
   chicken stock
¼ cup (90 g) honey or
   seeded mustard
¼ cup (60 g) reduced-fat sour cream

WARM CABBAGE SALAD
1 tablespoon olive oil
2 cups (160 g) shredded cabbage
   (red, white or a combination of both)
2 carrots, grated
3 spring onions, sliced
½ cup (125 ml) white wine vinegar

The sweetness of the honey and the tanginess of the mustard create a wonderful contrast in this dish.

1   Heat a large heavy-based frying pan over medium heat. Season the pork, then spray with olive oil and cook for 3–4 minutes each side or until cooked to your liking. Remove from the pan, cover with foil and keep warm.

2   Add the stock to the pan and stir to remove any caramelised bits of pork stuck on the base. Add the mustard and sour cream and stir until well combined and heated through.

3   Meanwhile, to make the salad, heat the olive oil in a large saucepan over medium heat. Add the cabbage, carrot and spring onion and cook, stirring, until the vegetables are just softened. Stir in the vinegar.

4   Divide the pork among four plates and drizzle with the honey-mustard sauce. Serve with the cabbage salad.

TIP Pork fillet is very lean and tender – cut it into thick slices and gently flatten with your fingers (on the cut side). The fillet can be replaced with pork schnitzel slices, but make sure you halve the cooking time. Experiment with different mustards – Dijon would make a nice change.

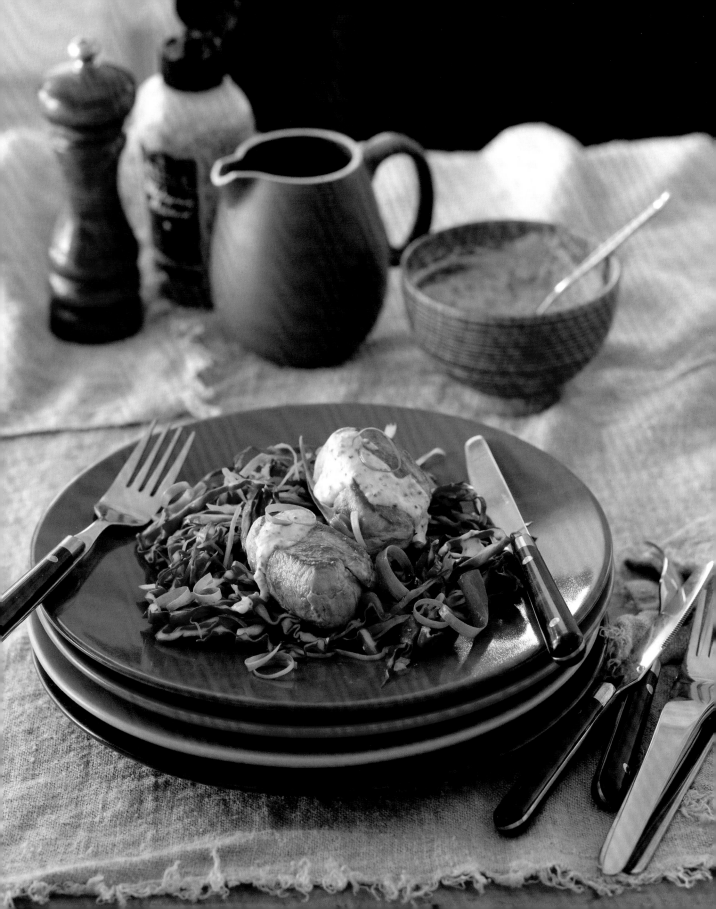

Pork cutlet with avocado, orange and beetroot salad

SERVES 4   **PREP** 15 mins + resting time   **COOK** 10 mins

2 tablespoons redcurrant jelly
   or cranberry sauce
4 × 200 g pork cutlets,
   trimmed of fat

AVOCADO, ORANGE & BEETROOT
SALAD
1 avocado, thickly sliced
2 oranges, segmented
700 g tinned baby beetroots,
   drained and halved
100 g rocket (arugula)
¼ cup roughly chopped mint
½ red (Spanish) onion,
   finely sliced
1 tablespoon olive oil
2 teaspoons lemon juice

1 Preheat a grill plate or barbecue grill to high. Rub redcurrant jelly into the pork using your fingers, then transfer immediately to the grill plate and cook for 4 minutes each side, or until browned and cooked through. Set aside for 5 minutes.

2 Place avocado, orange, beetroot, rocket, mint and onion in a bowl and toss lightly. Drizzle with oil and lemon juice.

3 Serve pork cutlets with salad alongside.

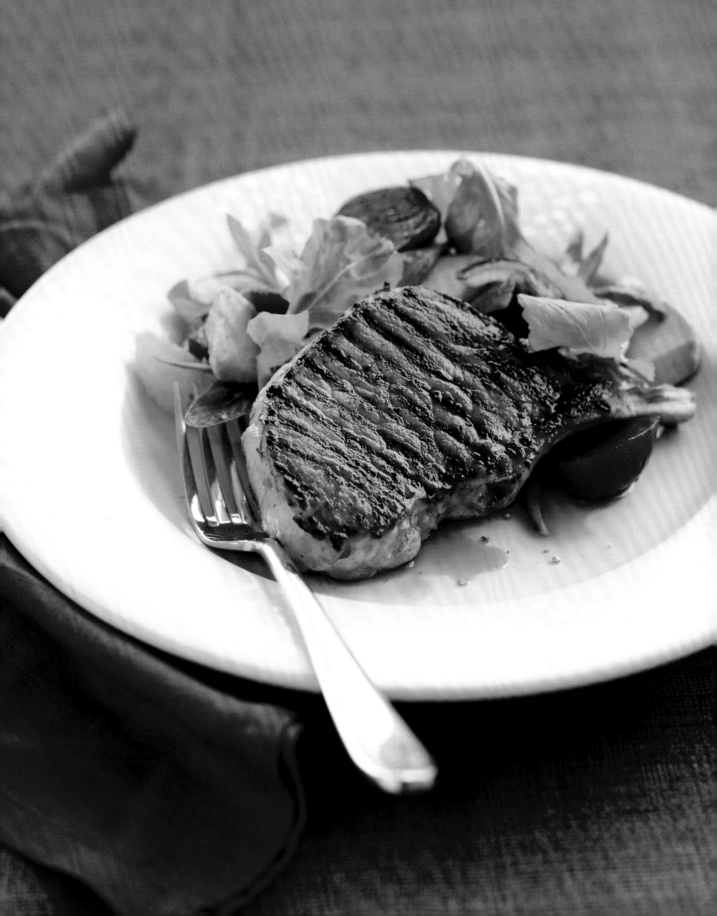

Apricot chicken

SERVES 4   PREP 15 mins   COOK 40 mins

2 tablespoons plain flour
1 tablespoon Moroccan spice mix
800 g chicken thigh cutlets,
    trimmed and skin removed
1 tablespoon olive oil
1 onion, chopped
3 cloves garlic, crushed
4 sprigs thyme
1 × 400 ml tin apricot nectar
90 g dried apricots
½–1 cup (125–250 ml) salt-reduced
    chicken stock
2 tablespoons red wine vinegar

**Moroccan cooking often includes fruit in savoury dishes, so
the spice blend works perfectly here with the chicken, dried
apricots and sweet apricot nectar.**

1   Combine the flour and spice mix in a large bowl, then sprinkle over
the chicken to coat lightly.

2   Heat the olive oil in a large heavy-based saucepan over medium–high
heat and brown the chicken on both sides. Remove and set aside.

3   Add the onion and garlic to the pan and stir until softened. Add the
thyme, apricot nectar, apricots and half the stock and bring to a simmer.
Return the chicken to the pan and simmer for 20 minutes or until
cooked through, adding more stock if necessary. Stir in the vinegar.

4   Serve with rice from your daily bread allowance and steamed
vegetables.

> **TIP** You can make your own Moroccan spice mix by combining
> a teaspoon each of ground cumin, ginger, coriander, cinnamon and
> paprika. Otherwise, look for it in the spice section at the supermarket.

Asian chicken, tomato and pineapple hotpot

SERVES 4   PREP 20 mins   COOK 12 mins

2 stalks lemongrass, trimmed
¼ cup (60 ml) fish sauce
1.25 litres salt-reduced chicken stock
800 g skinless chicken breast fillets,
    cut into 2 cm pieces
250 g sugar snap peas, trimmed
½ small ripe pineapple, peeled,
    cored and cut into 1.5 cm pieces
400 g cherry tomatoes, halved
200 g bean sprouts
2 spring onions, trimmed and
    thinly sliced on the diagonal
1 red chilli, thinly sliced
¼ cup (60 ml) lime juice
2 tablespoons caster sugar
    or powdered sweetener
handful mint and coriander
    (cilantro)leaves (optional)

The sweet and sour flavours of this delicate lemongrass-infused hotpot are typically South-East Asian. Be sure to serve the delicious broth too.

1   Bruise the lemongrass stalks, then tie each in a knot. Place in a large saucepan, then add the fish sauce and chicken stock and bring to simmering point over low heat. Add the chicken and sugar snaps, then cook for 3 minutes.

2   Add the pineapple, tomato and bean sprouts, then cook for 4–5 minutes or until the sprouts have softened slightly and the chicken is cooked through. Stir in the spring onion, chilli, lime juice and sugar or sweetener, then divide among warmed large bowls. Top with herbs, if using, then serve.

TIP You can use lemon juice instead of lime juice if you prefer.

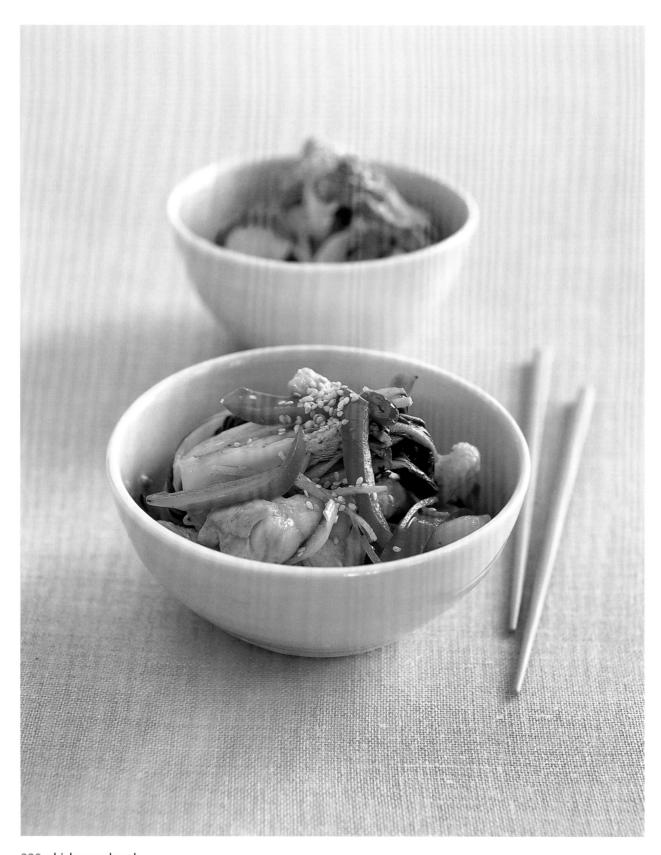

1 SERVE =
2 units protein
1 unit vegetables
1 unit fats

Stir-fried ginger chicken with sesame bok choy

SERVES 4   PREP 15 mins   COOK 20 mins

2 teaspoons sesame seeds
2 small bunches bok choy (pak choi),
　halved and washed
1 tablespoon sesame oil
800 g skinless chicken breast,
　cut into thick strips
1 × 3 cm piece ginger, julienne
1 clove garlic
1 small red chilli, finely sliced
1 onion, quartered
½ red capsicum (pepper),
　seeded and sliced
$^1/_3$ cup (80 ml) dry sherry
　(or Chinese rice wine)
2 tablespoons soy sauce

1   Heat a small non-stick frying pan over medium heat. Add sesame seeds and toss for 5 minutes, or until lightly toasted. Set aside.

2   Bring a little water to a simmer in a wok. Put bok choy into a bamboo steamer and place steamer in wok. Cover wok and steam bok choy for 2–3 minutes. Remove from steamer and set aside.

3   Heat a wok or large frying pan over medium heat. Add 1 teaspoon of the sesame oil and heat until smoking, then add chicken. Stir-fry for 6–8 minutes, or until chicken is cooked and golden. Remove from wok and set aside. Wipe out wok with paper towel.

4   Return wok to heat and add remaining sesame oil. When oil is smoking, add ginger, garlic, chilli, onion and capsicum and stir-fry for 2 minutes. Return chicken to wok. Add sherry and soy sauce and stir to combine. Add bok choy and toss through.

5   Serve sprinkled with toasted sesame seeds and with a side serve of rice from your daily bread allowance, if desired.

Pork cutlets with fennel, celery and white wine

SERVES 4   PREP 25 mins   COOK 25 mins

1 tablespoon olive oil
4 × 300 g pork cutlets, trimmed of fat
1 onion, thinly sliced
3 sticks celery, finely chopped
1 large bulb fennel, trimmed
   and thinly sliced
1 teaspoon fennel seeds
1 cup (250 ml) dry white wine
1½ cups (375 ml) salt-reduced
   chicken stock
2 tablespoons chopped oregano
   or 2 teaspoons dried oregano
2½ tablespoons capers
small handful snipped chives
   (optional)
1 tablespoon lemon juice
1 tablespoon tapenade (optional)

These braised vegetables are a great accompaniment to pork, but would work equally well with chicken or fish.

1 Heat the oil in a large, heavy-based casserole dish or deep frying pan over medium heat. Add the pork cutlets and cook for 2 minutes on each side or until browned, then remove and set aside on a plate.

2 Add the onion, celery and fennel to the dish or pan, then reduce the heat to low–medium and cook, stirring often, for 5–6 minutes or until the vegetables start to soften.

3 Add the fennel seeds, white wine and stock, season with salt and pepper and bring to simmering point. Cover, then cook over medium heat for 10 minutes or until the vegetables are soft. Stir in the oregano, capers, chives (if using) and lemon juice.

4 Add the cutlets to the dish, cover and cook for 5–6 minutes or until the pork is just cooked through. Divide among warmed plates, then add a teaspoon of tapenade to each plate (if using) and serve immediately.

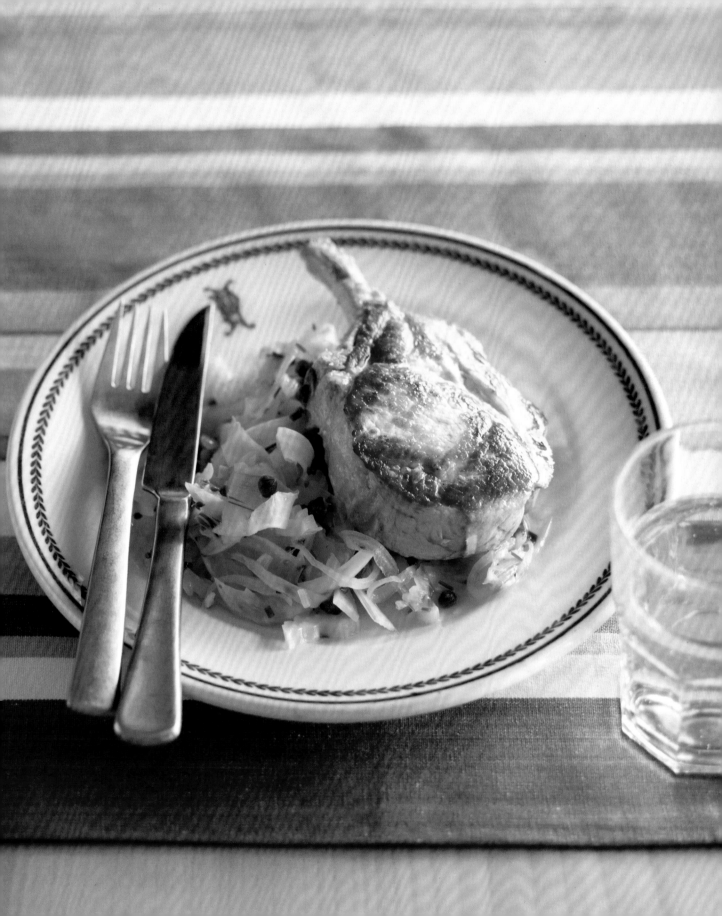

Chicken tagine

SERVES 4　PREP 15 mins　COOK 40 mins

1½ tablespoons olive oil
800 g chicken thigh fillets,
　trimmed of fat and cut
　into 5 cm pieces
1 onion, finely chopped
6 cloves garlic, crushed
2 sticks celery, thinly sliced
3 teaspoons ground coriander
1 teaspoon ground ginger
1 × 400 g tin chopped tomatoes
60 g dried apricots,
　roughly chopped
2 teaspoons grated lemon zest
2 tablespoons lemon juice
1 cinnamon stick
2 cups (300 g) diced pumpkin (squash)
1 cup (250 ml) salt-reduced
　chicken stock
3 tablespoons chopped coriander
　(cilantro), plus extra sprigs
　to garnish

A tagine is the name for a Moroccan stew and the conical-shaped terracotta dish it is traditionally cooked in. Don't worry if you don't have a tagine – the recipe works just as well in a heavy-based saucepan.

1　Heat the olive oil in a medium saucepan over medium heat. Add the chicken in batches and cook for 5 minutes or until golden. Remove and set aside. Add the onion, garlic and celery to the pan and cook for 5 minutes or until the onion has softened.

2　Add the ground coriander and ginger and saute for a further 1 minute, then add the chopped tomatoes, apricot, lemon zest, lemon juice, cinnamon, pumpkin and stock.

3　Return the chicken to the pan and bring the mixture to the boil, then reduce the heat and simmer for 20 minutes or until the chicken and pumpkin are cooked through. Season to taste and stir in the coriander. Garnish with extra coriander and serve with couscous from your daily bread allowance and steamed vegetables.

TIP　Add a finely sliced red chilli at the beginning of step 2 if you like a bit of heat in your food. The pumpkin can easily be replaced with sweet potato, for a slightly different flavour.

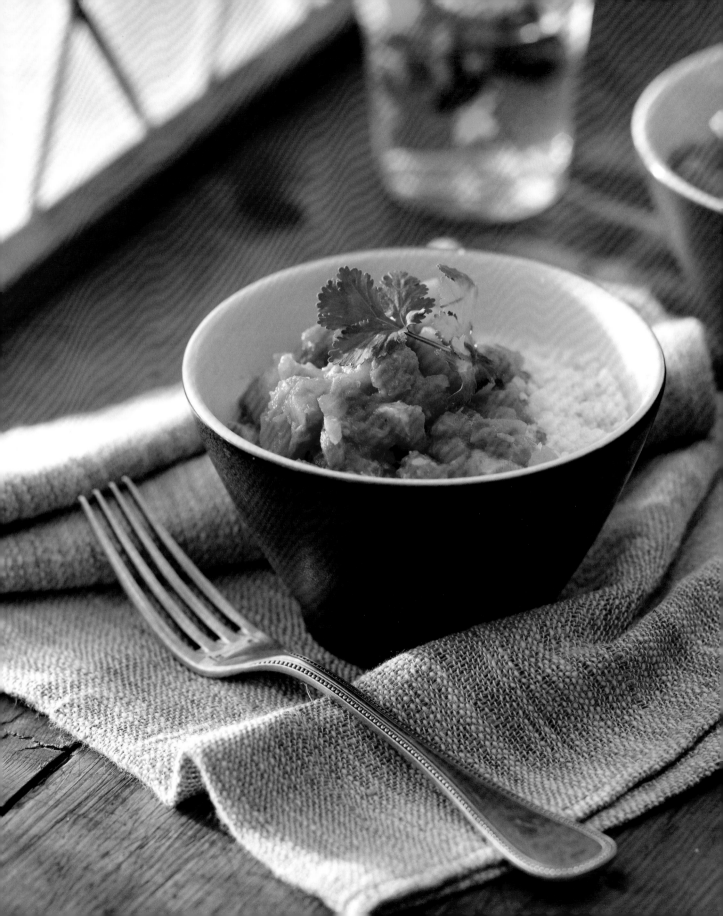

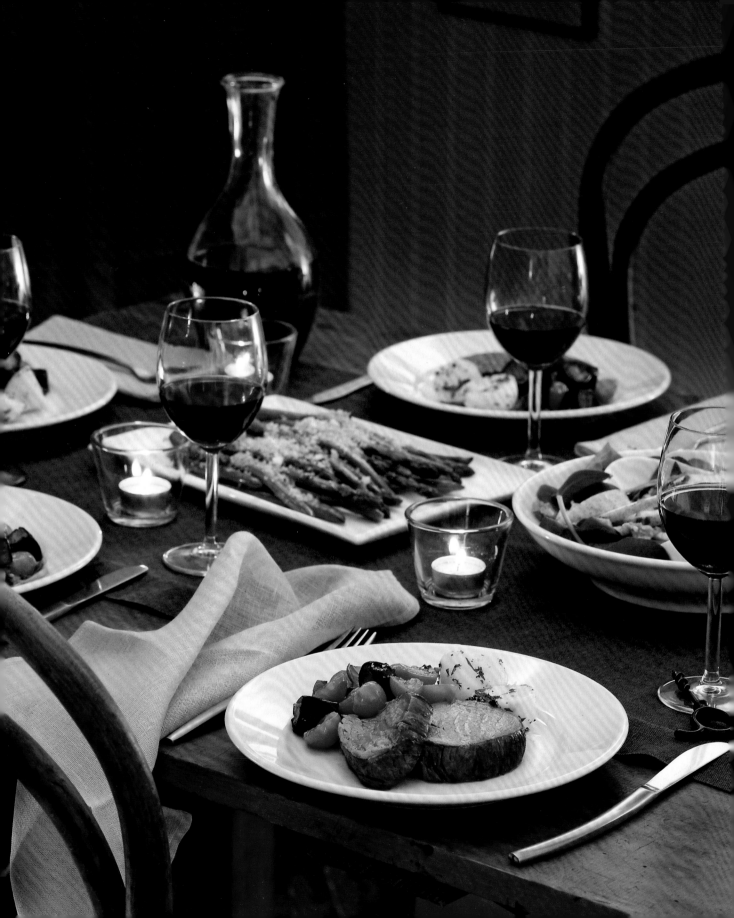

beef and veal

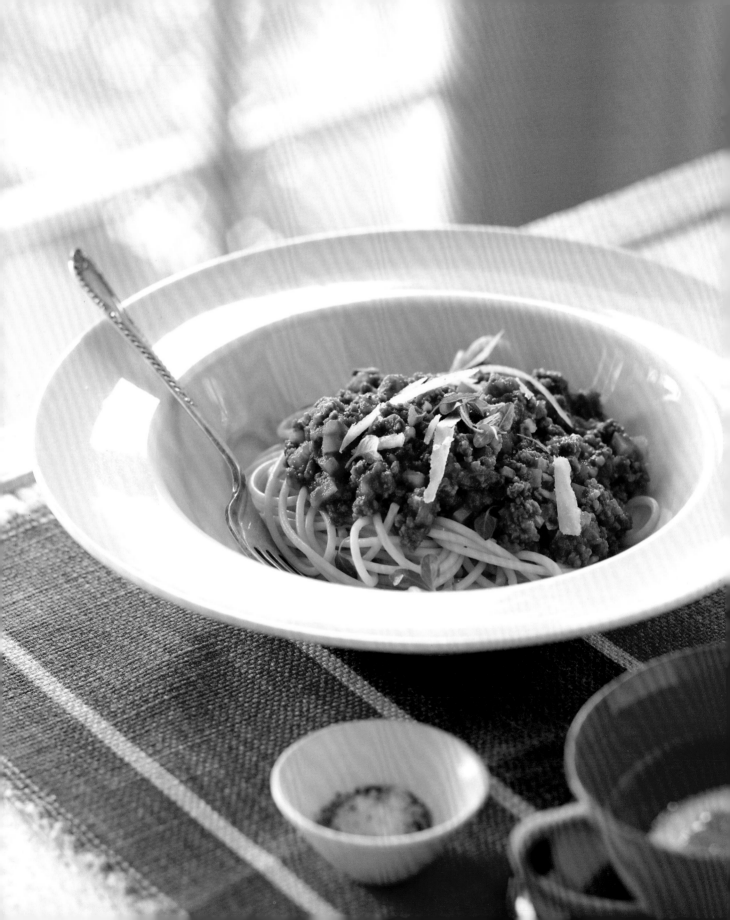

Bolognese

SERVES 4   PREP 10 mins   COOK 30 mins

1 tablespoon olive oil
1 onion, finely chopped
400 g lean minced beef
2 cloves garlic, crushed
1 carrot, finely diced
1 stick celery, finely diced
100 g mushrooms, finely diced
½ cup (125 ml) red wine
700 ml salt-reduced tomato passata
2 × 400 g tins chopped tomatoes
1–2 teaspoons reduced-fat
   beef stock powder
2 teaspoons dried oregano
2 bay leaves

An old-time favourite, Bolognese sauce is wonderfully versatile and may be served in a number of different ways. For something a little different, replace the minced beef with lean minced lamb and feel free to add extra vegetables.

1 Heat the olive oil in a large saucepan over medium heat and cook the onion until softened. Add the minced beef and cook until starting to brown, breaking up any lumps with the back of a wooden spoon. Add the garlic, carrot, celery and mushrooms and cook, stirring, for 5 minutes or until softened.

2 Pour in the wine and bring to the boil. Add the remaining ingredients and simmer, uncovered, for 25–30 minutes or until thickened. See below for serving suggestions.

TIP The quantities can easily be doubled to make extra portions of Bolognese sauce, which can be frozen for a later date.

1 SERVE =
2 units bread
1 unit dairy

SPAGHETTI BOLOGNESE

Cook 2 cups (170 g) spaghetti or your favourite pasta according to the packet instructions. Drain. Divide among four plates, and top with Bolognese sauce. Garnish with shaved parmesan and flat-leaf (Italian) parsley or oregano leaves.

1 SERVE =
2 units bread
1 unit dairy

PASTICCIO (PASTA BAKE)

Place 4 cups (360 g) cooked pasta, such as penne, in the base of a 4 litre baking dish and pour over the Bolognese sauce. To make a white sauce, blend 2 tablespoons cornflour with 2 cups (500 ml) reduced-fat milk. Pour into a small saucepan and cook, stirring constantly, over low heat until thickened. Pour the white sauce over the Bolognese. Top with 100 g grated reduced-fat cheese and bake in a preheated 180°C oven for 35–40 minutes or until golden.

1 SERVE =
2 units bread
½ unit dairy

CANNELLONI

Fill 200 g cannelloni tubes with the Bolognese. Pour the remaining Bolognese into the base of a 2 litre baking dish and arrange the stuffed cannelloni on top, pushing down as you go so they are slightly submerged. Top with 100 g grated reduced-fat cheese and bake in a preheated 180°C oven for 30 minutes or until golden on top.

Beef and vegetable pasta bake

SERVES 4   **PREP** 15 mins   **COOK** 1 hour 10 mins

2 tablespoons olive oil
800 g lean minced (ground) beef
1 red (Spanish) onion, diced
2 teaspoons dried mixed herbs
1 red capsicum (pepper),
   seeded and finely diced
1 × 400 g tin chopped tomatoes
1 cup (250 ml) salt-reduced beef stock
250 g rigatoni, cooked
2 zucchini (courgettes), diced
1 cup (120 g) frozen peas
100 g grated reduced-fat
   cheddar cheese

1   Heat half the oil in a large heavy-based saucepan over high heat. Add mince in two batches and cook for 5 minutes, or until just browned. Transfer to a large bowl. Add remaining oil to pan, along with onion, and cook for 5 minutes, or until onion is soft. Return mince to pan, add dried herbs, capsicum, tomatoes and stock and bring to a boil. Reduce heat and simmer for 35 minutes. Stir in pasta, zucchini and peas, then carefully pour into a 2 litre ovenproof dish.

2   Meanwhile, preheat oven to 200°C. Sprinkle cheese over pasta bake, transfer to oven and cook for 10 minutes, or until cheese is golden. Serve with a mixed-leaf salad.

1 SERVE =
2 units protein
1½ units vegetables
1 unit fats

Cinnamon, basil and pumpkin 'lasagne'

SERVES 4   PREP 20 mins   COOK 1 hour

olive oil spray
1 onion, finely chopped
2 sticks celery, finely chopped
800 g lean minced beef, pork or veal
1 teaspoon ground cinnamon
2 tablespoons tomato paste (puree)
1 × 400 g tin chopped tomato
handful basil leaves, torn (optional)
800 g pumpkin (squash), peeled,
   seeded and thinly sliced
basil leaves (optional), to serve

Healthy and hearty, this dish is far easier to make than traditional lasagne. Add 100 g parmesan from your dairy allowance if you like: grate it, then scatter some over each layer of meat.

1 Preheat the oven to 180°C.

2 Heat a large heavy-based non-stick frying pan over medium heat. Once hot, spray with olive oil, then add the onion and celery and cook, stirring often, for 3–4 minutes or until the vegetables are just starting to soften. Add the mince and cinnamon and cook, stirring, for 4–5 minutes or until the mince is browned. Stir in the tomato paste and chopped tomato, bring to simmering point and cook for 10 minutes or until the mixture thickens slightly. Remove from the heat, stir through the basil (if using) and season with salt and pepper.

3 Transfer half the mince mixture to a 2 litre roasting tin or baking dish, spreading it evenly over the base. Add half the pumpkin slices, overlapping them to cover the mince. Repeat with the remaining mince and pumpkin, then cover the dish tightly with foil and bake for 20 minutes. Remove the foil and bake for another 20 minutes or until the pumpkin is very tender.

4 Leave to stand for 5–10 minutes to cool slightly, then serve scattered with basil leaves (if using).

TIP While the cooking time here may seem long, the beauty of this dish is that once it's in the oven, it requires almost no attention. You can also freeze this for up to 8 weeks, so make a double batch to have some on hand for when time is short.

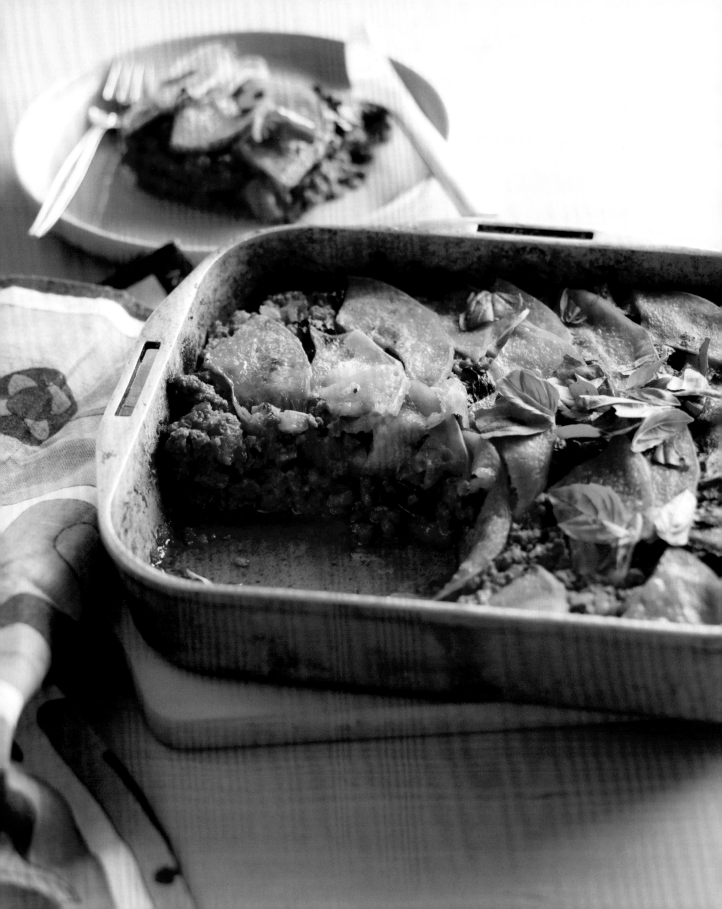

Veal parmigiana

SERVES 4   PREP 10 mins   COOK 15 mins

800 g thin veal steaks,
 trimmed of fat
2 tablespoons plain flour
2 tablespoons olive oil
700 ml salt-reduced tomato passata
1 teaspoon dried oregano
2 tablespoons chopped basil,
 plus extra leaves to serve
1 cup (100 g) grated reduced-fat
 mozzarella

Lightly pan-fried veal with a rich tomato sauce and golden melted cheese – what's not to like?

1 Preheat the grill to high.

2 Coat the veal lightly with the flour and season with a little salt and pepper.

3 Heat the olive oil in a large non-stick frying pan over medium heat. Brown the steaks for about 2 minutes each side (it is fine if they are still pink in the middle). Place in a single layer in a shallow ovenproof dish.

4 Combine the passata, oregano and basil in a medium saucepan and warm over medium heat or in the microwave. Pour the sauce over the veal, sprinkle with the grated cheese and place under the grill until the cheese has melted.

5 Sprinkle with the extra basil leaves and serve with a salad or steamed vegetables to the side.

TIP If the veal steaks are too thick, cover with plastic wrap and flatten them with a rolling pin.

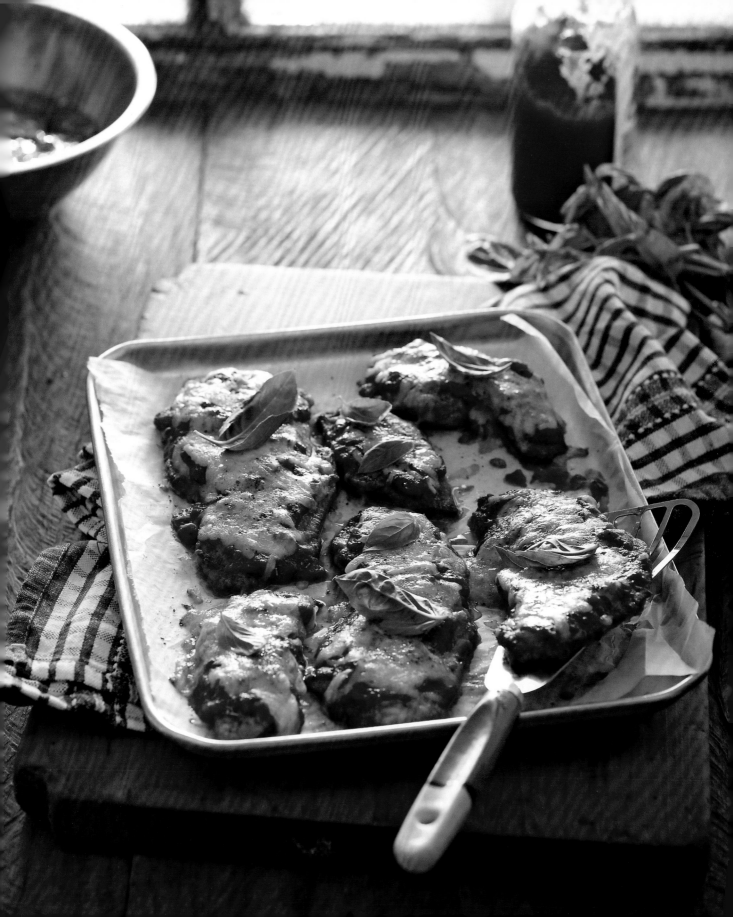

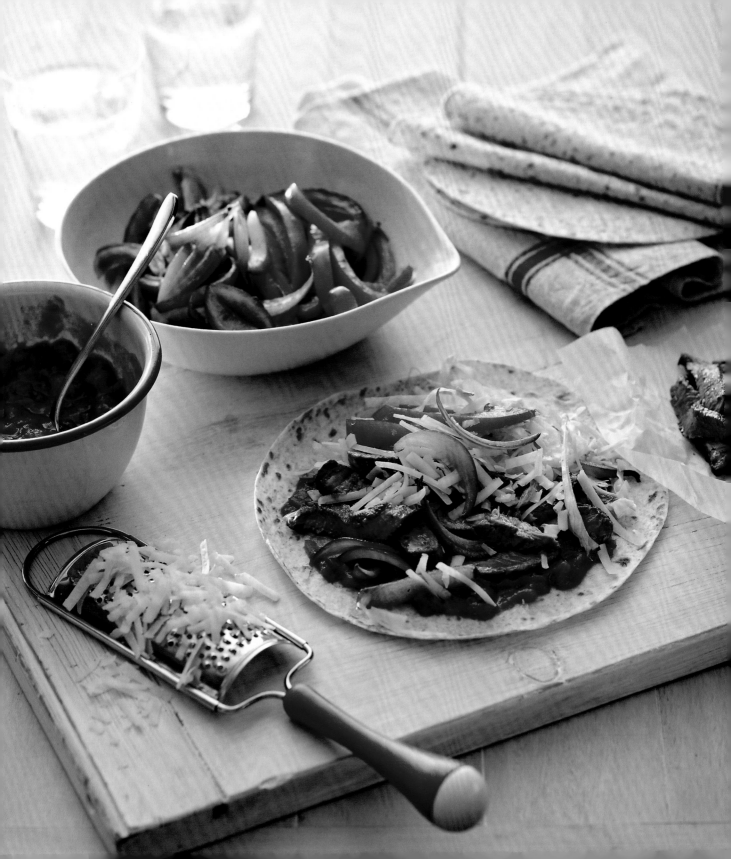

1 SERVE =
2 units protein
2 units bread
½ unit dairy
1 unit vegetables
1 unit fats

Beef fajitas

SERVES 4   PREP 20 mins + marinating time   COOK 10 mins

800 g rump or skirt steak
2 red capsicums (peppers),
    seeded and sliced
1 red (Spanish) onion, sliced
8 wholemeal wraps
shredded iceberg lettuce, to serve
ready-made tomato salsa, to serve
100 g grated reduced-fat cheddar

MARINADE
1 tablespoon olive oil
¼ cup (60 ml) lime juice
2 teaspoons ground cumin
1 teaspoon dried oregano
2 teaspoons brown sugar

Kids love a hands-on approach to eating, so these sizzling fajitas are sure to be popular. Best of all, everyone can choose their own filling ingredients.

1   Combine the marinade ingredients in a bowl, add the steak and rub the marinade all over. Cover and marinate in the refrigerator for 2 hours or overnight.

2   Drain the steak. Heat a frying pan over medium heat and cook the steak for about 2 minutes each side. Remove and set aside to rest. Add the capsicum and onion to the pan and cook, stirring, until they start to colour and soften. Cut the steak into thin slices.

3   Warm the wraps in the microwave and top with the lettuce, steak, vegetables, salsa and grated cheese. Roll up and serve immediately.

TIP You can also make chicken fajitas based on this recipe – just substitute trimmed chicken or thigh breast fillet for the beef steak.For a quick homemade salsa, combine 4 diced tomatoes, ½ finely chopped onion and the juice of 1 lemon. Add a little finely sliced chilli to taste.

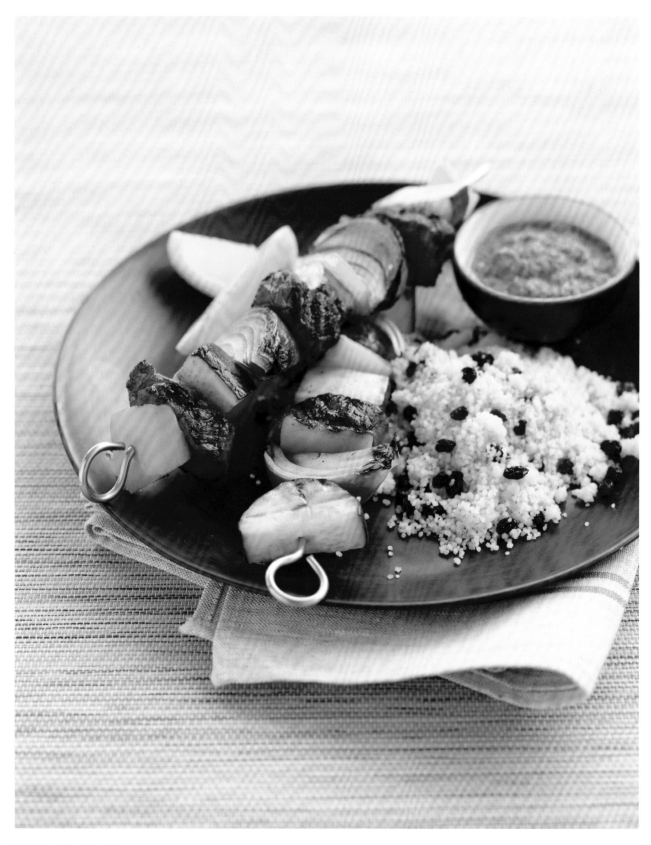

Beef kebabs with currant couscous and harissa

SERVES 4   PREP 25 mins + soaking time   COOK 10 mins

2 red (Spanish) onions, quartered
1 yellow capsicum (pepper),
    cut into 2 cm dice
2 small zucchini (courgettes),
    halved lengthways and then
    cut into 2 cm pieces
800 g beef rump, cut into cubes
1 tablespoon lemon juice
1 tablespoon olive oil
¾ cup couscous (makes 1$^1/_3$ cups
    cooked couscous)
¼ cup currants
1½ cups (375 ml) boiling water
2 teaspoons extra-virgin olive oil
1 lemon, cut into wedges

HARISSA
(makes approx. 2 cups; store
    leftovers in the fridge)
1 teaspoon ground coriander
1 teaspoon ground cumin
½ teaspoon ground fennel
½ teaspoon ground cinnamon
4 roasted red capsicums (peppers),
    chopped (to roast your own
    capsicums, see page 416)
¼ cup roughly chopped mint
2 cloves garlic, roughly chopped
1 small red chilli, chopped
finely grated zest and juice of 1 lime
2 tablespoons olive oil

1   To make the harissa, place all ingredients in a food processor and blend until smooth. Set aside.

2   If using bamboo skewers, soak in hot water for 30 minutes before use. Preheat a grill plate or barbecue grill to high. Thread vegetables and beef alternately onto 8 skewers. Drizzle with lemon juice and olive oil. Cook kebabs for 2 minutes each side – 8 minutes in total – or until meat is cooked and vegetables are browned. Set aside for 5 minutes.

3   Meanwhile, place couscous and currants in a heatproof bowl. Pour over boiling water and extra-virgin olive oil, cover with plastic wrap and allow to sit for 5 minutes. Fluff up with a fork.

4   Divide couscous and skewers among plates and serve with 2 tablespoons of harissa per person and a lemon wedge or two.

1 SERVE =
2 units protein
2 units vegetables
½ unit fats

Spiced beef skewers with Chinese salad

SERVES 4   **PREP** 30 mins   **COOK** 12 mins

800 g beef rump, sirloin or other
   lean beef, trimmed of fat and
   cut into 1.5 cm pieces
1½ teaspoons ground cumin
1 teaspoon chilli powder,
   or to taste
12 bamboo skewers, soaked
   in hot water for 30 minutes
vegetable oil spray

CHINESE SALAD

200 g snowpeas (mange-tout),
   trimmed and very thinly sliced
2 carrots, cut into fine matchsticks
200 g bean sprouts
1 large cucumber, cut into
   fine matchsticks
400 g kohlrabi (about ½ kohlrabi),
   or daikon radish (about ½ daikon
   radish), cut into fine matchsticks
1 small red (Spanish) onion,
   very thinly sliced

SOY DRESSING

¼ cup (60 ml) white vinegar
¼ cup (60 ml) salt-reduced
   light soy sauce
1 tablespoon caster sugar
   or powdered sweetener
2 cloves garlic, crushed
2 teaspoons sesame oil

Kohlrabi has a taste and texture similar to turnip, and is delicious in this salad – it's well worth picking up if you see it at your greengrocer.

1   Place the beef in a bowl and add the cumin and chilli powder. Toss to coat well, then cover and set aside.

2   To make the Chinese salad, bring a saucepan of water to the boil. Add the snowpeas and cook for 1–2 minutes or until just wilted, then remove to a bowl with a slotted spoon and set aside. Add the carrot and sprouts to the pan of boiling water and cook for 2 minutes or until softened, then drain and add to the bowl with the snowpeas. Add the remaining ingredients to the bowl and toss to combine well.

3   To make the dressing, place all the ingredients in a bowl and whisk to combine well. Pour over the vegetables and toss to combine.

4   Thread the beef onto the skewers. Heat a large heavy-based non-stick frying pan over medium–high heat. Once hot, spray with vegetable oil, then, working in batches if necessary, cook the beef for 7–8 minutes, turning often, for medium–rare or until cooked to your liking.

5   Serve the beef skewers with the salad alongside.

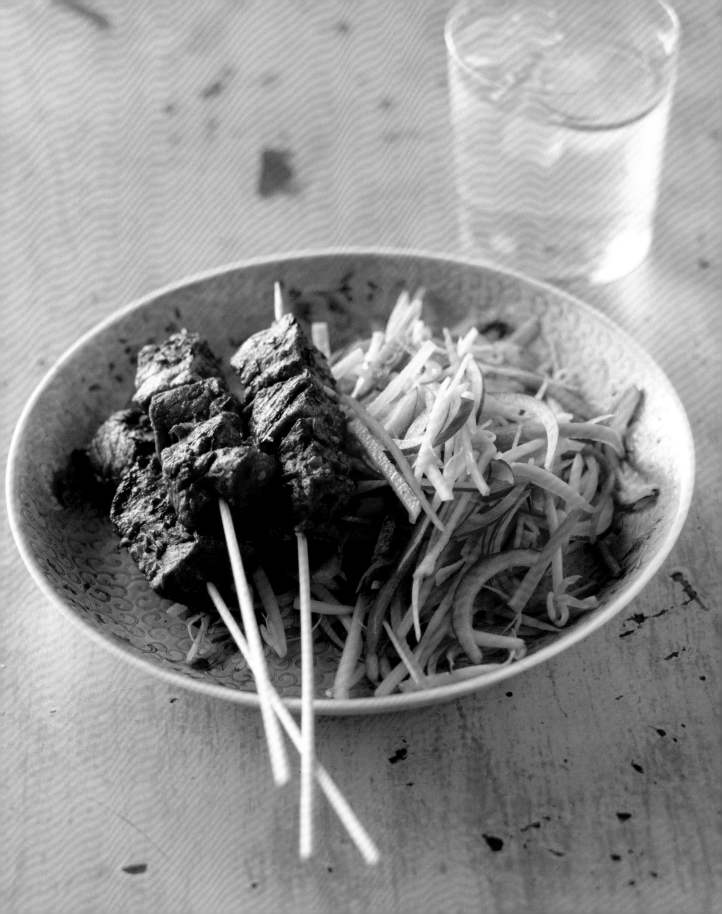

1 SERVE =
2 units protein
1 unit bread
1½ units vegetables
1 unit fats

Roast beef and vegetables with salsa verde

SERVES 4   PREP 20 mins   COOK 1 hour

800 g piece roasting beef,
    trimmed of fat
olive oil spray
4 potatoes, peeled and halved
4 cloves garlic, skin on
300 g pumpkin (squash),
    peeled and cut into
    3 cm chunks
2 bulbs baby fennel, halved
4 small onions, peeled
    and left whole
1 tablespoon olive oil
5 small vine-ripened tomatoes,
    left whole

SALSA VERDE
handful of chopped flat-leaf
    (Italian) parsley
½ cup (40 g) chopped basil
1 tablespoon capers, rinsed,
    drained and finely sliced
4 anchovy fillets, finely sliced
1 clove garlic, crushed
1 teaspoon Dijon mustard
2 tablespoons red wine vinegar
1 tablespoon extra virgin olive oil

Roast beef and a generous array of roast vegetables are given a lift with the fresh, tart flavours of homemade salsa verde.

1 Preheat the oven to 200°C.

2 Heat a medium frying pan over high heat. Season the beef with salt and pepper and spray with olive oil. Sear on all sides until well browned, then place in a large roasting tin.

3 Toss the potato, garlic, pumpkin, fennel and onions in the olive oil and arrange around the beef in the roasting tin. Roast for 40 minutes or until cooked to your liking. Remove the beef and set aside to rest, loosely covered with foil.

4 Add the tomatoes to the roasting tin and return to the oven for 10 minutes or until just cooked.

5 Meanwhile, combine all the salsa verde ingredients in a medium bowl.

6 Slice the beef and serve with the pan juices, vegetables and salsa verde.

TIP Add extra beef to the roasting tin (allow an additional 15 minutes per 500 g) and use it for lunch the next day – in a salad or sandwich. Eye fillet would be perfect for this recipe, but of course it can be expensive, so sirloin, scotch fillet and rump are also suitable.

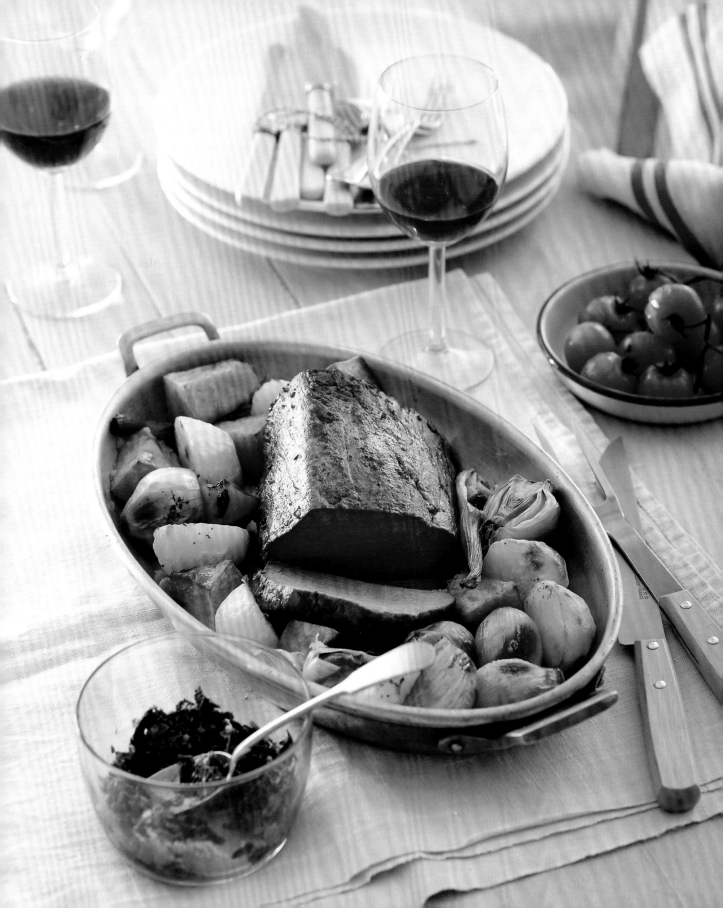

1 SERVE =
2 units protein
1½ units vegetables
1½ units fats

Roast beef with beetroot, pumpkin and carrot

SERVES 4   **PREP** 15 mins + resting time   **COOK** 35 mins

1 × 800 g sirloin, most fat removed
1½ tablespoons olive oil
4 carrots, cut into 3 cm chunks
4 beetroots, peeled and cut
   into quarters
200 g butternut pumpkin,
   peeled and cut into 4 pieces
12 cloves garlic, skins on
2 sprigs rosemary, leaves only

1   Preheat oven to 200°C.

2   Heat a heavy-based frying pan over high heat. Coat meat with 2 teaspoons of the oil and sear on all sides. Transfer to a baking dish, fat-side up. Cook in oven for 30 minutes for medium–rare, or until done to your liking.

3   Meanwhile, place vegetables in a separate baking dish. Drizzle over the remaining oil, lightly season, and toss to coat. Sprinkle rosemary over vegetables, then roast for 35 minutes.

4   Remove meat from oven, cover loosely with foil and set aside to rest for 10 minutes before carving. Serve with roasted vegetables.

Classic roast beef

SERVES 4   **PREP** 15 mins + resting time   **COOK** 40 mins

1 tablespoon Dijon mustard
1 kg lean topside roast
freshly ground black pepper
2 tablespoons olive oil
4 small onions, peeled
500 g pumpkin, peeled and
   cut into large chunks
3 parsnips, peeled and
   cut into large chunks
2 sprigs rosemary, leaves picked
300 g green beans

1   Preheat oven to 180°C.

2   Using your hands, rub mustard all over beef. Season
    with pepper. Heat oil in a flameproof baking dish
    over high heat. Add beef and sear on all sides. Place
    onions, pumpkin and parsnips in baking dish around
    beef and sprinkle with rosemary. Roast for 35 minutes,
    or until done to your liking. Transfer meat to a plate,
    cover lightly with foil and allow to rest for 10 minutes.

3   Meanwhile, bring a small saucepan of water to a boil.
    Add beans and cook for 5–6 minutes, then drain.

4   Slice beef and serve with roasted vegetables
    and beans.

Beef provençal casserole

SERVES 4   **PREP** 15 mins   **COOK** 2 hours 45 mins

2 tablespoons olive oil
2 onions, finely chopped
200 g field mushrooms, sliced
2 cloves garlic, crushed
800 g diced lean beef
2 tablespoons plain flour
1 × 400 g tin diced tomatoes
1 cup (250 ml) red wine
1 cup (250 ml) beef stock
½ red capsicum (pepper),
   seeded and sliced
1 tablespoon chopped flat-leaf
   (Italian) parsley
1 tablespoon chopped oregano

1   Preheat oven to 170°C.

2   Heat 2 teaspoons of the oil in a large, heavy-based
    frying pan over high heat. Add onion, mushrooms
    and garlic and saute for 5 minutes, or until soft.
    Transfer to a large, ovenproof dish.

3   Toss meat in lightly seasoned flour. Heat remaining oil
    in frying pan and cook beef, in 2 batches, until well-
    browned. Transfer to onion and mushroom mixture.

4   Add tomato, wine, stock and capsicum to frying pan
    and bring to a gentle boil, scraping up any bits of beef
    stuck to bottom of pan. Add to casserole dish. Cover
    and transfer to oven for 1½–2 hours. Remove lid and
    cook for a further 30 minutes, or until meat is tender.
    Stir through herbs and season to taste.

1 SERVE =
2 units protein
1½ units vegetables
1 unit fats

Provençal beef pot roast

SERVES 4   PREP 20 mins   COOK 1 hour 10 mins

2 teaspoons olive oil

1 × 800 g piece beef topside, trimmed of fat

8 salad onion bulbs, trimmed with root end intact

1 bunch Dutch (baby) carrots, trimmed

½ cup (80 g) pitted black olives (optional)

2 tablespoons tomato paste (puree)

2 sprigs rosemary

3 wide strips orange zest, removed with a vegetable peeler

2 cups (500 ml) red wine

1 cup (250 ml) salt-reduced beef stock

250 g green beans, trimmed

Enjoy the French flavours of this delicious, melt-in-the-mouth dish. It only takes a few minutes to throw together at the end of the day, then bubbles away on the stove while you put your feet up. Topside is an economical cut that requires long, slow cooking to become tender.

1 Heat the oil in a heavy-based saucepan large enough to hold the meat and vegetables snugly. Add the beef and cook, turning, for 5 minutes or until browned all over.

2 Add the onions, carrots, olives (if using), tomato paste, rosemary, orange zest, wine and stock, then bring to simmering point. Reduce the heat to low, cover with a tight-fitting lid and cook for 50 minutes. Turn the beef over, add the green beans to the pan, then cover and cook for 15 minutes or until the meat and vegetables are tender.

3 Transfer the meat to a board and cut into thin slices, then divide the meat and vegetables among warmed plates. Remove the rosemary and orange zest from the pan and spoon the sauce over the meat and vegetables, then serve.

TIP If your piece of topside is larger than 800 g, adjust the cooking time accordingly, and save the leftovers to have with a salad the next day.

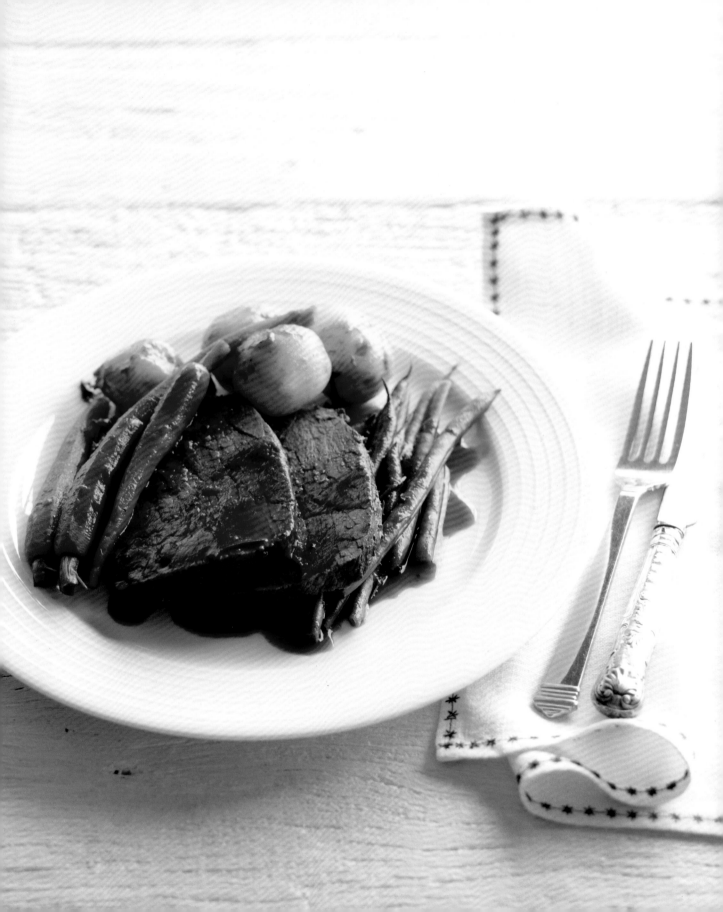

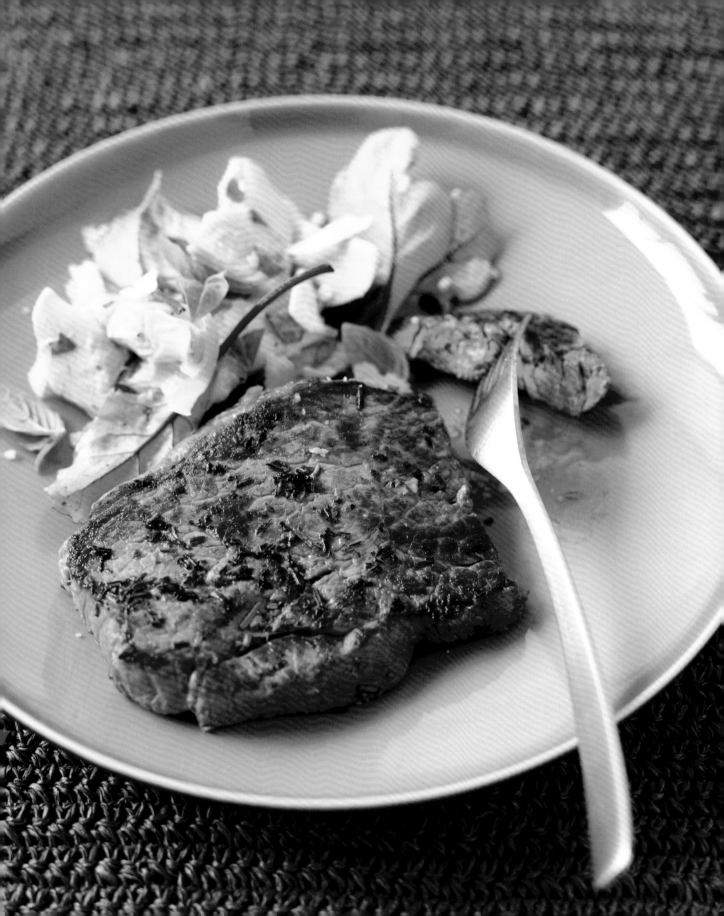

Barbecued steak with artichoke and herb salad

SERVES 4   PREP 15 mins + resting time   COOK 10 mins

1 tablespoon chopped rosemary
1 clove garlic, crushed
1 tablespoon olive oil
4 × 200 g rump steaks,
   trimmed of fat

ARTICHOKE & HERB SALAD
1 × 340 g jar marinated artichoke
   hearts, drained
1 tablespoon lemon juice
1 tablespoon olive oil
½ cup coarsely grated parmesan
¼ cup chopped basil
2 tablespoons chopped flat-leaf
   (Italian) parsley
2 cups salad leaves
freshly ground black pepper,
   to taste

1   Preheat a grill plate or barbecue grill to high.

2   In a small bowl, mix rosemary, garlic and olive oil. Rub into steaks using your fingers. Cook steaks for 4 minutes each side, or until done to your liking. Remove from heat, cover with foil and set aside to rest for 5–10 minutes.

3   To make the salad, mix all ingredients. Serve steak with salad and your favourite steamed vegetables.

Lemon cumin veal cutlets with parsnip mash and baby green beans

SERVES 4   PREP 10 mins + marinating time   COOK 35 mins

finely grated zest of 1 lemon
2 teaspoons ground cumin
1 tablespoon olive oil
1 clove garlic, crushed
4 × 200 g veal cutlets
400 g baby green beans

PARSNIP MASH
6 small parsnips (700 g), peeled
   and cut into large pieces
1 tablespoon light margarine
½ cup (125 ml) reduced-fat milk

1 Place lemon zest, cumin, oil and garlic in a large bowl and mix well. Add the veal cutlets and turn to coat thoroughly. Cover bowl and refrigerate for 30 minutes.

2 Meanwhile, place parsnips in a saucepan and cover with cold water. Bring to a boil and cook for 15 minutes, or until tender. Drain and place in a food processor with margarine and milk, and blend until smooth. Season to taste.

3 Preheat a grill plate or barbecue grill to high. Cook cutlets for 4 minutes each side, or until done to your liking.

4 Bring a saucepan of water to the boil. Place beans in a steamer and cook for 5 minutes.

5 Serve cutlets with parsnip mash and steamed baby green beans. Baby carrots make a delicious side dish to this.

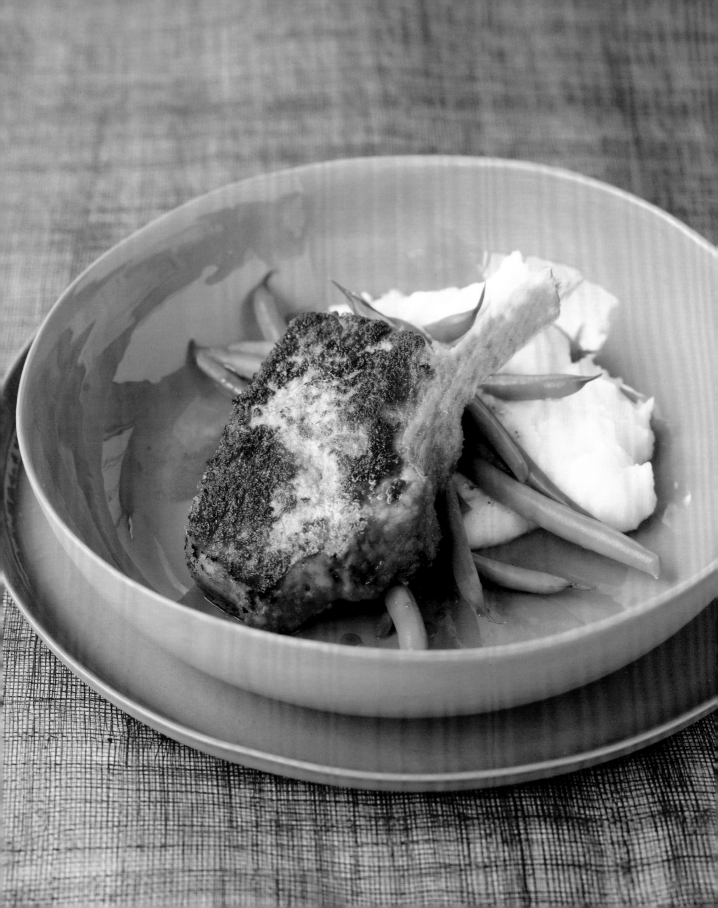

Veal cutlets with tomato risotto

SERVES 4   PREP 10 mins   COOK 45 mins

olive oil spray
4 × 200 g veal cutlets
2 teaspoons capers,
    rinsed and drained
lemon wedges, to serve
    (optional)

TOMATO RISOTTO
1 tablespoon olive oil
1 onion, finely diced
2 cloves garlic, crushed
1 cup (200 g) short-grain rice
1 zucchini (courgette),
    finely diced
1½ cups (375 ml) salt-reduced
    chicken stock
1 × 400 g tin chopped tomatoes
50 g parmesan, shaved or grated

The tomato risotto is baked in the oven, making it fuss-free and easy to do. It's a good match for the juicy veal cutlets – perfect with the piquant capers and a squeeze of lemon.

1 Preheat the oven to 200°C.

2 To make the risotto, heat the olive oil in a 1.5 litre flameproof casserole dish and cook the onion for about 5 minutes or until soft. Add the garlic, rice and zucchini and stir until the rice is well coated with oil. Add the stock and tomatoes and bring to a simmer, then cover and bake in the oven for 35 minutes.

3 About 10 minutes before serving time, spray a large frying pan with olive oil and heat over high heat. Season the veal cutlets with salt and pepper, then add them to the pan and cook for 3–4 minutes each side, or until cooked to your liking.

4 Sprinkle the parmesan over the risotto and serve with the veal cutlets, capers and lemon wedges (if using), and your choice of salad and vegetables to the side.

TIP Lamb or veal steaks also work wonderfully here, if you are looking for a cheaper option. The risotto can be simmered on the stovetop, if preferred. To boost the vegetable content, add a cup or so of finely diced vegetables with the rice and zucchini.

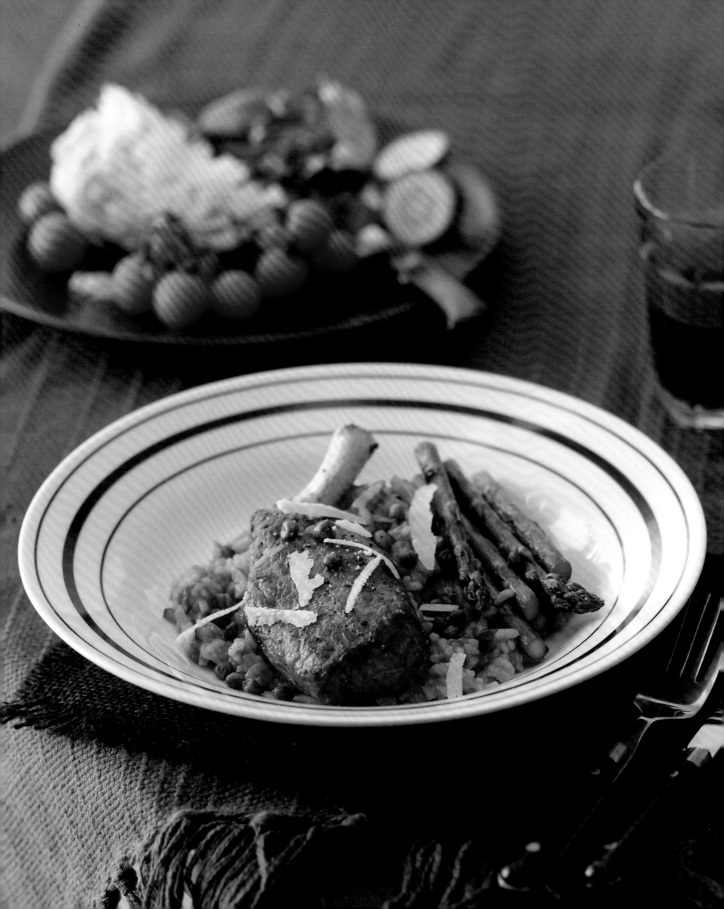

1 SERVE =
2 units protein
½ unit dairy
½ unit vegetables*
* or 1½ units with serving suggestion

Individual meatloaves

SERVES 4　PREP　20 mins　COOK　35 mins

olive oil spray
700 g lean minced beef
2 eggs, lightly beaten
1 onion, finely chopped
3 cloves garlic, crushed
1 tablespoon tomato paste (puree)
1 small green capsicum (pepper),
　finely chopped
1 zucchini (courgette), grated
2 teaspoons Cajun spice mix
3 tablespoons chopped flat-leaf
　(Italian) parsley
2 teaspoons finely grated
　lemon zest
50 g grated parmesan
salt-reduced tomato ketchup,
　to serve (optional)

These mini versions are a new take on an old favourite. Of course, the mixture works just as well as a traditional meatloaf – just spoon the mixture into a loaf tin and bake for 45 minutes.

1　Preheat the oven to 180°C. Spray eight ½ cup (125 ml) mini loaf tins or muffin holes with olive oil.

2　Combine all the ingredients, except the parmesan and ketchup, in a large bowl and mix thoroughly with your hands. Divide the mixture among the tins or muffin holes and sprinkle with the parmesan.

3　Bake for 35 minutes or until cooked through. Serve with tomato ketchup if you like, and a green salad to the side.

TIP　You can replace the minced beef with lean minced lamb or a combination of lean minced veal and pork. Leftovers can be sliced and used to fill sandwiches or served with salad for lunch the following day.

Bourguignon-style beef casserole

SERVE 4   PREP 15 mins   COOK 1 hour 40 mins

1 tablespoon olive oil
100 g lean rindless bacon, diced
700 g lean stewing beef, trimmed
   of fat and cut into 3 cm pieces
8 baby onions, peeled and left whole
2 carrots, diced
2 sticks celery, diced
4 cloves garlic, crushed
200 g button mushrooms
1 cup (250 ml) red wine
1 cup (250 ml) salt-reduced beef stock
2 tablespoons tomato paste (puree)
2 strips orange zest
3 sprigs thyme
2 teaspoons cornflour (cornstarch)
   (optional)

You'll feel as if you've been whisked away to Provincial France as you indulge in this hearty meal. It is a wonderful dish for a long Sunday lunch with family and friends.

1 Preheat the oven to 160°C.

2 Heat the olive oil in a flameproof casserole dish over medium heat and brown the bacon and beef in batches. Remove from the dish. Add the onions, carrot and celery and cook, stirring, for 5 minutes until lightly coloured, then stir in the garlic, mushrooms, wine, stock, tomato paste, orange zest and thyme.

3 Bring to the simmer, then cover and bake in the oven for 1½ hours. If a thicker sauce is desired, blend the cornflour with a little water and stir through the casserole as soon as it has been removed from the oven, until it has thickened. Serve with a large bowl of steamed vegetables.

TIP Make a double batch and freeze in serving sizes, for an easy weeknight meal. This casserole also works beautifully with the same quantity of trimmed leg of lamb in place of the beef.

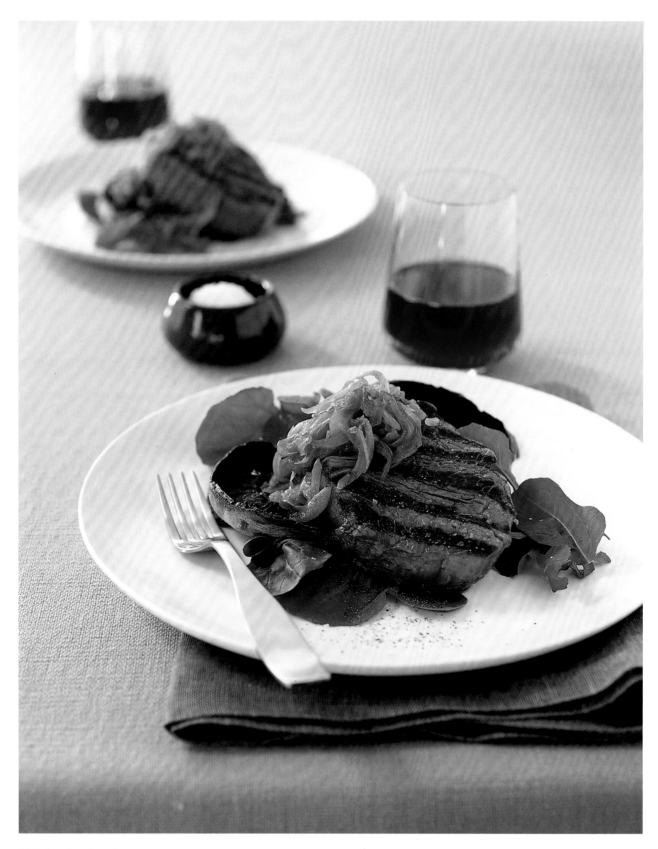

1 SERVE =
2 units protein
1½ units vegetables
½ unit fats

Char-grilled beef fillet with mushrooms and caramelised onion

SERVES 4   PREP   10 mins + resting time   COOK   1 hour

3 onions, finely sliced
2 teaspoons olive oil
2 teaspoons balsamic vinegar
8 field mushrooms, peeled
  and stems removed
½ cup (125 ml) white wine
1 × 800 g beef fillet
100 g rocket (arugula) leaves

1   Preheat oven to 180°C.

2   Cook onions in oil in a saucepan over medium heat, stirring occasionally, for 30 minutes, or until soft. Add balsamic vinegar and cook for a further 5 minutes, or until mixture is sticky. Season to taste.

3   Heat a large non-stick frying pan over high heat and sear fillet on all sides. Transfer meat to a baking dish.

4   Place mushrooms in a second baking dish, then pour over wine and lightly season. Cover with foil. Place both dishes in oven and bake for 15 minutes. Remove beef from oven, cover with foil and set aside to rest for 10 minutes. At the same time, remove foil from mushrooms and bake for a further 10 minutes.

5   Cut meat into four pieces and serve with rocket leaves, caramelised onions and mushrooms.

Veal saltimbocca with tomatoes and zucchini

SERVES 4   **PREP** 15 mins   **COOK** 15 mins

600 g veal escalopes
200 g lean ham slices
8 sage leaves
2 tablespoons olive oil
100 ml white wine
400 g zucchini (courgettes), sliced
2 cloves garlic, crushed
2 tomatoes, diced
3 tablespoons shredded basil
1 teaspoon balsamic vinegar
small basil leaves, extra, to garnish

This attractive recipe is a great one to prepare when entertaining friends at short notice, or to make you feel a little special midweek.

1 Spread a large piece of plastic wrap on your work surface. Place the veal escalopes on top and cover with second piece of plastic wrap. Using a rolling pin, flatten the escalopes to a thickness of about 5 mm. Season with salt and pepper.

2 Lay a slice of ham over each escalope, and place a sage leaf on top. Fold the overlapping edges of ham under and secure with a cocktail stick.

3 Heat 1 tablespoon of the olive oil in a non-stick frying pan over high heat. Add the veal, ham-side down, and cook for 2 minutes each side until browned. Reduce the heat and add the wine. Cook for about 2 minutes or until the liquid has evaporated. Transfer the escalopes to serving plates and remove the cocktail sticks.

4 Meanwhile, heat the remaining oil in a saucepan over medium heat. Add the zucchini and cook for about 2–3 minutes or until coloured and just tender. Add the garlic and cook for 1 minute. Stir in the tomato and basil and cook until heated through. Remove the pan from the heat and stir in the balsamic vinegar. Season to taste. Garnish with the extra basil leaves and serve with the veal saltimbocca.

TIP Did you know saltimbocca means 'jump in your mouth' in Italian? You can replace the lean ham slices with slices of pancetta or prosciutto for a more authentic Italian flavour.

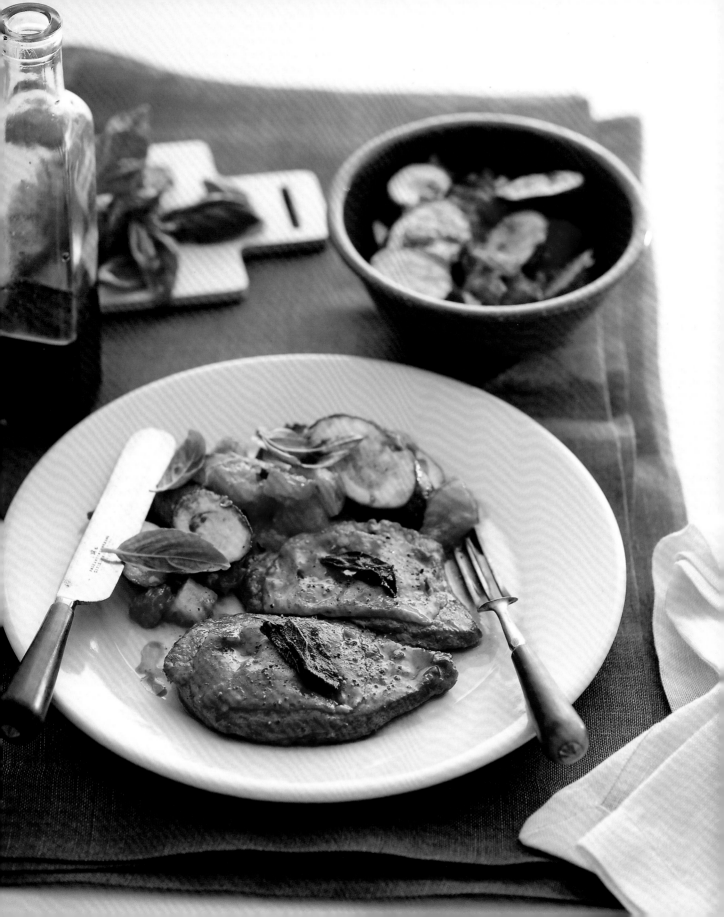

Veal escalopes with fennel, spinach and olives

SERVES 4   PREP 15 mins   COOK 5 mins

800 g veal loin, cut into 8 slices
2 tablespoons plain flour
2 tablespoons olive oil
1 bulb fennel, finely sliced
1 red (Spanish) onion,
    finely sliced
250 g baby spinach
12 kalamata olives
3 lemons
freshly ground black pepper

1 Spread a large piece of plastic wrap on your work surface. Place veal slices on top and cover with a second piece of plastic wrap. Using a rolling pin, flatten slices to 5 mm thickness. Lightly dust escalopes with flour.

2 Heat half the oil in a large frying pan over medium heat. Cook escalopes for 2 minutes each side, or until golden.

3 Meanwhile, place fennel, onion, spinach leaves and olives in a large bowl. Drizzle with remaining olive oil and the juice of 1 lemon, and season with pepper. Serve salad with veal steaks and the remaining lemons cut into wedges.

Fragrant Vietnamese beef with bok choy

SERVES 4   PREP 20 mins   **COOK** 1 hour 15 mins

1 tablespoon vegetable oil

800 g oyster blade steak, trimmed of fat, cut into large pieces

4 small onions, peeled leaving root end intact, quartered

6 Dutch (baby) carrots (about 400 g)

2 star anise

1 × 3 cm piece ginger, peeled and sliced

2 stalks lemongrass, trimmed and bruised

2 tablespoons tomato paste (puree)

2 cups (500 ml) salt-reduced beef stock

¼ cup (60 ml) fish sauce

1 × 400 g tin chopped tomato

4 baby bok choy, quartered lengthways

This aromatic braise can be quickly thrown together when you get home from work and left to cook while you unwind.

1 Heat the oil in a large heavy-based saucepan or casserole dish over medium heat. Add the beef and cook, turning occasionally, for 5–6 minutes or until well browned, then remove to a plate. Add the onion, carrots and star anise and cook, stirring, for 3–4 minutes or until the vegetables start to soften.

2 Return the beef to the pan, then add all the remaining ingredients except the bok choy. Bring to simmering point, then cover and cook over low heat for 1 hour or until the meat is tender. Remove the lemongrass, then add the bok choy, cover and cook for 8–10 minutes or until the bok choy is tender.

3 Divide the meat, vegetables and sauce among plates and serve.

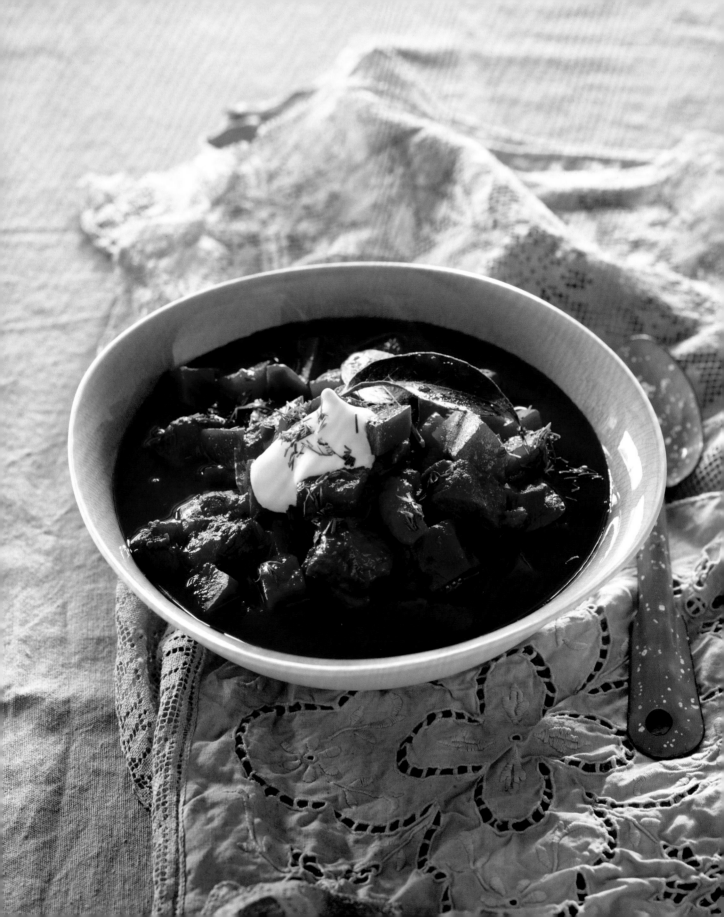

1 SERVE =
2 units protein
2 units vegetables
1 unit fats

Beef, parsnip and beetroot borscht

SERVES 4   PREP 30 mins   COOK 45 mins

1 tablespoon olive oil

800 g beef chuck steak or other
   stewing steak, trimmed of fat,
   cut into 1 cm pieces

1 onion, finely chopped

2½ tablespoons tomato paste (puree)

4 beetroot (about 700 g), peeled
   and cubed

2 parsnips, peeled and cubed

2 teaspoons caraway seeds

1 bay leaf, bruised

1.25 litres salt-reduced beef stock

⅓ cup (80 g) reduced-fat
   Greek-style yoghurt

1½ tablespoons chopped dill

The addition of beef to this classic Russian dish makes it a hearty meal in a bowl to stave off the chill of a winter's night.

1   Heat the oil in a large saucepan over medium heat, then add the beef and onion and cook, stirring, for 5–6 minutes or until the meat has browned. Add the tomato paste, vegetables, caraway seeds, bay leaf and stock and bring to simmering point, stirring to combine well.

2   Reduce the heat to low and cook for 45 minutes or until the meat and vegetables are very tender. Divide among large bowls, then spoon over the yoghurt, sprinkle with the dill and serve immediately.

Japanese beef, mushroom and eggplant stir-fry

SERVES 4   PREP 15 mins   COOK 15 mins

2 tablespoons mirin
1 tablespoon salt-reduced soy sauce
$1/_3$ cup (80 ml) teriyaki sauce
1 × 3 cm piece ginger, peeled
   and chopped
1 tablespoon vegetable oil
400 g button mushrooms, halved
6 Japanese eggplants (aubergines),
   trimmed and cut on the diagonal
   into 5 mm thick pieces
6 spring onions, trimmed
   and finely chopped
800 g beef stir-fry strips
1 teaspoon cornflour
2 teaspoons sesame seeds (optional)

Stir-fries are such a quick and easy weeknight staple, and so healthy and delicious. Mirin is a sweet Japanese cooking wine, often added to marinades and sauces, available from most supermarkets.

1   Combine the mirin, soy sauce, teriyaki sauce and ginger in a bowl and set aside.

2   Heat half the oil in a large non-stick wok over medium–high heat, add the mushroom and eggplant and stir-fry, tossing the wok often, for 5–6 minutes or until the vegetables are cooked through. Remove to a bowl.

3   Add the remaining oil, almost all of the spring onion (reserving a small handful for the garnish), and the beef to the wok, then stir–fry for 5 minutes or until the meat is nearly cooked through. Return the mushroom mixture to the wok and add the reserved sauce, tossing to combine well. Cook for 2–3 minutes or until the liquid comes to simmering point.

4   Combine the cornflour with 1 tablespoon water in a small bowl, then add to the wok, stirring it into the sauce. Cook for another 30 seconds or until the liquid boils and thickens slightly, then divide among bowls. Scatter over the reserved spring onion and the sesame seeds (if using), then serve.

TIP You can buy pre-cut beef stir-fry strips from your butcher.

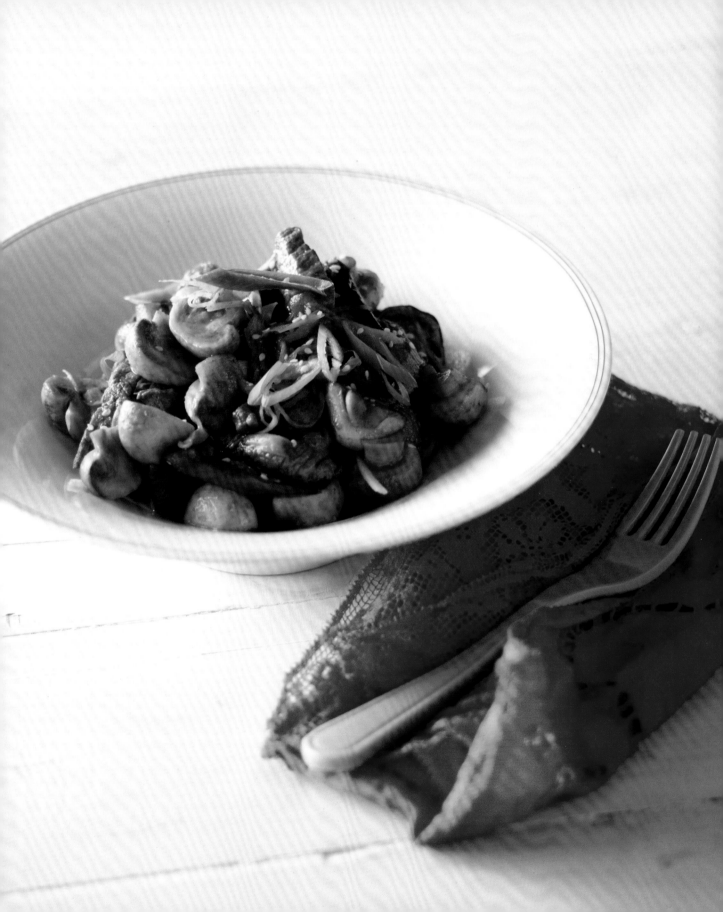

1 SERVE =
2 units protein
1 unit vegetables
1 unit fats

Thai beef salad

SERVES 4   PREP 10 mins + resting time   COOK 10 mins

800 g rump steak
1 tablespoon olive oil
100 g baby spinach leaves
1 red capsicum (pepper),
   seeded and finely sliced
1½ cups (120 g) bean sprouts
4 spring onions (scallions),
   finely sliced
½ cup coriander (cilantro) leaves
2 tablespoons chopped mint

DRESSING
2 tablespoons lime juice
1 tablespoon fish sauce
1 tablespoon soy sauce
1 clove garlic, crushed
1 red chilli, seeded and chopped

1 Heat a grill plate or barbecue grill to hot.

2 Brush meat with oil and cook for 3–4 minutes each side for medium–rare, or until cooked to your liking. Place steaks in a warm place, or cover with foil, and set aside for 5 minutes to rest.

3 Meanwhile, mix all dressing ingredients in a small bowl.

4 Slice meat across the grain into thin strips.

5 Place beef and remaining ingredients in a large bowl. Pour dressing over salad, then toss gently and serve immediately.

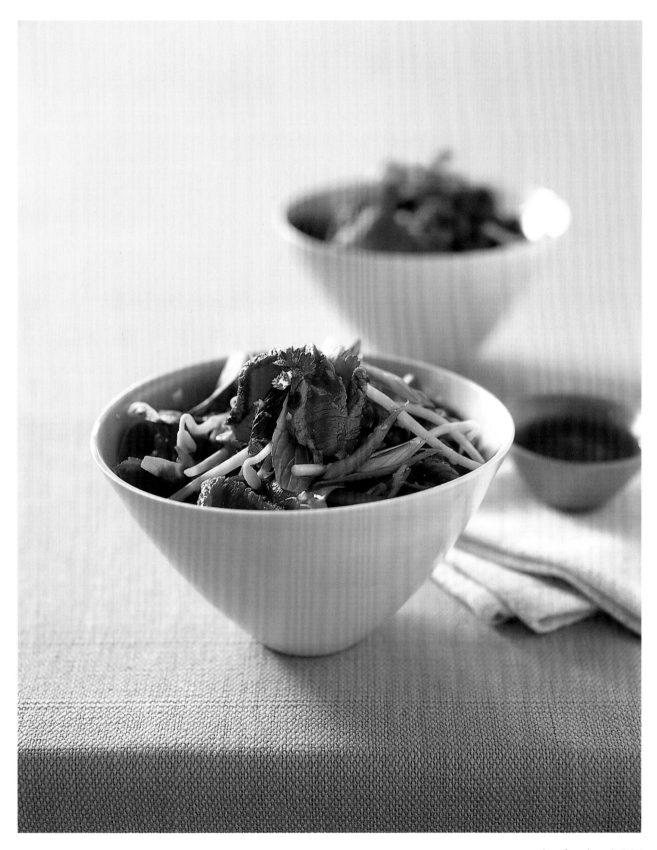

Meatballs in tomato and basil sauce

SERVES 4   PREP 20 mins   COOK 40 mins

MEATBALLS

700 g lean minced (ground) beef
2 eggs
¼ cup (70 g) tomato paste
1 tablespoon dried oregano
1 onion, finely chopped
2 tablespoons chopped flat-leaf
  (Italian) parsley
2 tablespoons olive oil

SAUCE

1 teaspoon olive oil
1 clove garlic, crushed
2 tablespoons chopped
  red capsicum (pepper)
2 × 400 g tins crushed tomatoes
½ cup (125 ml) beef stock
freshly ground black pepper
¼ cup basil, torn

1 To make the meatballs, mix all ingredients except oil in a large bowl. Roll tablespoonfuls of mixture into balls and set aside. Heat oil in a large frying pan over high heat. Carefully add half the meatballs and cook, turning occasionally, for 8–10 minutes, or until cooked through. Remove from pan and drain on paper towel. Repeat with remaining uncooked meatballs. Do not overcrowd pan when cooking or meatballs will stew.

2 For the sauce, heat oil in a small saucepan over medium heat. Add garlic and capsicum and cook, stirring occasionally, for 3 minutes, or until capsicum is soft. Add tomato and stock, then reduce heat to low and simmer for 5 minutes. Add pepper to taste, basil and meatballs and simmer for a further 8–10 minutes.

3 Serve with salad or vegetables.

Stir-fried beef and broccolini in oyster sauce

SERVES 4   PREP 15 mins   COOK 15 mins

1–1½ tablespoons vegetable oil
800 g lean beef, thinly sliced
3 cloves garlic, crushed
350 g broccolini, trimmed
1 red capsicum (pepper), sliced
6 spring onions, cut into 3 cm pieces
½ cup (125 ml) salt-reduced
   chicken stock
2 tablespoons oyster sauce

A hybrid blend of broccoli and Chinese kale, broccolini is a delicious, tender vegetable with thinner stalks than regular broccoli. If you can't find it, regular broccoli works just as well in this dish.

1 Heat a tablespoon of the oil in a wok or large frying pan over high heat. Stir-fry the beef in batches, adding more oil if necessary. Drain on paper towel.

2 Add the garlic and vegetables to the wok and stir-fry until just starting to soften. Add the stock, oyster sauce and beef and toss until heated through. Serve with steamed rice from your daily bread allowance.

1 SERVE =
2 units protein
1 unit bread
½ unit vegetables*
1 unit fats
* or 1½ units with serving suggestion

Teriyaki beef with egg noodles

SERVES 4   PREP 15 mins   COOK 15 mins

2 teaspoons sesame oil
2 teaspoons vegetable oil
4 × 200 g beef steaks, trimmed
    of fat and thinly sliced
2 small onions, sliced
3 cloves garlic, crushed
1 × 3 cm piece ginger, grated
150 g mushrooms, sliced
¼ cup (60 ml) teriyaki sauce
coriander (cilantro) leaves,
    to serve (optional)

NOODLES
1¹⁄₃ cups (160 g) cooked
    egg noodles, still hot
1 red capsicum (pepper),
    cut into thin strips
6 spring onions, sliced
1 teaspoon sesame oil

Ready in 30 minutes, this is a terrific meal to throw together at the end of a busy day.

1 Heat the oils in a wok or large non-stick frying pan over high heat. Stir-fry the beef in batches, then remove from the wok and drain on paper towel.

2 Add the onion, garlic and mushrooms to the wok or pan and stir-fry for 2–3 minutes. Return the beef to the wok, add the teriyaki sauce and mix until heated through. If the mixture is too dry, add a little water.

3 To prepare the noodles, combine all the ingredients. Divide among four noodle bowls and top with the teriyaki beef and coriander leaves (if using). Serve with steamed Asian greens.

TIP To make chicken teriyaki, simply replace the beef with the same quantity of chicken breasts. Teriyaki sauce is a blend of soy sauce and sweet rice wine, and is great for marinating meat and vegetables. It is available in supermarkets and Asian grocers.

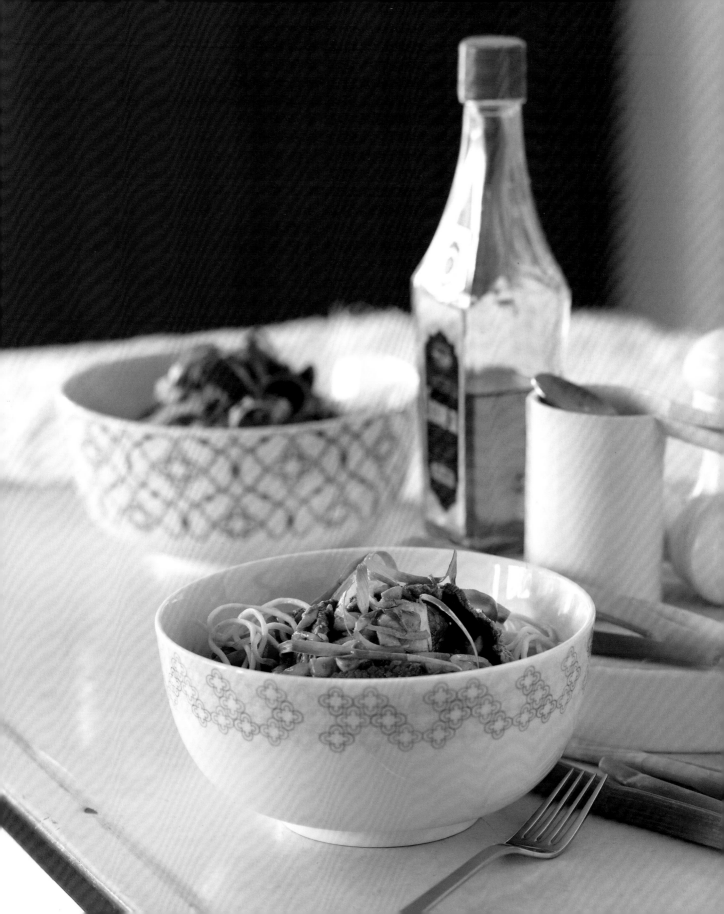

1 SERVE =
2 units protein
¼ unit vegetables*
2 units fats
* or 1¼ units with serving suggestion

Beef goulash

SERVES 4   PREP 20 mins   COOK 1¾ hours

2 tablespoons olive oil
800 g lean stewing steak, trimmed
   of fat, cut into 3 cm pieces
2 onions, sliced
1 red capsicum (pepper),
   seeded and chopped
2 cloves garlic, crushed
1 tablespoon sweet paprika
1 teaspoon caraway seeds
2 tablespoons tomato paste (puree)
3 sprigs thyme
1 litre salt-reduced beef stock
1 tablespoon plain flour

Goulash is a delicious dish originating from Eastern Europe, perfect for a cold winter's day.

1 Heat the olive oil in a large heavy-based saucepan over high heat and brown the beef in batches. Remove and set aside.

2 Add the onion, capsicum and garlic to the pan and cook, stirring, for 5 minutes or until softened. Stir in the paprika, caraway seeds and tomato paste and cook for 1 minute, then add the thyme and stock. Return the beef to the pan. Bring to the boil, then reduce the heat, cover and simmer for 1½ hours or until the beef is tender.

3 Blend the flour with a little water and add gradually to the pan, stirring constantly, until the sauce has thickened. Serve the goulash with rice, barley, mashed potato or pasta noodles from your daily bread allowance and steamed green vegetables.

TIP The goulash can be prepared the day before, stored in the refrigerator and then gently reheated. You can also divide it into meal-sized portions and freeze. It will then be ready to thaw and reheat at the end of a busy day, or to have as a nutritious lunch to take to work. You could use chuck, gravy, skirt or round cuts of beef for this dish. Sweet paprika adds a prominent flavour to this dish that is not spicy, and therefore child-friendly.

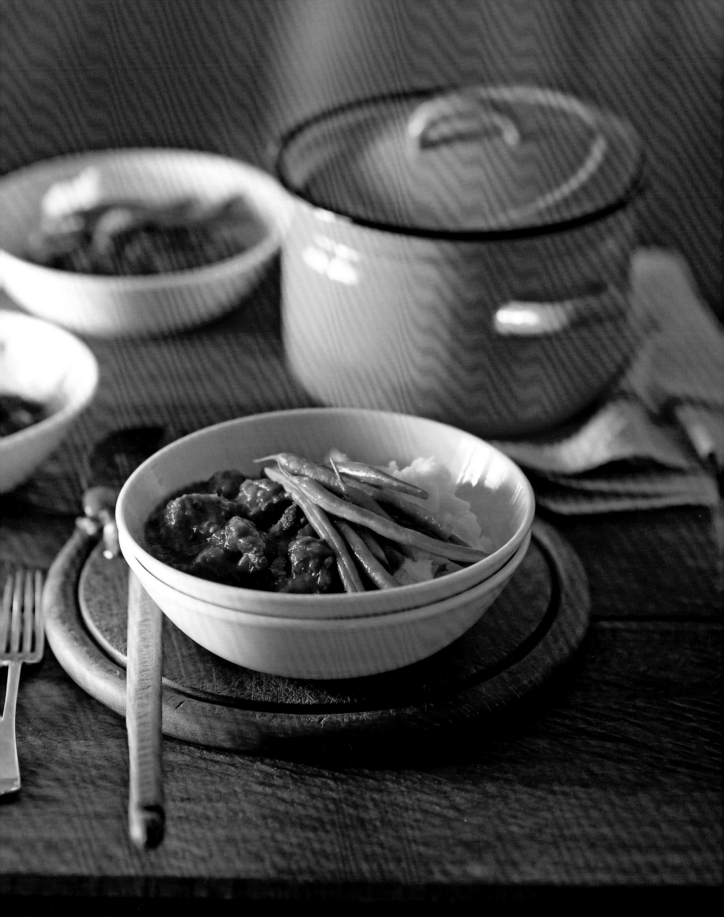

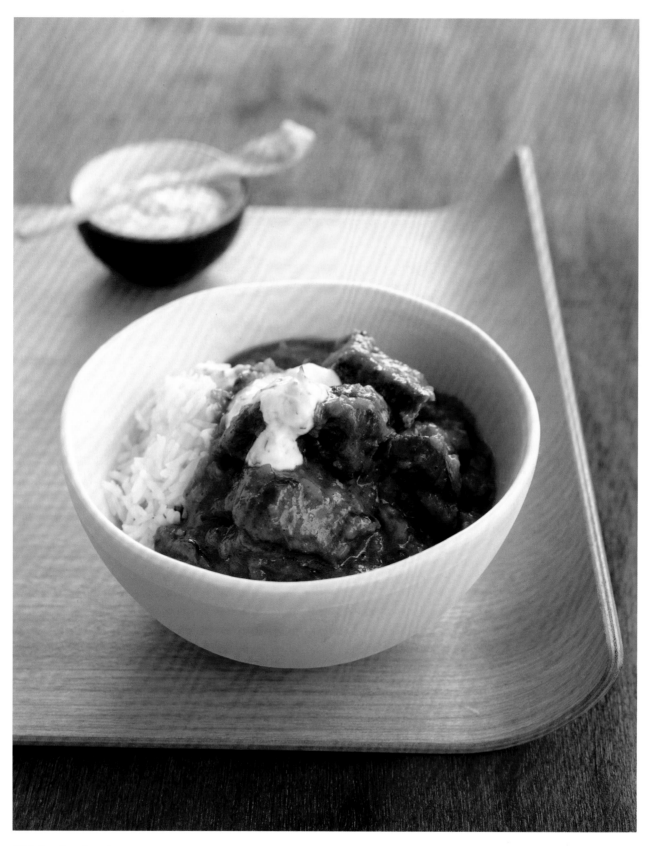

Beef vindaloo

SERVES 4 PREP 20 mins COOK 2 hours

1 teaspoon chilli powder
1 teaspoon ground cumin
½ teaspoon ground white pepper
2 tablespoons freshly grated ginger
2 cloves garlic, crushed
1 teaspoon ground turmeric
1 tablespoon olive oil
2 onions, chopped
800 g lean beef, cut into 4 cm pieces
1 stick cinnamon
½ teaspoon ground cardamom
½ teaspoon ground nutmeg
2 cups (500 ml) cold water
1 green chilli, finely sliced
¼ cup (60 ml) white wine vinegar
2 teaspoons brown sugar
¾ cup (150 g) rice (makes approx.
    1⅓ cups cooked rice)

1 Mix chilli powder, cumin, pepper, ginger, garlic and turmeric in a small bowl, and set aside.

2 Heat oil in a large heavy-based saucepan over medium heat. Add onions and cook for 10 minutes, or until golden. Add beef in batches and cook for 10 minutes, or until beef is lightly browned. Return all meat to the pan, add the mixed spices plus the cinnamon, cardamom and nutmeg, and cook for 2 minutes, or until fragrant. Add water (it should just cover beef) and chilli, and bring to a boil. Reduce heat and simmer for 1 hour. Stir in vinegar and sugar and cook for a further 20 minutes.

3 Meanwhile, cook rice for 10–15 minutes in boiling water, then drain. Serve rice and curry with Yoghurt Sauce (see page 536) and lots of fresh steamed vegetables.

1 SERVE =
2 units protein
¼ unit dairy
1 unit fats
* 1 unit vegetables with serving
suggestion

Beef rogan josh

SERVES 4   PREP 15 mins + marinating time   COOK 1 hour

800 g diced stewing beef,
   trimmed of fat
200 g reduced-fat natural yoghurt
1 tablespoon vegetable oil
1 onion, chopped
1 cinnamon stick
5 cardamom pods, bruised
1 teaspoon chilli powder, or to taste
1 teaspoon ground turmeric
3 cloves garlic, crushed
1 × 5 cm piece ginger, grated
3 tomatoes, diced
2 tablespoons tomato paste (puree)
4 tablespoons chopped coriander
   (cilantro), plus extra to garnish
2 teaspoons garam masala

**Rogan josh is an aromatic North Indian curry. Not only
is it much healthier to make your own (rather than having
takeaway), you can also tailor the heat to suit your own taste.
This curry is also delicious with lamb.**

1   Combine the beef and yoghurt in a bowl and set aside for 30 minutes.

2   Heat the oil in a frying pan or medium saucepan with a tight-fitting
lid over medium heat. Add the onion and cook, stirring, for about
10 minutes until golden. Add the spices, garlic and ginger and stir
until fragrant. Stir in the beef and marinade, tomato and tomato paste.

3   Cover and cook over low heat for 40 minutes, checking from time
to time and adding a little water if it starts to stick. When the beef
is tender, add the coriander and garam masala. Garnish with extra
coriander and serve with steamed rice from your daily bread
allowance and steamed vegetables to the side.

TIP Although this is a mild curry, you can remove the chilli so
it's absolutely kid-friendly. Likewise, you can increase the chilli
taccording to taste.

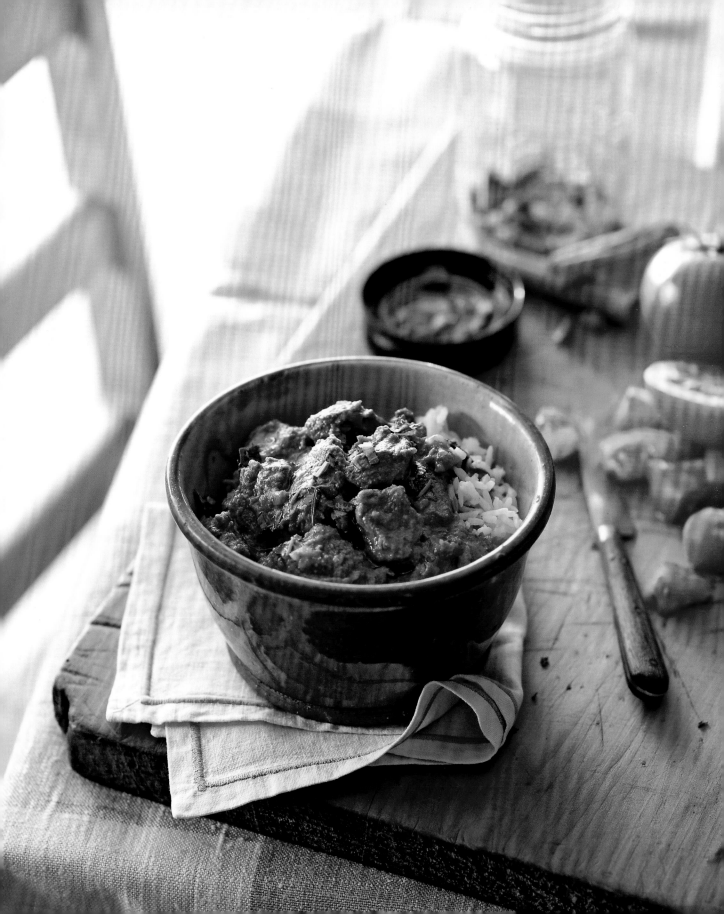

Beef stroganoff

SERVES 4   PREP 10 mins   COOK 35 mins

1 tablespoon vegetable oil
800 g lean beef strips
1 large onion, finely sliced
1 clove garlic, crushed
400 g button mushrooms, sliced
¾ cup (180 ml) salt-reduced
  beef stock
1 tablespoon Worcestershire sauce
1 tablespoon cornflour (cornstarch)
  mixed with 2 tablespoons cold water
100 g reduced-fat natural yoghurt
¼ cup roughly chopped flat-leaf
  (Italian) parsley

1 Heat oil in a large non-stick frying pan over medium heat. Add beef strips in batches and cook for 5 minutes, or until browned. Return all meat to pan, add onion, garlic and mushrooms and cook for 10 minutes, or until vegetables are soft. Stir in stock, Worcestershire sauce and cornflour mixture and bring to a boil. Reduce heat and simmer, covered, for 10 minutes. Stir in yoghurt and parsley, and season to taste.

2 Serve with rice or pasta from your daily bread allowance and steamed vegetables.

1 SERVE =
2 units protein
1½ units vegetables
1½ units fats

Chimichurri steak with cos salad

SERVES 4   PREP 20 mins   COOK 5 mins

4 × 200 g beef steaks, trimmed of fat
olive oil spray

CHIMICHURRI SAUCE

1 cup (20 g) flat-leaf (Italian)
   parsley leaves
4 cloves garlic, roughly chopped
1 red (Spanish) onion, diced
2 teaspoons dried oregano
1 teaspoon sweet paprika
2 tablespoons olive oil
¼ cup (60 ml) red wine vinegar
¼ teaspoon chilli flakes (optional)

SALAD

1 cos lettuce, quartered and
   cut into 5 mm slices
4 roma (plum) tomatoes,
   cut into wedges
1 red (Spanish) onion, thinly sliced
1 red capsicum (pepper), cut into
   thin strips
2 tablespoons red wine vinegar
½ teaspoon Dijon mustard
2 teaspoons olive oil

Chimichurri sauce is a popular accompaniment to grilled meats in Argentina. Simple to make, yet richly flavoured, it is sure to become a regular weeknight hit.

1   To prepare the chimichurri sauce, combine all the ingredients and a generous pinch of salt and pepper in a food processor. Pulse to form a coarse paste. Coat the steaks with half the sauce (save the rest for later) and leave the meat to marinate while you make the salad.

2   To prepare the salad, combine all the vegetables in a bowl. Mix together the vinegar, mustard and olive oil in a screw-top jar and shake well. Pour over the salad and toss to combine.

3   Heat a chargrill or heavy-based frying pan over high heat. Spray with olive oil and cook the steaks for 2–3 minutes each side or until cooked to your liking.

4   Top the steaks with the remaining chimichurri sauce and serve with the salad.

TIP The chimichurri sauce flavours become richer and more intense over time, so if you can, prepare it the night before you plan to use it. Be careful not to cross-contaminate the portion of chimichurri sauce reserved as a sauce to serve. The raw meat should not make contact with it as the sauce will not be cooked.

Parmesan and herb veal rolls with red wine sauce and mixed vegetables

SERVES 4   PREP 25 mins   COOK 25 mins

1 tablespoon olive oil

2 onions, finely chopped

2 cloves garlic, crushed

1 tablespoon finely chopped
   flat-leaf (Italian) parsley

1 tablespoon chopped oregano
   or basil leaves

50 g parmesan, grated

8 semi-dried tomatoes, drained
   and chopped

4 × 200 g veal or beef scaloppine,
   halved (or cut into thirds if
   very large)

12 Dutch (baby) carrots, trimmed
   and halved lengthways

1 large head broccoli, trimmed
   and cut into florets

300 g green beans, trimmed

RED WINE SAUCE

1 cup (250 ml) red wine

½ cup (125 ml) salt-reduced chicken
   or beef stock

2½ teaspoons Dijon mustard

2½ teaspoons cornflour (cornstarch)

The rich flavours of this quick red wine sauce will transform a simple grilled or barbecued steak into something more special. Vary the vegetables depending on what is in season.

1 Heat half the olive oil in a saucepan over medium heat, then add the onion and garlic and cook, stirring, for 4–5 minutes or until softened. Remove from the heat and transfer to a bowl, then stir in the herbs, parmesan and semi-dried tomato. Season to taste with salt and pepper, then set aside to cool.

2 Lay the meat out on a board. Divide the onion mixture among the pieces of meat, placing it down the middle of each piece in a neat row. Roll each piece of meat up around the filling, then secure with toothpicks.

3 Heat the remaining olive oil in a large non-stick frying pan over medium heat, then add the meat. Cover the pan, reduce the heat to low–medium and cook, turning the rolls often, for 10 minutes or until cooked through. Remove the rolls to a warmed plate and cover with foil to keep warm. Reserve the pan.

4 Meanwhile, bring a large saucepan of water to the boil. Add the carrots and cook for 3 minutes, then add the broccoli and beans and cook for another 3 minutes or until the vegetables are tender. Drain well.

5 To make the sauce, place the reserved pan over low–medium heat, then add the wine, stirring and scraping the base of the pan with a wooden spoon to remove any stuck-on bits. Bring to the boil and cook, stirring, for 1–2 minutes or until reduced slightly. Combine the stock, mustard and cornflour in a small bowl, whisking until smooth, then add this mixture to the simmering wine, whisking constantly until smooth and thickened slightly.

6 Remove the toothpicks from the rolls, then season with pepper and serve with the vegetables and the sauce spooned over.

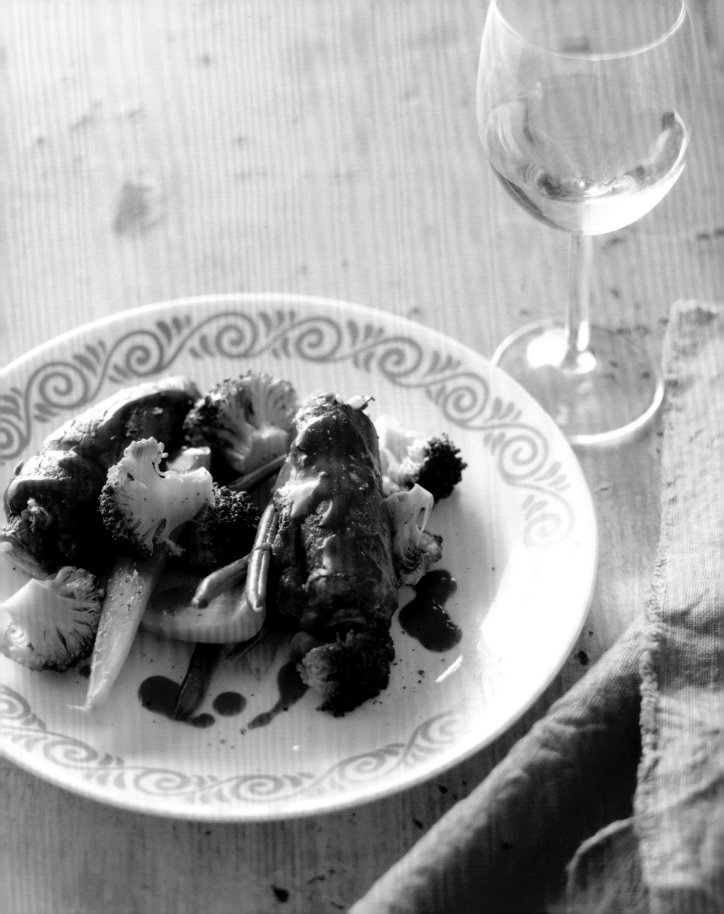

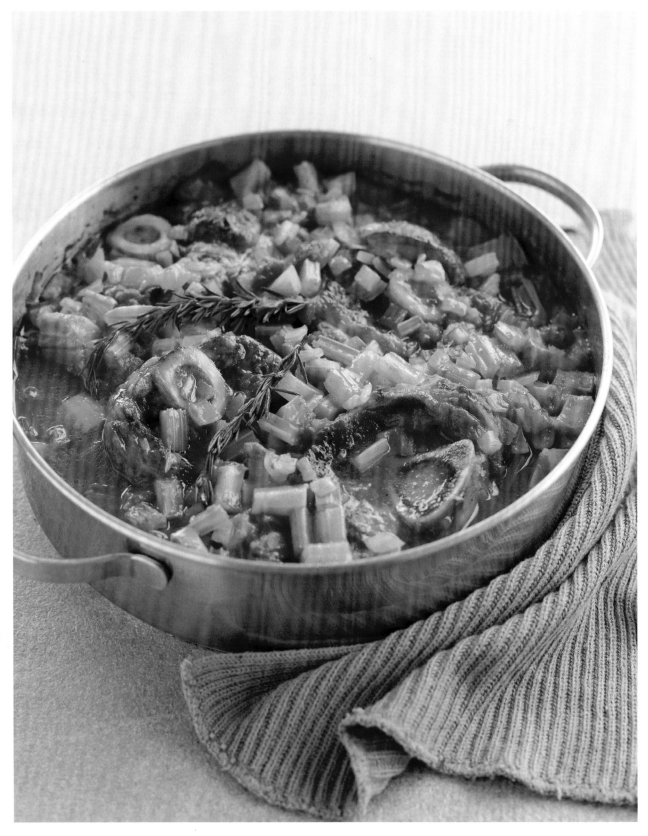

1 SERVE =
2 units protein
1 unit vegetables
2 units fats

Osso bucco with lemon and parsley

SERVES 4   PREP 15 mins   COOK 2 hours

2 kg large veal osso bucco (200 g
    meat per person)
2 tablespoons canola oil
1 onion, diced
2 carrots, roughly chopped
2 sticks celery, roughly chopped
1 clove garlic, sliced
1 tablespoon tomato paste
1 cup (250 ml) white wine
2 sprigs rosemary
2 cups (500 ml) chicken stock
1 × 400 g tin chopped tomatoes
2 teaspoons cornflour (cornstarch)
    mixed with 2 tablespoons cold water
2 tablespoons roughly chopped
    flat-leaf (Italian) parsley
2 tablespoons finely grated lemon zest

1   Heat a large heavy-based saucepan over high heat. Coat veal with
    half the oil and cook, in batches, for 10 minutes, or until browned.
    Transfer to a large ovenproof casserole.

2   Preheat oven to 180°C.

3   Heat the remaining oil in a saucepan over medium heat. Add
    onion, carrots, celery and garlic and cook for 5 minutes, or until
    vegetables are soft and lightly coloured. Add tomato paste, wine,
    rosemary, stock, tomatoes and cornflour and stir to combine. Pour
    vegetables and sauce over the veal. Cover with foil and bake for
    1 hour. Remove foil and bake for a further 30 minutes. Remove from
    the oven and sprinkle parsley and lemon zest over the osso bucco.
    Serve with steamed vegetables.

Soy and ginger beef with broccolini

SERVES 4   PREP 10 mins   COOK 40 mins

1 litre water
1 litre salt-reduced beef stock
$^1/_3$ cup (80 ml) light soy sauce
2 cloves garlic, sliced
1 × 4 cm piece fresh ginger, sliced
juice of 1 lime
1 bunch coriander (cilantro),
   stalks and leaves separated
800 g lean beef fillet
2 bunches broccolini, trimmed
4 spring onions (scallions),
   sliced on an angle

1 Bring water, stock, soy sauce, garlic, ginger, lime juice and coriander
   stalks to a boil in a large heavy-based saucepan. Reduce heat and
   simmer for 10 minutes. Add beef and cook for 20 minutes. Remove
   beef and set aside for 10 minutes.

2 Meanwhile, strain stock and transfer to a clean saucepan. Return
   to a boil, then add broccolini and simmer for 3 minutes. Turn off the
   heat, add the spring onions and allow to infuse for 1 minute. Finely
   slice the meat.

3 Strain the vegetables, reserving the stock, and transfer to serving
   bowls. Add sliced beef and a little of the stock. To serve, scatter with
   coriander leaves and offer extra steamed greens.

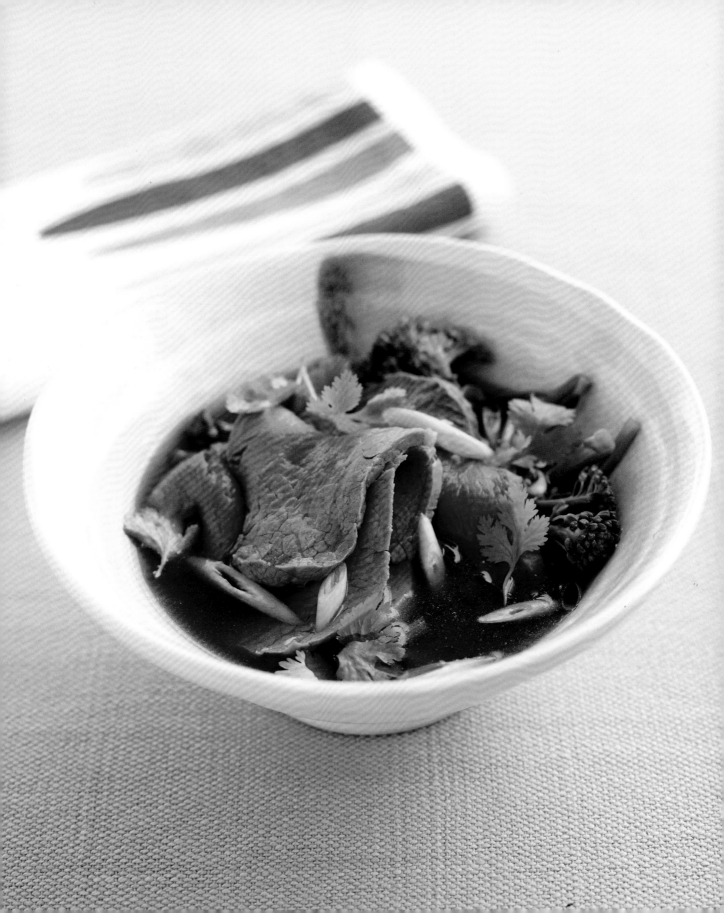

Poached beef salad with Vietnamese dressing

SERVES 4 PREP 10 mins + infusing time COOK 15 mins

2 cups (500 ml) beef stock
1 star anise
2 strips orange zest
1 × 400 g piece sirloin (approx.
    50 mm thick)
150 g mixed salad leaves
2 tablespoons shredded mint leaves
2 tablespoons shredded coriander
    (cilantro) leaves
60 g snowpea sprouts
½ red onion (Spanish),
    finely sliced
1 carrot, julienne
½ red capsicum (pepper),
    seeded and finely sliced

DRESSING
1 tablespoon olive oil
3 teaspoons fish sauce
2 teaspoons rice wine vinegar
½ clove garlic, chopped
1 × 2 cm piece lemongrass,
    thinly sliced
1 red chilli, finely sliced

1 Bring stock to a boil in a saucepan. Add star anise and orange zest, then reduce heat to simmer and allow to infuse for a few minutes. Add meat and bring to the boil. Remove from heat and set aside to gently cook for 15 mintues – meat should remain rare in the centre – then drain and set aside.

2 Whisk all dressing ingredients together in a bowl. Place remaining ingredients in a bowl, then pour dressing over and toss to combine.

3 Slice meat across the grain into thin strips. Serve meat with salad on the side.

Beef and eggplant 'cannelloni'

SERVES 4   **PREP** 20 mins   **COOK** 1 hour 10 mins

2 tablespoons olive oil
800 g lean minced (ground) beef
1 onion, finely diced
1 clove garlic, crushed
2 tablespoons tomato paste
2 cups (500 ml) salt-reduced
   beef stock
1 × 250 g packet frozen spinach,
   defrosted
freshly ground black pepper
2 large eggplants (aubergines),
   thinly sliced lengthways
olive oil spray
700 ml tomato passata
   (tomato puree)
50 g grated parmesan

1 Heat half the oil in a large heavy-based saucepan over high heat. Add mince in two batches and cook for 5 minutes, or until just browned. Transfer to a large bowl. Add remaining oil to pan, along with onion and garlic, and cook for 10 minutes, or until golden. Return mince to pan, add tomato paste and stir well. Add stock and bring to a boil. Reduce heat and simmer for 35 minutes. Stir in spinach and season with freshly ground black pepper.

2 Meanwhile, preheat oven to 200°C. Lightly spray eggplant slices with oil and bake for 15 minutes, or until golden.

3 Lay eggplant slices on your work surface and spoon beef mixture down the centre of each. Roll up eggplant slices. You should now have 12 eggplant 'cannelloni'. Transfer to an ovenproof dish, pour over tomato passata and sprinkle with parmesan. Bake for 10 minutes.

4 Serve with a crisp side salad.

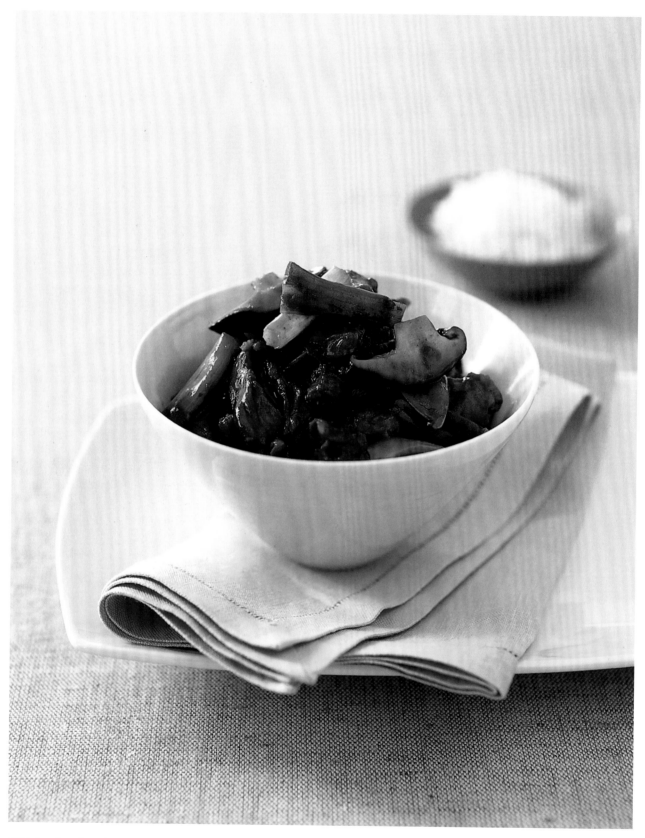

Beef, shiitake mushroom and snowpea stir-fry

SERVES 4   PREP 15 mins   COOK 20 mins

2 teaspoons cornflour (cornstarch)
½ cup (125 ml) beef stock
2 tablespoons soy
1 teaspoon sesame oil
800 g sirloin, finely sliced
1 tablespoon peanut oil
1 clove garlic, finely chopped
1 × 2 cm piece fresh ginger, grated
150 g shiitake mushrooms, halved
4 spring onions (scallions),
     cut into 2 cm pieces
100 g snowpeas (mange-tout)

1 In a cup, mix cornflour, stock, soy and sesame oil.

2 Combine beef, peanut oil, garlic and ginger in a large bowl.

3 Heat a wok or large frying pan over high heat. When wok is hot, stir-fry beef mixture in batches until browned. Set aside. Add mushrooms to wok and stir-fry for 2 minutes. Add spring onions and snowpeas and toss to combine. Stir cornflour mixture, then pour into wok and stir over high heat until sauce has thickened. Return beef to wok to heat through.

4 Serve with rice from your daily bread allowance, if desired.

VARIATIONS

Many, many ingredients go with beef, and almost everything can be stir-fried. Toss the following combinations in your wok: beef, garlic, ginger, capsicum (pepper), chilli, green beans and black bean sauce; beef, garlic, basil, snowpeas (mange-tout), broccoli and soy sauce; beef, ginger, shiitake mushrooms, baby bok choy (pak choi) and hoi sin.

Tex-Mex chilli beef

SERVES 4   PREP 15 mins   COOK 50 mins

1 tablespoon olive oil
1 onion, finely chopped
2 cloves garlic, crushed
600 g lean minced beef
1–2 teaspoons chilli powder
2 teaspoons paprika
3 teaspoons ground cumin
1 teaspoon dried oregano
¼ cup (70 g) tomato paste (puree)
1½ cups (375 ml) salt-reduced
  beef stock
1 × 400 g tin chopped tomatoes
1 × 400 g tin kidney beans,
  rinsed and drained
120 g diced avocado
2 tomatoes, finely diced
1 red (Spanish) onion, finely diced
⅓ cup (80 g) extra light sour cream
3 tablespoons roughly chopped
  coriander (cilantro)

This is another recipe that can be served in a number of different ways. These days, there are healthier versions of tortillas available at supermarkets – use these to make burritos, enchiladas and quesadillas with your Tex-Mex chilli beef.

1 Heat the olive oil in a large saucepan over medium heat and cook the onion for 2–3 minutes or until softened. Add the garlic and beef and cook, stirring to break up any lumps with the back of a wooden spoon, for 5 minutes or until the meat is browned. Stir in the chilli powder, paprika, cumin and oregano and cook for 1–2 minutes or until fragrant.

2 Add the tomato paste, stock, tomato and beans and bring to the boil, then reduce the heat and simmer for 40 minutes or until thickened and cooked through. Season to taste.

3 Combine the avocado, tomato and red onion in a medium bowl.

4 Divide the chilli beef among four bowls and top each portion with a little avocado salad, a tablespoon of sour cream and a sprinkling of coriander. Serve with rice from your daily bread allowance.

TEX-MEX LETTUCE CUPS
Spoon the chilli beef mixture into 8 large iceberg lettuce leaves, top with 4 sliced or diced tomatoes and 100 g grated reduced-fat cheese and serve.

ENCHILADAS
Spoon the chilli beef mixture onto 8 warm tortillas, top with 2 cups (120 g) shredded lettuce, 4 sliced or diced tomatoes and 100 g grated reduced-fat cheese and roll up.

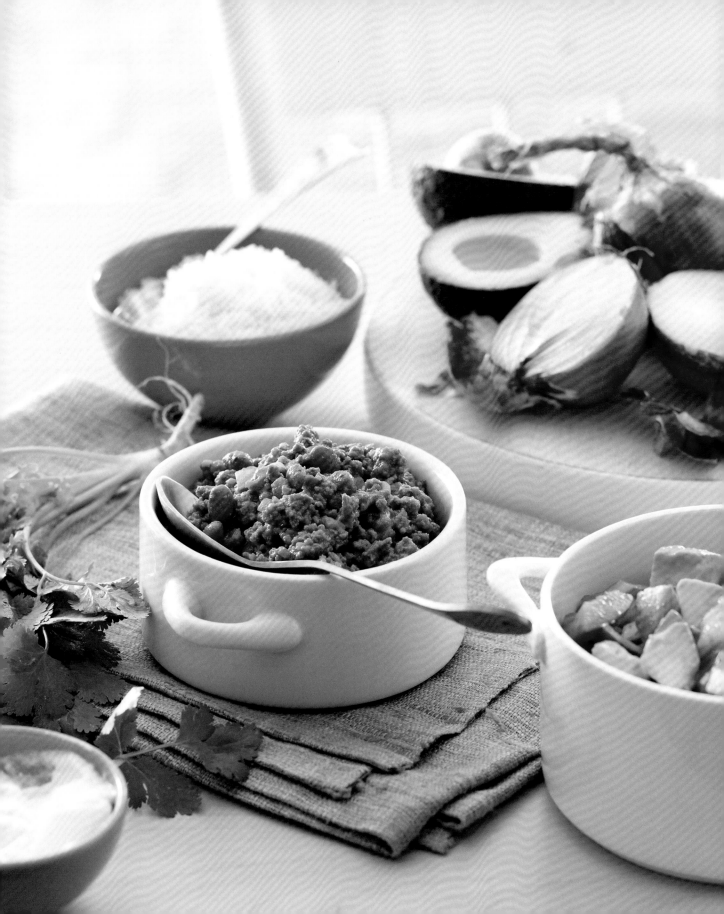

Thai-style beef and bean stir-fry

SERVES 4   PREP 15 mins   COOK 5 mins

3 cloves garlic, roughly chopped

1–2 long red chillies, seeded and
thinly sliced

1 tablespoons chopped coriander
(cilantro) roots and stems

2 tablespoon vegetable oil

800 g beef fillet, trimmed of fat
and thinly sliced

200 g green beans, trimmed
and cut into short lengths

100 g mixed mushrooms

1 tablespoon light soy sauce

1 tablespoon oyster sauce

¼ cup (60 ml) salt-reduced
chicken stock

coriander (cilantro) leaves,
to serve (optional)

1 red chilli, extra, thinly sliced
(optional)

Give your local Thai takeaway a miss and whip up this homemade version instead. It's simple to prepare and much healthier than a bought version.

1 Combine the garlic, chilli and coriander roots and stems in a small food processor to make a paste.

2 Heat the oil in a wok or large frying pan over high heat. Add the garlic paste and beef slices and stir-fry for 2 minutes or until golden brown. Add the beans, mushrooms, sauces and stock and cook for 2 minutes or until the beans are just tender.

3 Garnish the stir-fry with coriander leaves and extra chilli (if using) and serve with steamed rice from your daily bread allowance.

TIP Coriander roots and stems are often discarded; however, they are full of flavour and can add a powerful boost to the taste of a meal. Try using oyster, shiitake or button mushrooms, or a combination of all three.

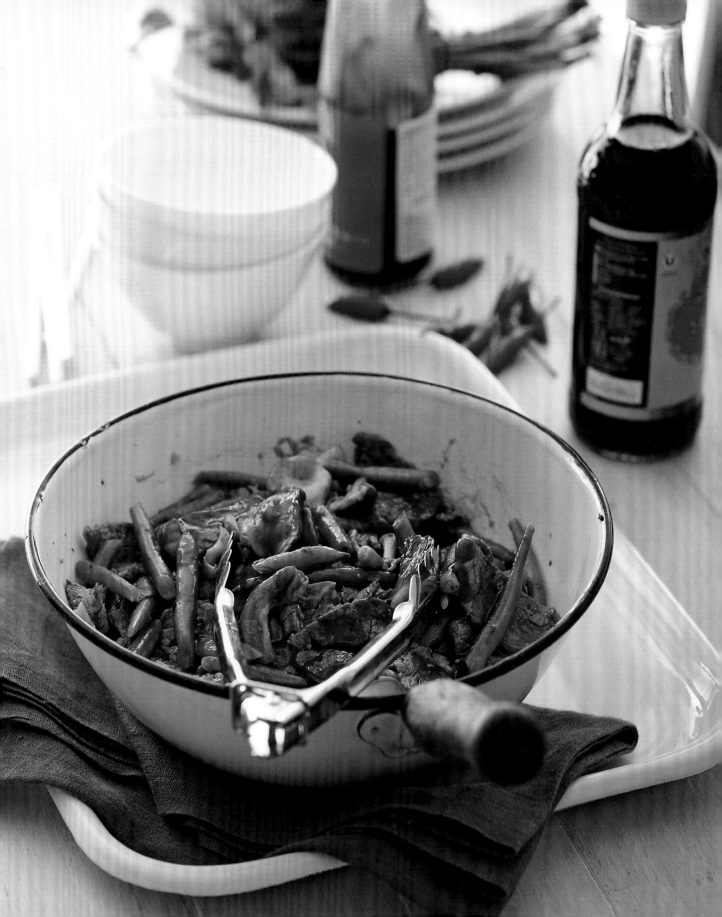

Veal rolls in tomato and red wine sauce

SERVES 4   PREP 20 mins   COOK 30 mins

4 × 200 g veal steaks, sliced
2 cloves garlic, finely chopped
2 teaspoons finely chopped flat-leaf
    (Italian) parsley
2 teaspoons finely chopped sage
2 teaspoons finely chopped basil
1 tablespoon olive oil
1 small onion, chopped
180 g button mushrooms, sliced
1 tablespoon tomato paste
200 ml water
½ cup (125 ml) red wine
4 Roma (plum) tomatoes, diced

1 Place veal on chopping board, cover with plastic wrap and pound with a mallet, or your fist, to a thickness of 5 mm. Lightly season and sprinkle with garlic, parsley, sage and basil. Roll each slice of veal up tightly, and secure with toothpicks.

2 Heat oil in a large, deep-sided frying pan over high heat. Add rolls and cook, turning occasionally, for 6 minutes, or until browned on all sides. Remove from pan and set aside.

3 Add onion and mushrooms to pan and cook over high heat for 1 minute. Mix tomato paste with water then add to pan with wine and tomato. Return veal rolls to pan, reduce heat to low and cook gently for 20 minutes, or until tender. Serve with your favourite steamed vegetables.

Sichuan pepper sirloin with broccoli and capsicum

SERVES 4   **PREP** 15 mins + resting time   **COOK** 15 mins

4 × 200 g sirloins, trimmed of fat
2 tablespoons Sichuan pepper, crushed
1 tablespoon vegetable oil
2 teaspoons sesame oil
1 small onion, sliced
1 clove garlic, finely chopped
400 g broccoli, cut into small florets
1 red capsicum (pepper), seeded and cut into strips
2 tablespoons soy sauce
1 tablespoon hoisin sauce
2 tablespoons water

1 Place sirloins on a large plate and sprinkle both sides of the meat with Sichuan pepper. Preheat a grill plate or barbecue grill to high and cook steaks for 4 minutes each side (for medium–rare), or until done to your liking. Transfer to a clean plate, lightly cover with foil and allow to rest for 5–10 minutes.

2 Meanwhile, heat a wok or large non-stick frying pan over high heat. Add oils and, when smoking, add onion and garlic and stir-fry for 2 minutes. Add broccoli and capsicum and cook for a further 2 minutes, stirring constantly. Add soy sauce, hoisin sauce and water and toss to coat. Serve vegetables alongside the peppered sirloins.

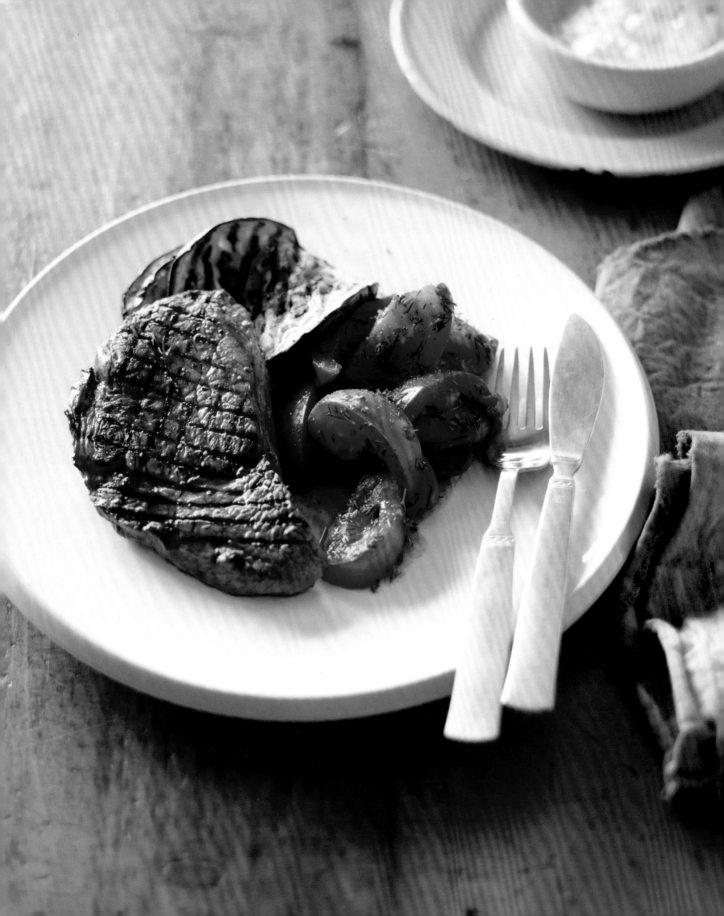

Steak with dill-stewed tomato, grilled eggplant and tzatziki

SERVES 4   PREP 15 mins   COOK 20 mins

500 g firm, ripe tomatoes,
   cut into wedges
2 tablespoons red wine, salt-reduced
   beef stock or water
1 bunch dill, chopped
1 eggplant (aubergine), trimmed
   and cut into 5 mm thick slices
olive oil spray
4 × 200 g beef steaks (rump, sirloin
   or eye fillet), trimmed of excess fat

TZATZIKI
1 Lebanese (small) cucumber, peeled,
   seeded and finely chopped
1 clove garlic, crushed
200 g reduced-fat Greek-style yoghurt

Grilling eggplant is a great alternative to frying as you need far less oil.

1 Combine the tomato and wine, stock or water in a saucepan, then cover and cook over low–medium heat for 5–6 minutes or until the tomato has just softened. Stir in the dill, season to taste with salt and pepper, then set aside.

2 To make the tzatziki, place the cucumber in a fine sieve and, using your hands, press down on the flesh to squeeze out as much excess liquid as possible. Combine the cucumber flesh with the garlic and yoghurt in a bowl, season to taste, then refrigerate until needed.

3 Heat a chargrill plate or a large frying pan over medium heat. Spray the eggplant lightly with olive oil, then, working in batches if necessary, cook the eggplant for 5–6 minutes, turning once, or until lightly charred and tender. Remove and set aside. Increase the heat to medium–high. Spray the steaks lightly with olive oil and cook for 3–4 minutes on each side for medium–rare or until cooked to your liking.

4 Serve the steaks with the grilled eggplant and tomato and the bowl of tzatziki to the side.

Seeded-mustard rack of veal with roasted vegetables

SERVES 4   PREP 20 mins + resting time   COOK 40 mins

500 g pumpkin, peeled and
   roughly chopped
2 carrots, cut into thick strips
2 zucchini (courgette), cut into
   large pieces
4 small brown onions, halved
2 tablespoons olive oil
2 tablespoons wholegrain mustard
4 spring onions (scallions),
   finely chopped
1 teaspoon finely grated orange zest
¼ cup (60 ml) orange juice
1.4 kg rack of veal (200 g meat
   per person), trimmed of fat

1 Preheat oven to 200°C.

2 Place pumpkin, carrot, zucchini and onions in a large, shallow baking
   dish, then add half the oil and toss to coat.

3 Mix the mustard, spring onion, zest, juice and remaining oil in a bowl.
   Place veal on a wire rack set over vegetables, and coat meat with
   mustard mixture. Roast, uncovered, for 40 minutes, or until veal is
   cooked to your liking. Remove meat from oven, cover loosely with
   foil and set aside to rest for 10 minutes before carving.

4 Serve veal with roasted vegetables.

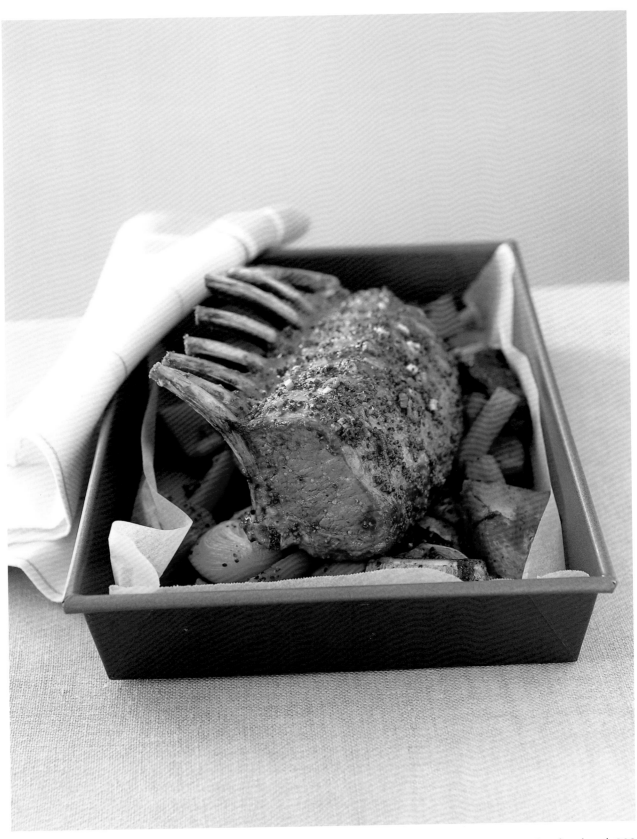

Beef fillet with cherry tomato and eggplant compote

SERVES 4   PREP 10 mins   COOK 35 mins

800 g beef fillet, trimmed of fat
olive oil spray
4 medium chat potatoes,
    quartered and steamed,
    to serve (optional)

CHERRY TOMATO AND
EGGPLANT COMPOTE
1 tablespoon extra virgin olive oil
4 baby eggplants (aubergines),
    thickly sliced
200 g cherry tomatoes, halved
2 cloves garlic, crushed
2 tablespoons finely shredded basil

The Mediterranean flavours in the compote are lovely with the beef, but would also go well with grilled tuna, chicken or lamb.

1 Preheat the oven to 190°C. Spray the fillet with olive oil and season to taste. Heat a grill plate or non-stick frying pan over high heat, add the fillet and brown on all sides. Transfer to a roasting tin and roast for 30 minutes or until cooked to your liking. Cover and rest for 10 minutes.

2 Meanwhile, to make the compote, heat the olive oil in a non-stick frying pan and cook the eggplant for 3–4 minutes or until golden. Add the tomato and garlic and cook for a further 2 minutes or until the tomato starts to soften. Stir in the basil.

3 Serve the steaks with the compote and a side of steamed chat potatoes, if liked.

1 SERVE =
2 units protein
1 unit vegetables
2 units fats

Veal scaloppine with caponata

SERVES 4   PREP 20 mins   COOK 35 mins

4 × 200 g veal loin steaks
2 lemons, cut into wedges

CAPONATA
1 eggplant (aubergine), diced
olive oil spray
2 tablespoons olive oil
1 clove garlic, crushed
1 red (Spanish) onion, chopped
1 red capsicum (pepper),
  seeded and diced
3 Roma (plum) tomatoes, chopped
½ cup roughly torn basil

1 Preheat oven to 200°C.

2 Tip eggplant onto a baking tray and lightly spray with oil. Transfer to oven and cook for 15 minutes, or until golden.

3 Heat half the oil in a large saucepan over high heat. Add garlic, onion and capsicum and cook for 5 minutes. Add eggplant and tomatoes and cook for a further 10 minutes. Season lightly and stir in basil.

4 Meanwhile, spread a large piece of plastic wrap on your work surface. Place veal steaks on top and cover with a second piece of plastic wrap. Using a rolling pin, lightly flatten steaks.

5 Heat remaining oil in a large non-stick frying pan over high heat. Add scaloppine and cook for 2 minutes each side, or until done to your liking. Serve with caponata and wedges of lemon, and offer a side salad.

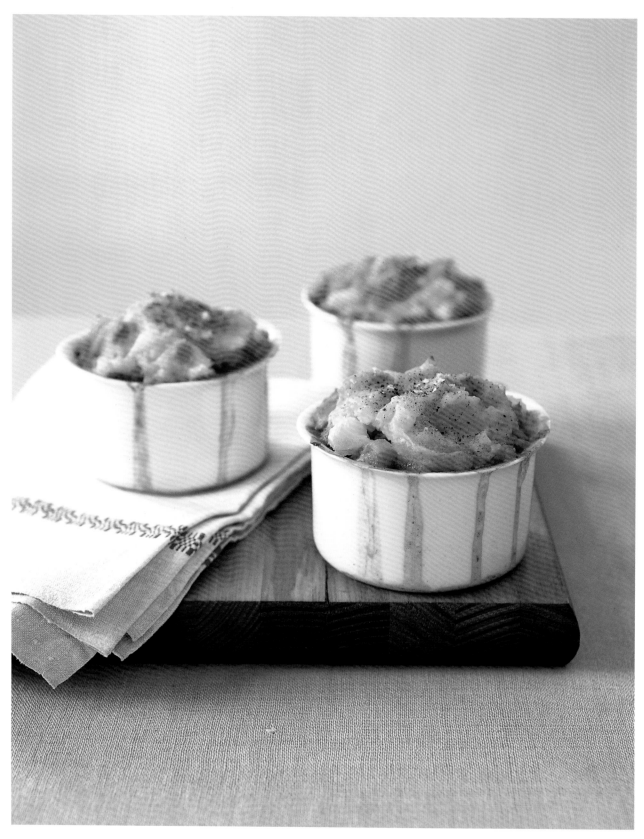

1 SERVE =
2 units protein
½ unit bread
1½ units vegetables
2 units fats

Beef and potato pie

SERVES 4   PREP 20 mins   COOK 1 hour 15 mins

800 g lean minced (ground) beef
2 tablespoons olive oil
2 onions, finely chopped
1 carrot, finely chopped
1 stick celery, finely chopped
2 cloves garlic
1 beef stock cube
½ cup (125 ml) hot water
1 tablespoon flour
½ cup (125 ml) red wine
4 ripe tomatoes, diced
1 tablespoon chopped rosemary
2 tablespoons chopped flat-leaf
    (Italian) parsley
2 sweet potatoes, peeled,
    boiled and drained
300 g pumpkin, peeled
    boiled and drained

1 Coat mince with half the oil. In a hot pan, brown mince in small batches. Set aside. Heat the remaining oil in a large saucepan over medium heat. Add onion, carrot, celery and garlic and cook for 4 minutes, or until soft. Dissolve stock cube in water, then add to pan with cooked mince along with vegetables, flour, wine, tomato and herbs. Bring to a boil, then simmer for 25 minutes.

2 Preheat oven to 180°C.

3 In a bowl, roughly mash sweet potatoes and pumpkin with a fork. Season to taste.

4 Spoon pie filling into a 1-litre capacity ovenproof casserole dish or 4 individual dishes. Top with mash, then bake for 20 minutes. Serve with a mixed-leaf salad.

1 SERVE =
2 units protein
1½ units bread
½ unit dairy
½ unit vegetables*
1 unit fats
* or 1½ units with serving suggestion

Cottage pie

SERVES 4   PREP 20 mins   COOK 1¼ hours

1 tablespoon olive oil
1 onion, finely diced
2 carrots, finely diced
800 g lean minced beef
¼ cup (70 g) tomato paste (puree)
2 cloves garlic, crushed
2 cups (500 ml) salt-reduced
   beef stock
2 tablespoons Worcestershire sauce
1 teaspoon dried oregano
2 teaspoons cornflour
1 cup (120 g) frozen peas
800 g potatoes, peeled and
   cut into chunks
¼ cup (60 ml) reduced-fat milk
100 g grated reduced-fat cheddar
   (optional)

Just the thing for a cosy evening at home, this pie can be prepared in advance then popped in the oven when it's nearly time to eat.

1 Preheat the oven to 180°C.

2 Heat the olive oil in a large saucepan over medium heat, add the onion and carrot and cook, stirring, for 5–10 minutes or until softened.

3 Increase the heat to high, add the mince and cook for 5 minutes or until browned, breaking up any lumps with the back of a wooden spoon. Add the tomato paste and garlic and cook for 1 minute, then stir in the stock, Worcestershire sauce and oregano. Simmer for 15–20 minutes or until the carrot is cooked through and the liquid has reduced.

4 Mix the cornflour with 1 tablespoon water to make a paste, then pour into the saucepan with the peas. Stir until thickened.

5 Meanwhile cook the potato in a large saucepan of boiling water for 15 minutes or until tender. Drain. Return to the saucepan and then mash with the milk. Season with a little salt and pepper.

6 Pour the beef mixture into a deep baking dish. Spread an even layer of the mashed potato on top and sprinkle with the cheddar (if using). Bake for 30–40 minutes or until golden. Serve hot, with vegetables to the side.

TIP If the sauce isn't thick enough at step 4, add another teaspoon of cornflour mixed with a teaspoon of water and stir through the beef mix until thickened to your liking. If you don't have dried oregano in your pantry, use 1 teaspoon of dried mixed herbs in its place.

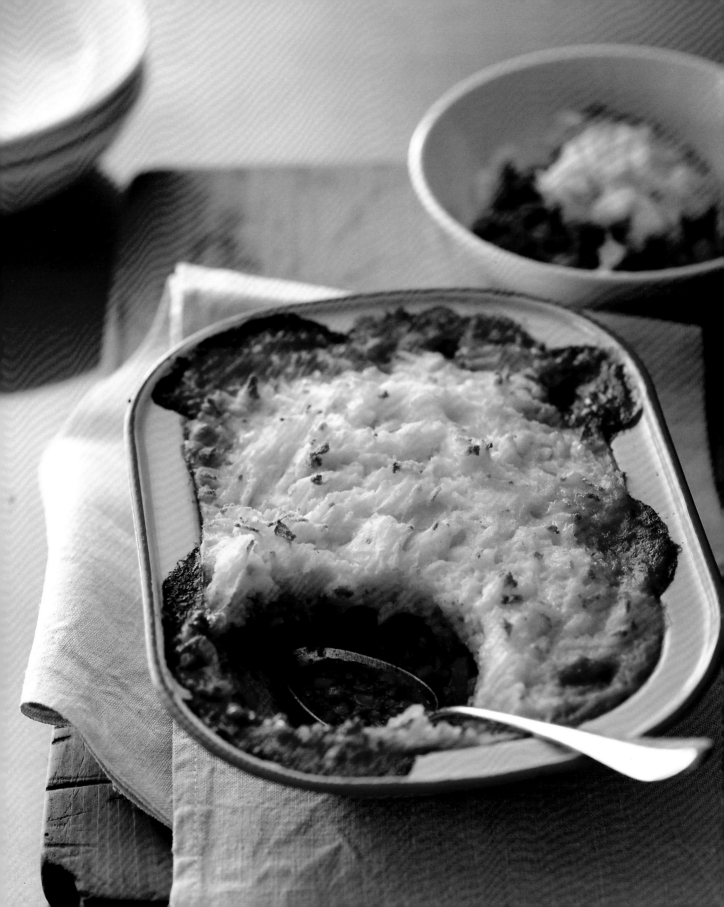

Beef and mushroom filo pie

SERVES 4   **PREP** 25 mins   **COOK** 1 hour 10 mins

2 tablespoons plain flour
800 g chuck or blade steak pieces
1 tablespoon olive oil
500 g field mushrooms, trimmed
   and coarsely chopped
2 tablespoons tomato paste (puree)
2 sprigs rosemary
1 cup (250 ml) salt-reduced beef stock
6 sheets filo pastry
olive oil spray

Who doesn't love a meat pie? This mushroom-laden version, with a delicious crunchy top, ticks all the right boxes and makes for a hearty dinner. Accompany this with green peas to increase your vegetable intake.

1   Preheat the oven to 180°C.

2   Combine the flour and beef in a large bowl and toss to coat well. Heat the oil in a large non-stick frying pan over medium heat, then add the beef and cook, stirring often, for 5–6 minutes or until browned all over. Transfer the beef to a 1.5 litre capacity baking dish, then add the mushrooms to the pan and cook, stirring, for 5–6 minutes or until softened a little. Add the mushrooms to the baking dish.

3   Add the tomato paste, rosemary and stock to the frying pan and stir until combined well. Bring the stock mixture to simmering point, then pour over the beef and mushrooms in the dish. Cover with a lid or tightly with foil and bake for 40 minutes. Remove from the oven and discard the rosemary.

4   Working with one sheet of pastry at a time, spray each piece lightly with olive oil, then use your hands to scrunch into a rosette shape and place on top of the meat mixture to cover. Return the dish to the oven and cook for another 15–20 minutes or until the pastry is golden, then serve immediately.

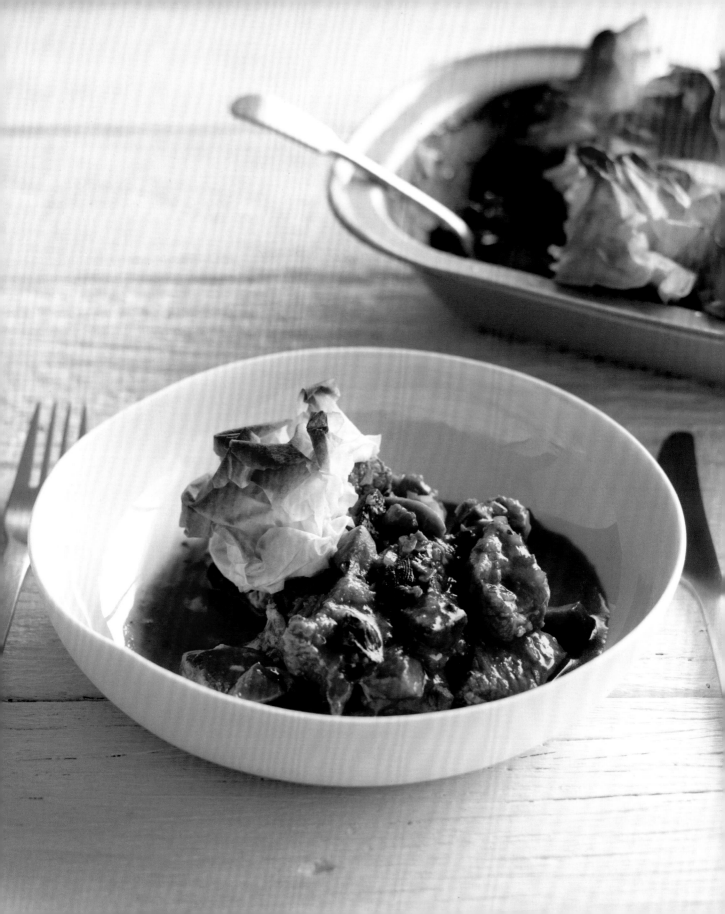

1 SERVE =
2 units protein
2 units bread
½ unit vegetables*
1 unit fats
* or 1½ units with serving suggestion

Beef burgers with salsa

SERVES 4   PREP 20 mins + chilling time   COOK 10 mins

700 g lean minced beef
1 tablespoon finely chopped thyme
1 onion, grated
3 cloves garlic, crushed
1 tablespoon tomato paste (puree)
1 tablespoon Worcestershire sauce
2 eggs, lightly beaten
1 tablespoon olive oil
4 wholemeal bread rolls,
   to serve (optional)

SALSA
1 × 400 g tin chopped
   tomatoes, drained
1 red capsicum (pepper),
   seeded and finely diced
1 small red (Spanish) onion,
   finely diced
½–1 teaspoon Tabasco sauce
   (to taste)
2 tablespoons finely chopped basil
1 tablespoon lemon juice, or to taste

Sink your teeth into this satisfying meal and enjoy the freshness of the tomato salsa, which is made in a flash.

1   Combine the beef, thyme, onion, garlic, tomato paste, Worcestershire sauce and egg in a large bowl. Form into four patties, then cover with plastic wrap and refrigerate for 30 minutes.

2   To make salsa, mix together all the ingredients.

3   Heat the olive oil in a heavy-based non-stick frying pan over medium heat. Add the burgers and cook for 5 minutes each side, flattening regularly.

4   Serve the burgers in the bread rolls (if using) with a dollop of salsa and a green salad.

TIP The salsa also makes a great dip, served with sliced vegetables or grilled flatbread. If you prefer a smoother texture, pulse all the ingredients in a food processor until the desired consistency is reached.

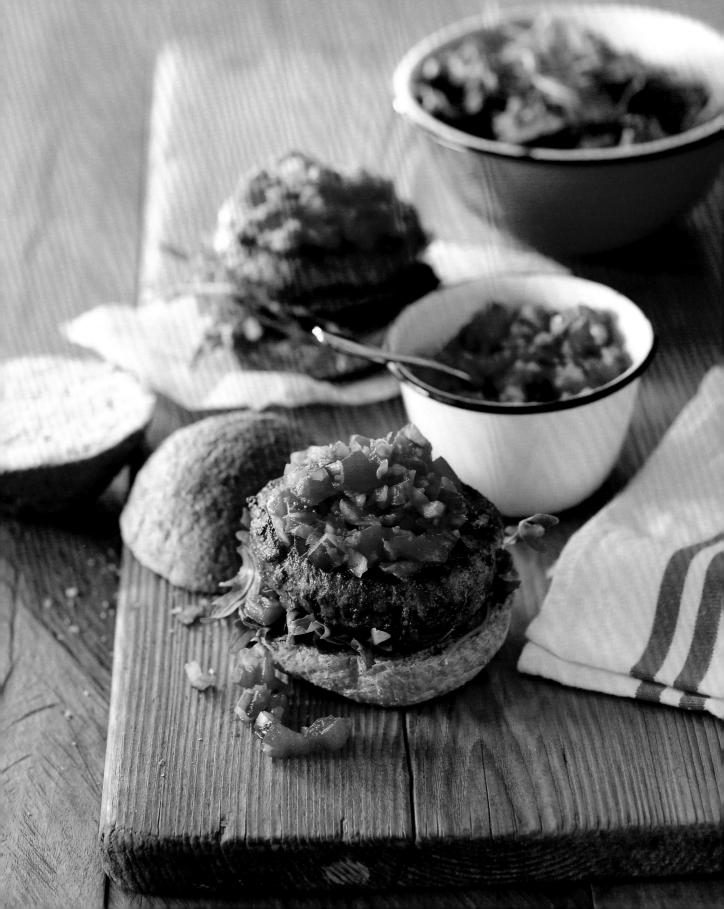

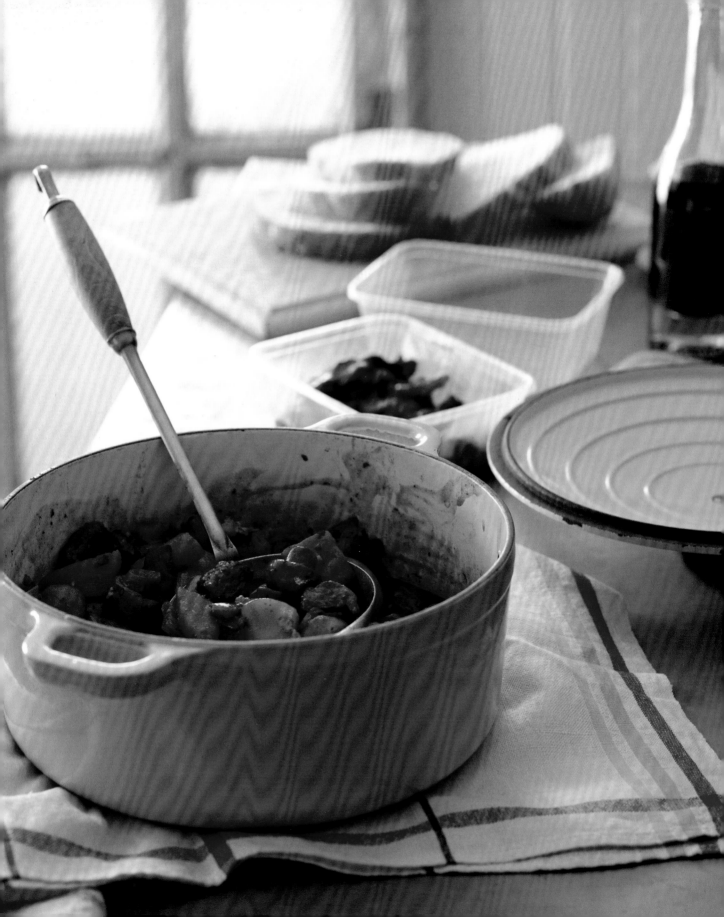

lamb

1 SERVE =
2 units protein
½ unit dairy
1½ units vegetables
1½ units fats

Slow-cooked lamb shoulder with pumpkin and feta salad

SERVES 4   PREP 20 mins   COOK 3 hours 40 mins

2 cloves garlic, crushed
grated zest and juice of 1 lemon
4 sprigs oregano, chopped
1 tablespoon extra virgin olive oil
800 g piece boned lamb shoulder,
    trimmed of fat (or use a shoulder
    with bone but allow for the weight
    of the bone)
½ cup (125 ml) salt-reduced
    chicken stock

SALAD
300 g pumpkin (squash),
    cut into 2 cm dice
olive oil spray
250 g cherry or small
    tomatoes, halved
100 g baby spinach leaves
1 tablespoon balsamic vinegar
2 teaspoons extra virgin olive oil
100 g reduced-fat feta, crumbled

This is the perfect meal for the weekend, when you have time to potter about in the kitchen. After long, slow baking, the lamb is meltingly tender.

1   Preheat the oven to 160°C.

2   Combine the garlic, lemon zest and juice, oregano and olive oil in a bowl. Add the lamb and coat well. Season with salt and pepper.

3   Place the lamb and marinade in a baking dish, add the stock and cover tightly with foil or a tight-fitting lid. Bake for 3 hours.

4   Meanwhile, to prepare the salad, line a baking tray with baking paper. Place the pumpkin on the tray, spray lightly with olive oil and season.

5   Remove the foil or lid from the lamb and increase the oven temperature to 240°C. Place the pumpkin in the oven. Pour almost all of the liquid out of the baking dish and return the lamb to the oven for 10–15 minutes, or until the lamb is crisp on the outside.

6   Remove the lamb from the oven, cover loosely with foil and rest for 15–20 minutes. Reduce the temperature to 180°C, add the tomatoes to the pumpkin and bake for a further 15–20 minutes or until cooked.

7   Combine the pumpkin, tomatoes, spinach, vinegar and olive oil, then sprinkle with the feta. Serve with the lamb, drizzled with the baking juices.

TIP If you like, marinate the lamb for several hours or overnight for even more flavour. Bring the lamb to room temperature before placing in the oven to ensure the meat is evenly cooked. It is important to rest the meat after cooking – it will be more tender and easier to cut. Play around with the flavour by using a variety of herbs – try rosemary or lemon thyme instead.

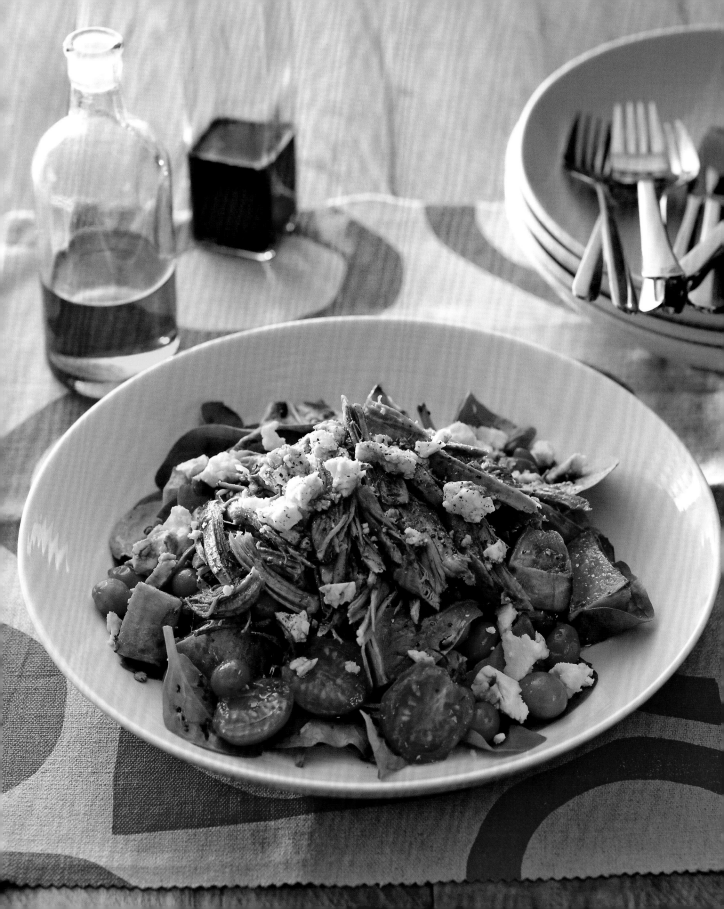

1 SERVE =
2 units protein
½ unit dairy
½ unit fruit
1 unit vegetables
2 units fats

Spiced lamb salad with orange, coriander and red onion

SERVES 4   **PREP** 15 mins + marinating time   **COOK** 6 mins

1 teaspoon ground cumin
juice and finely grated zest
   of 1 lemon
1 clove garlic, crushed
2 tablespoons olive oil
800 g lamb leg steaks
2 oranges, segmented
¼ cup roughly chopped
   coriander (cilantro)
½ red (Spanish) onion, finely sliced
100 g reduced-fat feta, crumbled
250 g baby spinach

1 Place cumin, lemon juice and zest, garlic and half the oil in a large dish and mix well. Add lamb, turning to coat thoroughly, then cover and set aside for 10 minutes.

2 Meanwhile, place remaining oil in a bowl, add oranges, coriander, onion, feta and spinach leaves and toss well.

3 Preheat a grill plate or barbecue grill to high. Add lamb and cook for 3 minutes each side, or until done to your liking. Serve with the salad.

Poached lamb with shaved fennel and grapefruit salad

SERVES 4   PREP 20 mins   COOK 50 mins + standing time

2.5 litres salt-reduced chicken stock
1 bay leaf
3 sprigs thyme
1 × 900 g boned rolled leg of lamb,
  trimmed of fat
2 pink grapefruit, peeled and
  all white pith removed
1 large bulb fennel, trimmed
  and very thinly sliced
1 red (Spanish) onion, thinly sliced
large handful watercress sprigs
large handful flat-leaf (Italian)
  parsley stalks (optional)
1 tablespoon extra virgin olive oil
1 tablespoon red wine vinegar

Cooking lamb this way results in moist, tender meat. Serve this with some steamed sugar snap peas for a delicious dinner.

1 Bring the stock, bay leaf and thyme to simmering point in a saucepan just large enough to hold the lamb snugly. Add the lamb, along with a little extra stock or water if necessary to just cover the lamb. Bring back to simmering point, then reduce the heat to low and cook for 45 minutes or until the lamb is just cooked through but still a little pink in the middle – do not allow the water to simmer too rapidly or the meat will be tough. Turn off the heat and leave the lamb for 20 minutes before removing it with a slotted spoon. When cool enough to handle, cut the lamb into 1 cm thick slices.

2 Holding the grapefruit over a large bowl, use a small serrated knife to cut segments from the grapefruit, letting the flesh and juices drop into the bowl. Place the remaining ingredients in the bowl and toss to combine well.

3 Divide the lamb and salad among plates and serve.

TIP Store any leftover lamb in the fridge to serve cold the next day with couscous and salad.

800 g lamb fillets

CHERMOULA PASTE

**1 teaspoon freshly ground
black pepper**

2 teaspoons ground cumin

2 teaspoons ground coriander

1 teaspoon cayenne pepper

**¼ cup loosely packed flat-leaf
(Italian) parsley leaves**

**¼ cup loosely packed coriander
(cilantro) leaves**

¼ cup loosely packed mint leaves

2 tablespoons lemon juice

**2 spring onions (scallions),
roughly chopped**

1 clove garlic, roughly chopped

SALSA

1 avocado, diced

**½ cup roughly chopped
coriander (cilantro)**

2 large tomatoes, diced

**4 spring onions (scallions),
finely sliced**

**1 roasted red capsicum (pepper),
chopped (to roast your own
capsicums, see below)**

1 tablespoon lemon juice

1 tablespoon olive oil

Chermoula lamb fillet with avocado and coriander salsa

SERVES 4   PREP 20 mins   COOK 6 mins

1 Process all paste ingredients finely. Rub paste into lamb fillets using your fingers, and set aside for 5 minutes. Meanwhile, preheat a grill plate or barbecue grill to high. Cook lamb for 3 minutes each side, or as liked. Put on a plate, cover with foil and set aside for 5 minutes.

2 Lightly toss all salsa ingredients, and season lightly to taste. Serve lamb fillet on salsa, with a mixed-leaf salad or your favourite greens.

TIP To roast capsicums, preheat oven to 180°C. Halve and seed capsicums and place, skin-side up, in a baking dish. Drizzle with a little olive oil and roast for 20 minutes. Remove from oven, cover with foil and allow to cool slightly. Peel off and discard skin.

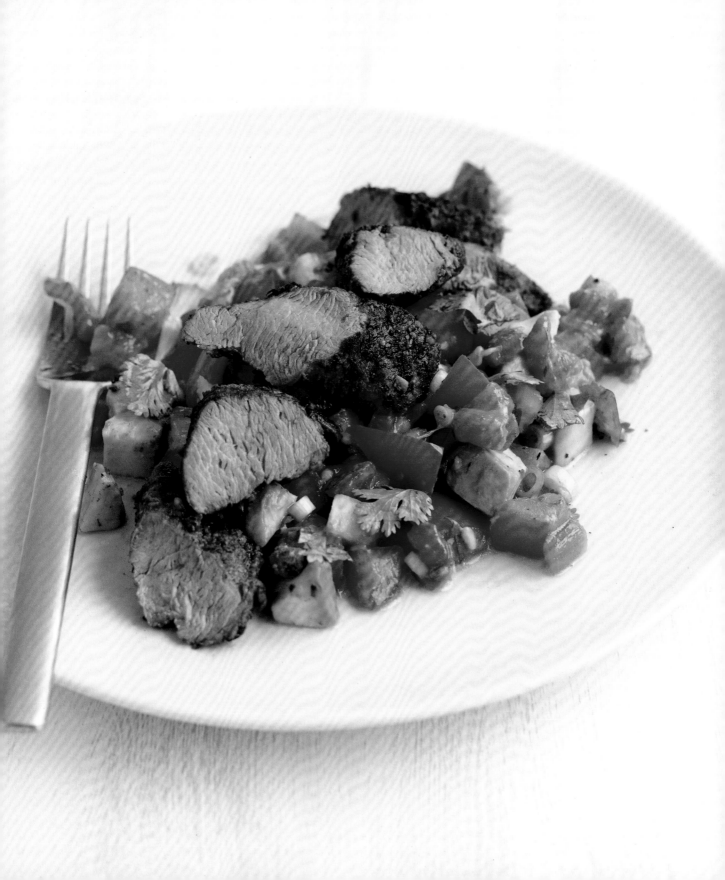

800 g lean lamb steaks, diced
1 tablespoon olive oil
2 cloves garlic, crushed
2 tablespoons lemon juice
1 teaspoon ground coriander
½ teaspoon ground turmeric
lemon wedges, to serve

HERBED YOGHURT

200 g reduced-fat natural yoghurt
1 tablespoon chopped coriander
   (cilantro)
1 tablespoon chopped mint
1 clove garlic, crushed

LEMON COUSCOUS

1 cup (200 g) couscous
1 cup (250 ml) salt-reduced
   chicken stock
2 teaspoons grated lemon zest
2 tablespoons chopped mixed herbs
   (such as coriander [cilantro]
   and mint)

Lamb skewers with lemon couscous and herbed yoghurt

SERVES 4   PREP 15 mins + marinating time   COOK 10 mins

Couscous is a fantastic side dish. It's ready in just a few minutes, and you can add all sorts of different flavourings to match the rest of the meal, such as grated lemon or lime zest, a touch of ground spice or a handful of finely chopped fresh herbs.

1 Combine the lamb, olive oil, garlic, lemon juice, ground coriander and turmeric in a bowl. Cover and set aside for 30 minutes or marinate in the refrigerator for longer if time permits.

2 To prepare the herbed yoghurt, combine all the ingredients in a bowl.

3 Preheat a chargrill or grill to medium. Thread the lamb onto skewers and cook for 2–3 minutes each side or until cooked to your liking.

4 Meanwhile, place the couscous in a heatproof bowl. Bring the stock to the boil and pour over the couscous, then cover and set aside for 5 minutes. Fluff up the couscous with a fork and stir in the lemon zest and and herbs.

5 Serve the lamb skewers with the couscous, herbed yoghurt, lemon wedges and salad or steamed vegetables.

TIP Soak wooden skewers in water for 30 minutes before threading on the lamb, to prevent scorching when grilling. If you don't want to use skewers, trimmed lamb chops or cutlets may be used in place of the steaks.

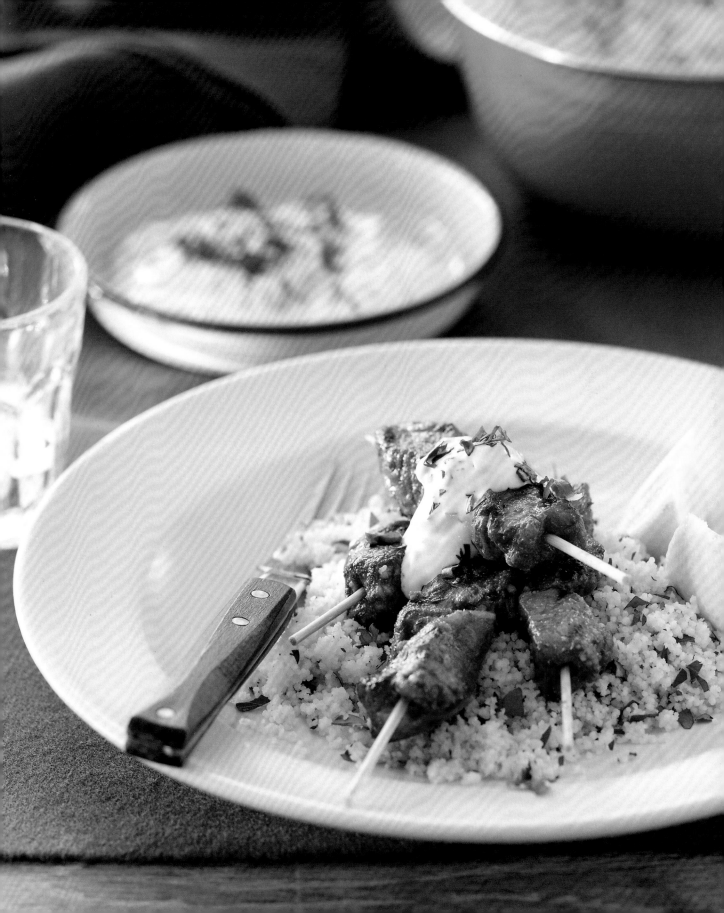

Indian lamb and spinach curry

SERVES 4   PREP 15 mins   COOK 1 hour

2 tablespoons olive oil
2 onions, finely sliced
2 cloves garlic, crushed
½ teaspoon cardamom seeds
1 teaspoon ground cinnamon
1 tablespoon garam masala
2 teaspoons turmeric
800 g lamb leg, cut into cubes
½ cup (140 g) reduced-fat
    natural yoghurt
1 × 400 g tin chopped tomatoes
1 × 250 g packet frozen
    spinach, defrosted
1 cup (250 ml) water
2 tablespoons finely shredded mint
½ cup coriander (cilantro) leaves,
    roughly chopped

1   Heat oil in a large heavy-based saucepan over high heat. Add onion and garlic and cook for 5 minutes, or until onion is golden. Add spices and lamb, then mix well and cook for 6–8 minutes, or until lamb begins to cook and change colour. Stir through yoghurt, then tomato. Add spinach and water, then reduce heat to medium and cook for 40 minutes, or until meat is tender.

2   Stir through mint and coriander and serve with rice from your daily bread allowance, if desired.

1 SERVE =
2 units protein
1 unit fats

Coriander and chilli lamb kebabs

SERVES 4 **PREP** 20 mins + soaking and marinating time **COOK** 10 mins

1 onion, chopped
2 cloves garlic, crushed
1 bunch coriander (cilantro),
  roughly chopped
2 tablespoons lemon juice
2 tablespoons white wine
1 tablespoon olive oil
1 teaspoon ground coriander
1 tablespoon garam marsala
2 small red chillies
1 teaspoon turmeric
800 g lamb fillets, cut into cubes

1 If using bamboo skewers, soak in hot water for 30 minutes prior to use.

2 Place all ingredients other than meat in a food processor and blend until well combined.

3 Thread meat onto 8 skewers and place in a shallow dish. Pour over marinade, turning kebabs to coat thoroughly. Cover with plastic wrap and allow to marinate for at least 30 minutes.

4 Heat a grill plate or barbecue grill to hot. Grill kebabs for 2 minutes each side – 8 minutes in total – or until done to your liking. (During cooking, brush kebabs with leftover marinade.)

5 Serve with a salad or vegetables.

VARIATIONS

Kebabs are a wonderful way to experiment with different meats, vegetables and marinades, since almost everything works. Choose your favourite type of meat or vegetables, turn to the Basics chapter, and go for your life.

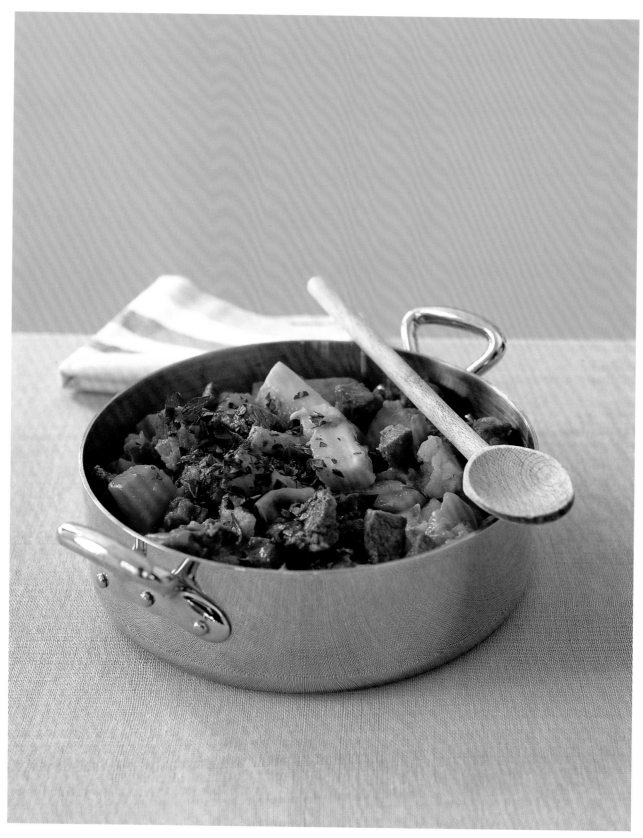

Italian lamb casserole

SERVES 4   PREP 20 mins   COOK 2 hours 10 mins

800 g lamb leg, cut into 3 cm cubes
2 tablespoons olive oil
1 onion, finely chopped
1 carrot, finely chopped
1 stick celery, finely chopped
2 cloves garlic, crushed
¼ cup (60 ml) red wine
2 tablespoons tomato paste
2 cups (500 ml) chicken stock
1 bay leaf
2 sprigs rosemary
water
2 parsnips, peeled and chopped
2 tablespoons flat-leaf
    (Italian) parsley

1 Preheat oven to 180°C.

2 Heat a large enamelled cast-iron casserole over high heat. Coat lamb with oil and cook, in small batches, for 5 minutes, or until browned. Remove from pan and set aside. Add onion, carrot and celery to pan and cook for 5 minutes, or until soft. Return lamb to pan, then add garlic, red wine and tomato paste and cook for a further 5 minutes. Add stock, bay leaf, rosemary and enough water to ensure lamb is covered. Cover with lid and bake in oven for 1 hour.

3 Add parsnip and cook for a further 40 minutes.

4 Serve sprinkled with parsley.

Italian lamb meatloaf

SERVES 4   **PREP** 15 mins + standing time   **COOK** 55 mins

700 g lean minced (ground) lamb
1 onion, finely diced
2 cloves garlic, finely chopped
1 teaspoon dried mixed herbs
3 Roma (plum) tomatoes, finely diced
2 tablespoons tomato sauce (ketchup)
¼ cup roughly chopped flat-leaf
   (Italian) parsley
70 g wholemeal breadcrumbs
2 eggs, lightly beaten
1 × 250 g packet frozen
   spinach, defrosted
¼ cup pine nuts, lightly toasted

1 Preheat oven to 180°C. Lightly grease a loaf tin.

2 In a large bowl, mix all ingredients using your hands. Season lightly. Press mixture into loaf tin, cover with foil and bake for 40 minutes. Remove foil and bake for a further 15 minutes, or until a brown crust forms. Tilt loaf tin and drain off any excess liquid, then allow meatloaf to stand for 10 minutes before cutting and serving.

Moroccan lamb with chickpeas and spinach

SERVES 4   PREP 15 mins   COOK 15 mins

1 tablespoon olive oil
1 onion, finely chopped
2 cloves garlic, crushed
700 g minced lamb
1 tablespoon Moroccan spice mix
3 tomatoes, diced
½ cup (125 ml) salt-reduced
   beef stock
130 g tinned chickpeas, rinsed
   and drained
½ cup (25 g) chopped mint
100 g baby spinach leaves
4 wholemeal pita breads
200 g reduced-fat natural
   yoghurt, mixed with
   1 tablespoon lemon juice

This versatile lamb recipe may be served in a couple of different ways, so it's perfect for leftovers. The quantities can easily be doubled.

1 Heat the olive oil in a non-stick frying pan over medium heat, add the onion and garlic and cook for 5 minutes or until softened. Increase the heat and add the mince, breaking up any lumps with the back of a wooden spoon. Cook until the mince is browned. Stir in the spice mix and cook for 1 minute, then add the tomato, stock and chickpeas. Cook until most of the liquid has evaporated, then stir in the mint.

2 Serve with the spinach leaves, pita bread and lemon yoghurt. Either use the pita bread as a wrap, or rip it into chip-sized pieces, toast under a grill or in the oven, and serve with the other ingredients, as you would with nachos.

1 SERVE =
2 units protein
1½ units vegetables
1½ units fats

Spiced lamb chops with ratatouille

SERVES 4   **PREP** 20 mins + refrigerating time   **COOK** 25 mins

800 g lamb loin chops,
trimmed of fat
1 tablespoon olive oil
lemon wedges

SPICE CRUST
1 tablespoon freshly ground
black pepper
2 teaspoons whole coriander seeds
1 teaspoon garam masala
2 cardamom pods, crushed
1 teaspoon chilli powder

RATATOUILLE
2 teaspoons olive oil
4 baby eggplants,
halved lengthways
1 onion, finely chopped
1 clove garlic, chopped
1 red capsicum (pepper),
seeded and sliced
1 zucchini (courgette), sliced
½ cup (125 ml) chicken stock
2 ripe tomatoes, diced
1 tablespoon chopped flat-leaf
(Italian) parsley
½ cup basil, torn

1   To make the spice crust, mix all spices well in a bowl. Coat chops with a little olive oil, then coat thoroughly in spice mixture. Cover with plastic wrap and refrigerate for 1 hour.

2   To make the ratatouille, heat oil in a large frying pan over medium heat. Add eggplant and cook for 4 minutes, or until golden. Add onion and garlic and saute until lightly coloured. Add capsicum and zucchini and cook for 1 minute, then add chicken stock and tomato. Bring to a boil and cook for a further 5 minutes. Add herbs and season to taste. Keep warm over heat.

3   Heat oil in a frying pan over high heat and cook chops for 3 minutes each side, or until done to your liking. Divide ratatouille between plates and top with chops and a wedge of lemon.

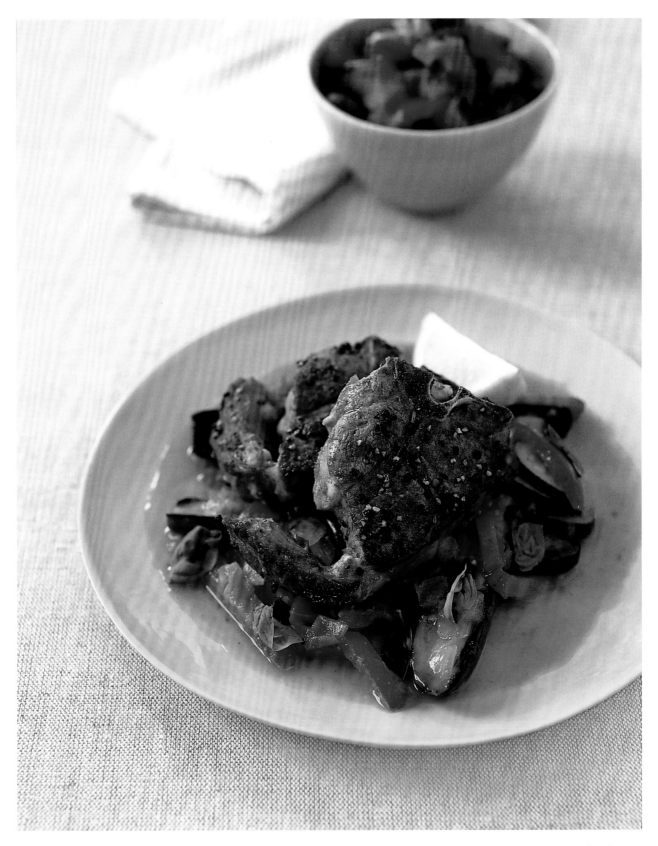

Moussaka

SERVES 4   PREP 20 mins   **COOK** 1 hour 10 mins

2 tablespoons olive oil
800 g lean minced (ground) lamb
1 large onion, diced
2 cloves garlic, crushed
2 teaspoons ground cinnamon
1 × 400 g tin chopped tomatoes
2 tablespoons roughly
   chopped oregano
1 cup (250 ml) salt-reduced
   chicken stock
4 eggplants (aubergines)
olive oil spray
100 g reduced-fat ricotta
¼ cup (60 ml) reduced-fat milk
100 g grated reduced-fat cheddar

1 Preheat oven to 200°C.

2 Heat oil in a large heavy-based saucepan over high heat. Cook lamb, in two batches, for 5 minutes, or until browned. Remove from pan and set aside. Heat remaining oil in pan. Add onion, garlic and cinnamon and cook for 5 minutes, or until onion is soft. Return meat to pan, add tomatoes, oregano and stock and bring to a boil. Reduce heat and simmer for 25 minutes.

3 Meanwhile, slice eggplants lengthways and spray both sides lightly with oil. Bake for 10 minutes, or until golden.

4 Spoon a quarter of the mince into a 2 litre baking dish, in an even layer. Cover with a third of the eggplant slices. Repeat layers, finishing with mince.

5 In a small bowl, mix ricotta, milk and cheese. Spoon over top of moussaka and bake for 30 minutes, or until golden brown. Serve with a crisp green salad.

Mongolian lamb

SERVES 4 PREP 10 mins + marinating time COOK 15 mins

2 tablespoons soy sauce

1½ tablespoons Chinese cooking
wine or sherry

4 × 200 g lamb steaks, trimmed
of fat and thinly sliced

½ cup (125 ml) salt-reduced chicken
stock, at room temperature

1 teaspoon cornflour (cornstarch)

1 tablespoon vegetable oil

1 teaspoon sesame oil

2 onions, cut into wedges

1 green capsicum (pepper),
cut into strips

4 cloves garlic, crushed

1 teaspoon grated ginger

1–2 red chillies, seeded and chopped

1 tablespoon oyster sauce

roughly chopped coriander (cilantro),
to serve

**You can still enjoy this popular takeaway dish by making this
lighter homemade version.**

1 Combine the soy sauce and Chinese cooking wine or sherry in
a large bowl, add the lamb and turn to coat. Cover and marinate
in the refrigerator for 30 minutes.

2 Slowly stir the stock into the cornflour, mixing well to smooth out
any lumps (it's important that the stock is cool when added to the
cornflour so that it doesn't thicken and turn lumpy). Set aside.

3 Remove the lamb from the bowl, reserving the marinade. Heat the oils
in a wok or large frying pan over medium heat and stir-fry the lamb in
batches until golden brown. Remove and set aside.

4 Add the onion and capsicum to the wok and stir-fry for 2 minutes. Add
the garlic, ginger and chilli and cook for 1 minute. Return the lamb to
the wok and add the cornflour mixture and oyster sauce. Stir gently
until the sauce has thickened. Sprinkle with coriander and serve with
steamed rice from your daily bread allowance and steamed vegetables.

TIP A little bit of sesame oil goes a long way so take care not to use
too much.

Lamb tagine

SERVES 4   PREP 20 mins   COOK 1 hour 50 mins

1 onion, roughly chopped
2 cloves garlic, roughly chopped
½ cup roughly chopped flat-leaf
    (Italian) parsley
½ cup roughly chopped
    coriander (cilantro)
1 green chilli, roughly chopped
2 teaspoons ground cinnamon
¼ cup (35 g) pitted dates,
    roughly chopped
2 teaspoons finely grated lemon zest
800 g lean lamb shoulder, trimmed
    of fat and cut into 2 cm pieces
1 tablespoon vegetable oil
1 cup (250 ml) water
1 × 400 g tin chopped tomatoes
¾ cup (150 g) couscous (makes
    1¹/₃ cups cooked couscous)
1 cup (250 ml) boiling water
1 teaspoon olive oil
100 g reduced-fat natural yoghurt

1   Blend onion, garlic, parsley, coriander, chilli, cinnamon, dates and
    lemon zest in a food processor until smooth. Set aside.

2   Heat a large heavy-based saucepan over high heat. Coat lamb with oil
    and cook, in small batches, for 5 minutes, or until browned. Return all
    lamb pieces to pan, add paste and stir to coat. Cook for 3–5 minutes,
    until aromatic. Add water and tomatoes and mix well. Bring to a boil,
    then reduce heat and simmer, covered, for 1½ hours, stirring
    occasionally. Season lightly.

3   Meanwhile, place couscous in a bowl and pour over boiling water and
    olive oil. Cover with plastic wrap and allow to sit for 5 minutes, or until
    water is absorbed. Fluff up with a fork.

4   Serve tagine with couscous, a dollop of yoghurt and lots of steamed
    vegetables.

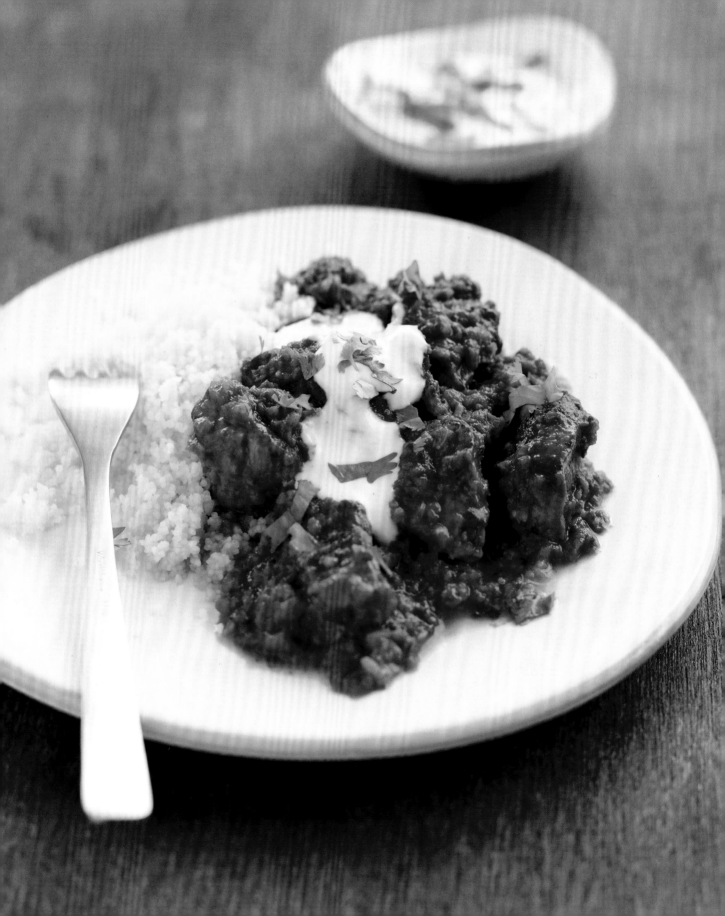

1 SERVE =
2 units protein
½ unit dairy
1½ units vegetables
2 units fats

Lamb, choko and snowpea green curry

SERVES 4   PREP 20 mins   COOK 25 mins

1 tablespoon vegetable oil
800 g lean lamb leg steaks,
   trimmed of fat, cut into
   2 cm pieces
1 onion, coarsely chopped
¼ cup (75 g) Thai Green Curry Paste
   (see page 541)
300 ml reduced-fat coconut-flavoured
   evaporated milk
100 ml salt-reduced chicken stock,
   plus a little extra if needed
2 tablespoons fish sauce
1 tablespoon lime juice
1 choko, peeled and cut
   into thin wedges
400 g snowpeas (mange-tout),
   trimmed

Choko is a green vegetable with a mild, refreshing flavour that is the perfect foil for the rich flavours of this Thai-style curry.

1 Heat half the oil in a large wok over medium–high heat, then add the lamb, in batches if necessary, and stir-fry for 3 minutes or until browned all over. Transfer to a bowl with any juices and wipe the wok clean.

2 Heat the remaining oil in the wok, then add the onion and stir-fry for 3 minutes. Add the curry paste and stir-fry for 1 minute or until fragrant. Return the lamb to the wok, then add the milk, stock, fish sauce, lime juice and choko, adding a little extra stock if necessary to just cover the meat. Bring the mixture to simmering point, then cook over low heat for 15 minutes or until the meat is tender.

3 Add the snowpeas, pushing them under the liquid to submerge. Cover the wok, then cook for 5 minutes or until the vegetables are tender. Serve.

TIP Replace the choko with thin wedges of peeled pumpkin if you prefer.

1 SERVE =
2 units protein
1 unit fats

Lamb and rosemary sausages

SERVES 4   PREP 20 mins   COOK 10 mins

750 g lean minced (ground) lamb
1 red (Spanish) onion, finely chopped
1 tablespoon chopped rosemary
1 tablespoon chopped flat-leaf
   (Italian) parsley
50 g wholemeal breadcrumbs
1 egg, lightly beaten
1 tablespoon olive oil

1   In a large bowl, mix all ingredients except olive oil. Season lightly. Form mixture into 8 equal portions, then roll each to form a sausage shape.

2   Heat oil in a large heavy-based frying pan over medium heat. Add sausages and cook, turning frequently, for 10 minutes, or until all sides are golden and sausages are cooked through. Serve with a salad, greens or pumpkin mash – or all three.

1 SERVE =
2 units protein
½ unit dairy
1 unit vegetables
1 unit fats

Polenta-crumbed lamb chops with zucchini and feta

SERVES 4   PREP 20 mins   COOK 10 mins

1 egg, lightly beaten
¼ cup (35 g) wholemeal plain flour
¼ cup (40 g) polenta
2 tablespoons finely chopped flat-leaf
   (Italian) parsley
800 g lamb chops
olive oil spray
1 tablespoon olive oil
2 zucchini (courgettes), diced
3 tomatoes, diced
1 red (Spanish) onion, diced
$1/_3$ cup shredded basil
50 g feta, crumbled into small pieces

1   Preheat a grill plate or barbecue grill to high. Pour egg onto a large dinner plate. Scatter flour over a second dinner plate. Combine polenta and parsley on a third dinner plate.

2   Crumb chops by coating them with flour, then dipping them in beaten egg, then coating them with the polenta and parsley mixture. Spray chops lightly with oil and grill for 5 minutes each side, or until golden.

3   Meanwhile, heat oil in a large non-stick frying pan over high heat. Add zucchini, tomatoes and onion and cook for 2 minutes. Stir in basil and feta, and season to taste. Serve with the chops.

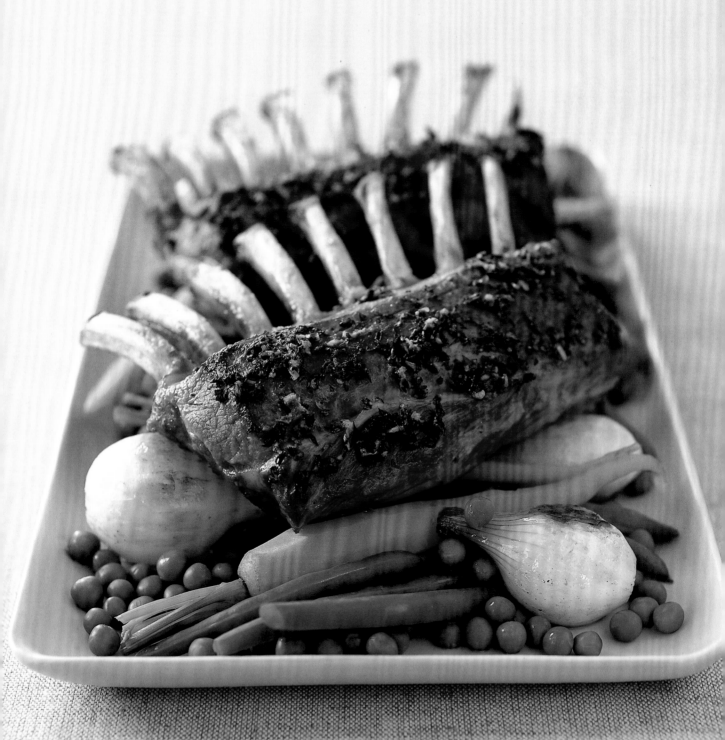

Baked rack of lamb with baby vegetables

SERVES 4   PREP 15 mins + resting time   COOK 40 mins

1 tablespoon olive oil

4 sprigs thyme, chopped

1 tablespoon chopped tarragon

1 tablespoon chopped flat-leaf (Italian) parsley

1 clove garlic

finely grated zest of 1 lemon

1.4 kg rack of lamb (200 g meat per person), trimmed of fat

200 g pearl (pickling) onions

200 g baby carrots

200 g green beans

200 g peas

1 Preheat oven to 200°C. In a bowl, mix half the oil with herbs, garlic and lemon zest.

2 Heat a large frying pan over high heat. Coat lamb in remaining oil and sear until golden on both sides. Transfer to a baking dish and rub herb mixture into rack. Add onions to dish and bake for 25 minutes. Remove meat from oven, cover loosely with foil and set aside to rest for 10 minutes.

3 Bring a large saucepan of lightly salted water to a boil. Cook carrots for 2 minutes, then add beans and peas and cook for a further 4 minutes. Drain and serve with lamb.

Pan-fried lamb steaks with minted pea puree

SERVES 4   **PREP** 15 mins + marinating time   **COOK** 20 mins

1 tablespoon olive oil
1 tablespoon lemon juice
1 teaspoon dried mint
800 g lamb steaks, trimmed of fat

MINTED PEA PUREE
300 g frozen peas
1 clove garlic, crushed
²/₃ cup (170 ml) salt-reduced
   chicken stock
small handful of finely chopped mint

This is a great example of how a few pantry staples can transform a straightforward meal into something special. If you can, marinate the steaks overnight to intensify the flavours.

1 Combine the olive oil, lemon juice and dried mint in a bowl. Add the lamb steaks and turn to coat. Cover and marinate in the refrigerator for 30 minutes, or longer if time permits.

2 To make the pea puree, combine the peas, garlic and stock in a medium saucepan. Bring to the boil, then reduce the heat and simmer for 15 minutes. Puree in a food processor. Season and stir in the mint.

3 Meanwhile, heat a non-stick frying pan over high heat and cook the lamb steaks for 3–4 minutes each side or until cooked to your liking. Rest for 5 minutes, then serve with the pea puree and steamed vegetables.

TIP You might like to leave the mint out of the puree if fussy children object to it. It will still taste delicious.

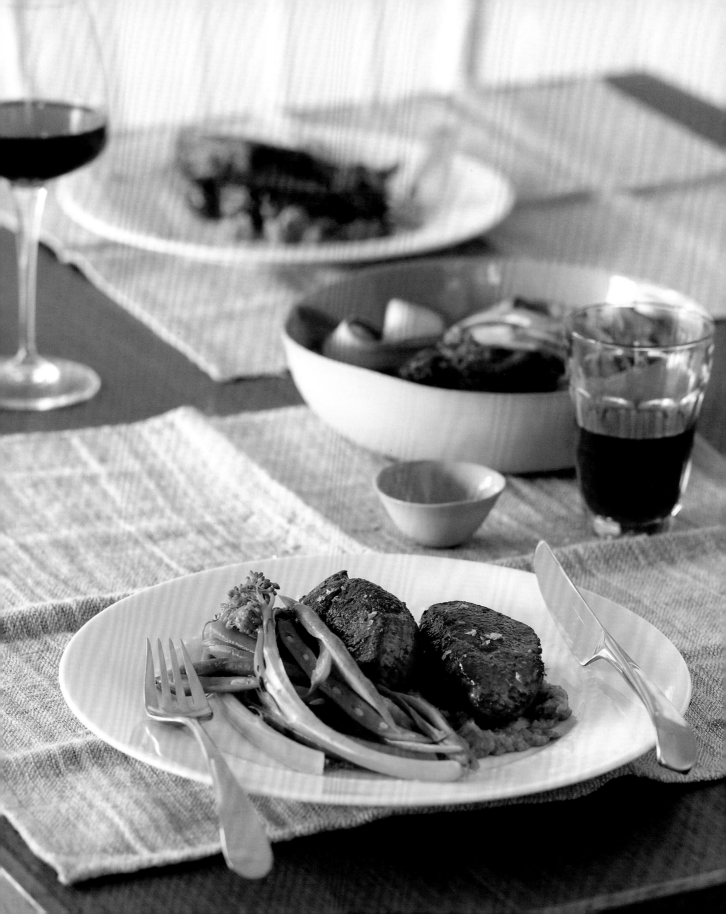

Barbecued lamb cutlets with minty yoghurt sauce

SERVES 4   PREP 15 mins + marinating time   COOK 5 mins

1 tablespoon olive oil
1 tablespoon Dijon mustard
¼ cup (60 ml) red wine vinegar
2 cloves garlic, crushed
1 teaspoon dried oregano
800 g lamb cutlets, trimmed of fat

MINTY YOGHURT SAUCE
100 g reduced-fat yoghurt
80 g reduced-fat Hummus
   (see page 530)
2 spring onions, finely sliced
2 tablespoons chopped mint

This impressive dish is super quick to throw together. Marinate the cutlets overnight if you like, for a more powerful flavour kick.

1   Combine the olive oil, mustard, vinegar, garlic and oregano in a large bowl. Toss the cutlets in the marinade, then cover and marinate in the refrigerator for 2 hours or overnight.

2   Heat a chargrill or barbecue to medium. Add the cutlets and cook for 2 minutes each side or until cooked to your liking.

3   Meanwhile, to make the yoghurt sauce, combine all the ingredients in a medium bowl.

4   Serve the cutlets with a dollop of sauce and a fresh green salad.

TIP For a budget alternative, try lamb or beef steaks in place of the lamb cutlets. They'll still taste great.

Lamb saag

SERVES 4   PREP 15 mins   COOK 1 hour

2 tablespoons vegetable oil
2 onions, sliced
2 cardamom pods, lightly crushed
1 stick cinnamon
1 tablespoon garam masala
2 cloves garlic, crushed
800 g lamb leg, cut into 3 cm cubes
2 tablespoons water, plus 1 cup
  (250 ml) extra water
1 green chilli, finely chopped
2 Roma (plum) tomatoes, diced
1 × 500 g packet frozen
  spinach, defrosted
2/3 cup (190 g) reduced-fat
  natural yoghurt

1 Heat oil in a large heavy-based saucepan over high heat. Add onions, cardamom pods and cinnamon and cook for 10 minutes, or until onions are soft and golden. Add garam masala, garlic, lamb and 2 tablespoons of water and cook for 10 minutes, or until lamb is browned and spices are fragrant. Reduce heat and add chilli, tomatoes, spinach, extra 1 cup of water and half the yoghurt, and simmer for 30–40 minutes, or until lamb is tender.

2 Serve with an extra dollop of yoghurt, plus rice from your daily bread allowance.

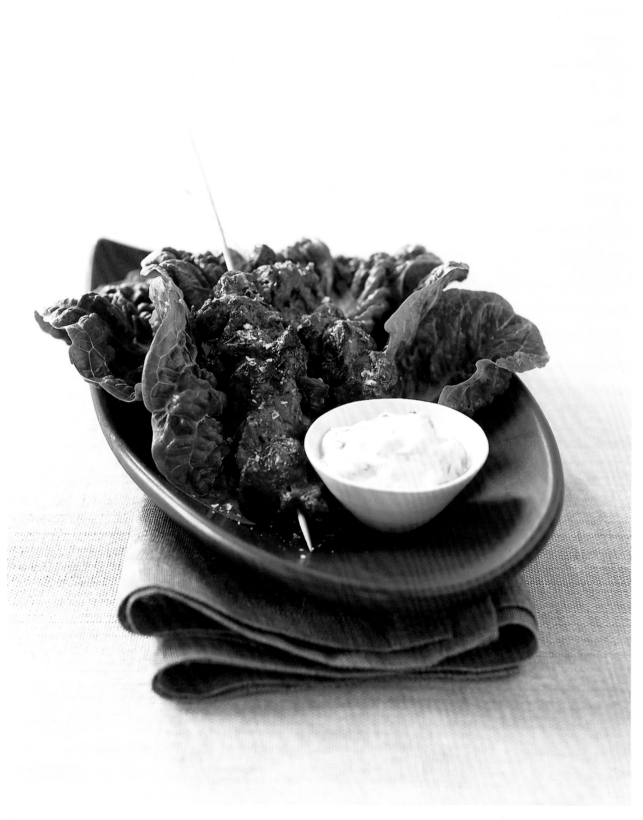

Greek-style lamb kebabs with tzatziki

SERVES 4   PREP 20 mins + soaking and marinating time   COOK 8 mins

800 g lamb fillets, cut into cubes

MARINADE
2 tablespoons dried oregano
1 tablespoon olive oil
1 clove garlic, crushed

TZATZIKI
1 clove garlic, crushed
200 g reduced-fat natural yoghurt
**1 Lebanese (small) or continental
    cucumber, finely grated**
½ red (Spanish) onion, finely diced
**1 tablespoon chopped flat-leaf
    (Italian) parsley**
1 tablespoon chopped mint

1 Mix marinade ingredients in a shallow dish. Add lamb, turning to coat thoroughly. Lightly season, then cover with plastic wrap and refrigerate for anywhere from 2 hours up to overnight – the longer you leave it, the better the result.

2 If using bamboo skewers, soak in hot water for 30 minutes prior to use.

3 Preheat grill plate or barbecue grill to high.

4 Thread lamb onto eight skewers. Grill for 2 minutes each side – 8 minutes in total – or until done to your liking.

5 Meanwhile, combine all tzatziki ingredients in a bowl and lightly season. Serve alongside kebabs and offer a salad.

1 SERVE =
2 units protein
½ unit fruit
2½ units vegetables
2 units fats

Herb and garlic lamb with green caponata

SERVES 4   PREP 25 mins   COOK 1 hour 20 mins

2 cloves garlic, crushed
2 teaspoons finely chopped rosemary
1 tablespoon finely chopped
    flat-leaf (Italian) parsley
4 anchovy fillets, drained of oil
    and finely chopped
1 × 1.5 kg lamb leg, trimmed of fat
olive oil spray

GREEN CAPONATA
1 tablespoon olive oil
1 onion, coarsely chopped
2 cloves garlic, chopped
4 sticks celery, cut into 1.5 cm pieces
1 eggplant (aubergine), trimmed
    and cut into 1.5 cm pieces
$1/_3$ cup (50 g) raisins
1 large green capsicum (pepper),
    trimmed, seeded and cut into
    2 cm pieces
3 zucchini (courgettes), trimmed
    and cut into 1 cm pieces
½ cup (75 g) stuffed green olives,
    coarsely chopped
1 tablespoon balsamic vinegar,
    or to taste

This lamb is so simple to prepare, and can be cooking away while you're making the caponata. Any leftover lamb will be delicious with a salad or in sandwiches the next day.

1   Preheat the oven to 180°C.

2   Combine the garlic, rosemary, parsley and anchovies in a small bowl. Using a sharp knife, make small, deep incisions all over the lamb. Use the garlic mixture to fill the incisions, creating more incisions if you have mixture left over. Spray a large flameproof roasting tin with olive oil, then add the lamb and cook over medium heat, turning often, for 5–6 minutes or until browned all over. Transfer to the oven and roast for 1 hour and 15 minutes or until the lamb is cooked through and tender.

3   Meanwhile, for the caponata, heat the oil in a large saucepan over medium heat. Add the onion, garlic, celery, eggplant and raisins and cook, stirring, for 5–6 minutes or until they start to soften, then add the capsicum. Cover and cook, stirring often, for 30 minutes or until the vegetables are soft. Add the zucchini, then cover and cook for another 10 minutes or until the zucchini is tender. Stir in the olives and vinegar.

4   Divide the caponata among warmed plates. Carve the lamb into chunks or slices, then serve with the caponata.

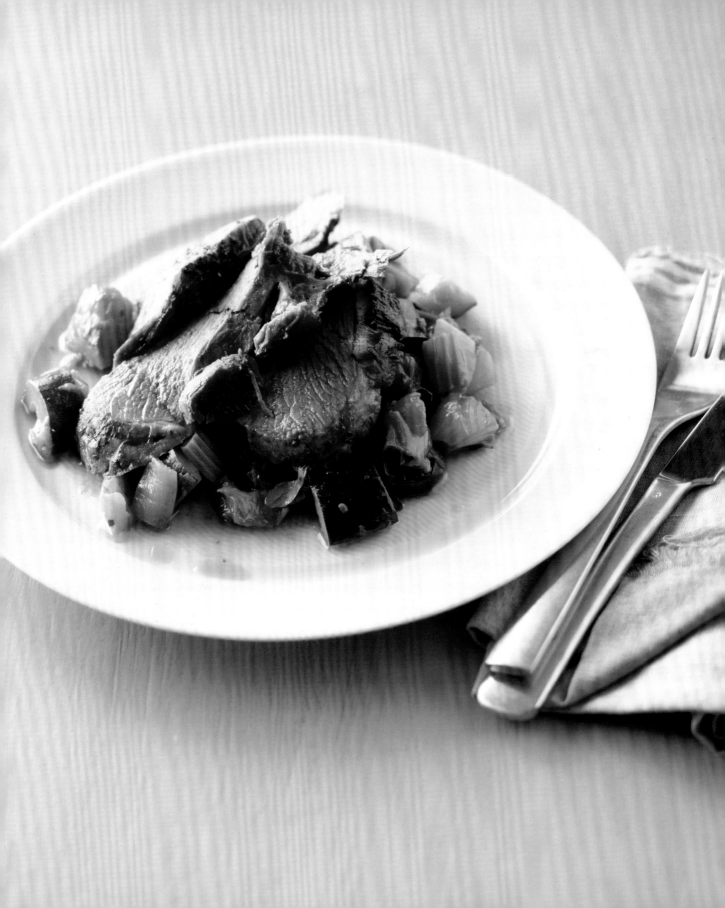

Lamb biryani

SERVES 4   PREP 20 mins + resting time   COOK 1 hour 15 mins

800 g lamb leg steaks, cut
    into 2 cm cubes
2 tablespoons vegetable oil
2 onions, finely sliced
2 cloves garlic, crushed
1 tablespoon finely chopped
    fresh ginger
1 green chilli, seeded and
    finely chopped
2 teaspoons garam masala
1 teaspoon ground turmeric
1 teaspoon ground cinnamon
½ teaspoon ground cardamom
½ teaspoon ground nutmeg
½ teaspoon cayenne pepper
1 bay leaf
½ cup (140 g) reduced-fat
    natural yoghurt
¼ cup (60 ml) lime juice
½ cup (100 g) basmati rice
¼ cup (40 g) sultanas
handful roughly chopped
    coriander (cilantro)
2 tablespoons roughly chopped
    toasted cashews

1 Heat a large heavy-based saucepan over high heat. Coat lamb in half the oil and cook, in batches, for 5 minutes, or until browned. Remove from pan.

2 Heat remaining oil in pan. Cook onions and garlic for 6 minutes. Add ginger, chilli, spices and bay leaf and cook for 2 minutes more. Stir through yoghurt and lime juice. Mix in lamb, then cover and simmer for 10 minutes. Mix in rice and ¾ cup water. Preheat oven to 180°C.

3 Transfer to an ovenproof dish and cover with foil. Bake for 30–40 minutes, or until rice is cooked. Set aside for 5 minutes. Stir through sultanas, garnish with coriander and cashews and serve with a green salad.

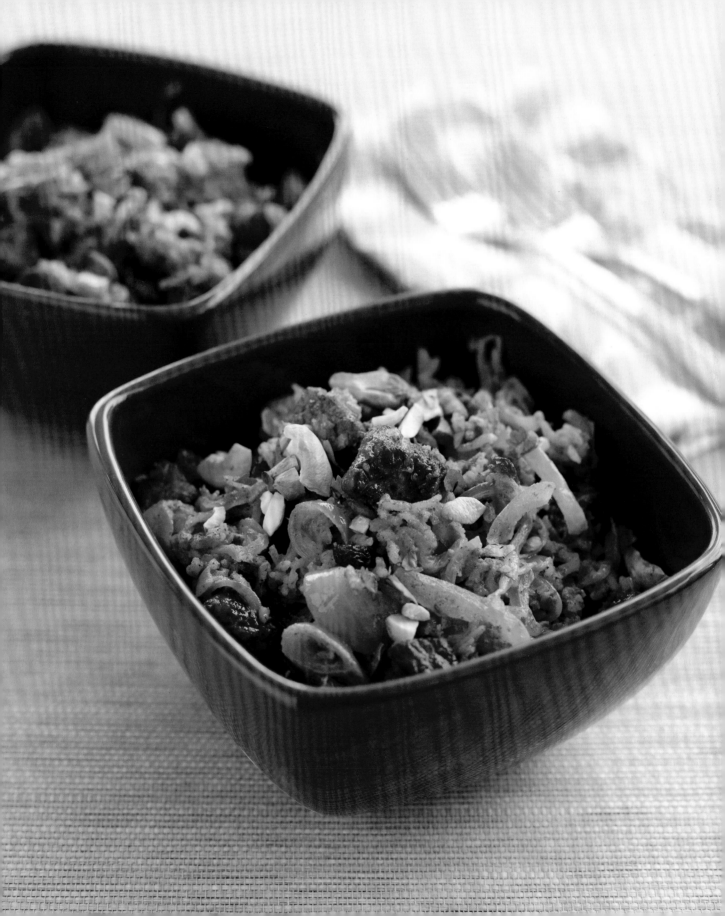

Lamb shanks

SERVES 4   PREP 15 mins   COOK 2 hours 20 mins

2 kg lamb shanks (200 g meat
    per person), on the bone
2 tablespoons olive oil
2 cloves garlic
2 onions, chopped
1 cup diced celery
1 cup (250 ml) white wine
3 cups (750 ml) chicken stock
1 tablespoon lemon zest
3 stalks parsley
2 bay leaves
¼ cup chopped flat-leaf
    (Italian) parsley

1 Preheat oven to 160°C.

2 Heat a large, enamelled cast-iron casserole over high heat. Coat shanks
   with oil and cook, turning occasionally, for 10 minutes, or until well-
   browned. Remove shanks to a plate.

3 Add garlic, onion and celery to the casserole and cook for 5 minutes,
   or until soft. Add wine, stock, lemon zest, parsley stalks and bay leaves
   and bring to a boil. Return shanks to casserole and lightly season.
   Cover with lid and cook, in the oven, for 1½–2 hours, or until meat
   begins to fall off the bone.

4 Check seasoning, then garnish with parsley. Serve with steamed
   vegetables.

1 SERVE =
2 units protein
1 unit vegetables

Lamb loin chops with asian coleslaw

SERVES 4   PREP 15 mins   COOK 10 mins

950 g lamb loin chops (200 g
   meat per person)
2 tablespoons plum sauce
2 cups (100 g) shredded
   Chinese cabbage
1 cup (80 g) bean sprouts
½ red capsicum (pepper),
   seeded and finely sliced
4 spring onions (scallions),
   finely sliced
1 carrot, coarsely grated
¼ cup shredded mint
¼ cup roughly chopped
   coriander (cilantro)
¼ cup (60 ml) soy sauce
2 tablespoons lime juice
1 tablespoon fish sauce
2 tablespoons sweet chilli sauce

1 Preheat a grill plate or barbecue grill to high. Brush chops with plum
   sauce, then cook, being careful not to burn the sauce, for 5 minutes
   each side, or until done to your liking.

2 Meanwhile, place remaining ingredients in a bowl and mix well.
   Cover bowl and set aside for 5 minutes to allow the flavours to infuse.
   Serve with the chops.

Spiced lamb fillets with broccolini

SERVES 4   PREP 15 mins   COOK 20 mins

2 cloves garlic
2 tablespoons olive oil
800 g lamb fillets
2 onions, sliced
2 tablespoons tomato paste
½ cup (125 ml) red wine
1½ tablespoons sultanas
½ small green chilli, chopped
1 tablespoon shredded mint
½ teaspoon paprika
1 tablespoon pine nuts
zest of 1 lemon
2 bunches broccolini

1 Place garlic and oil in a bowl. Add lamb and toss to coat thoroughly.

2 Heat a large frying pan over high heat. Brown lamb, in small batches, for 1–2 minutes, then remove from pan and set aside. Add onion to pan and cook for 5 minutes, or until soft. Stir through tomato paste, wine, sultanas, chilli, mint, paprika, pine nuts and lemon zest and cook for 2–3 minutes. Return meat to the pan to heat through.

3 Meanwhile, bring a small saucepan of lightly salted water to a boil. Blanch broccolini for 2–3 minutes, then drain.

4 Top lamb with onion mixture and serve broccolini alongside.

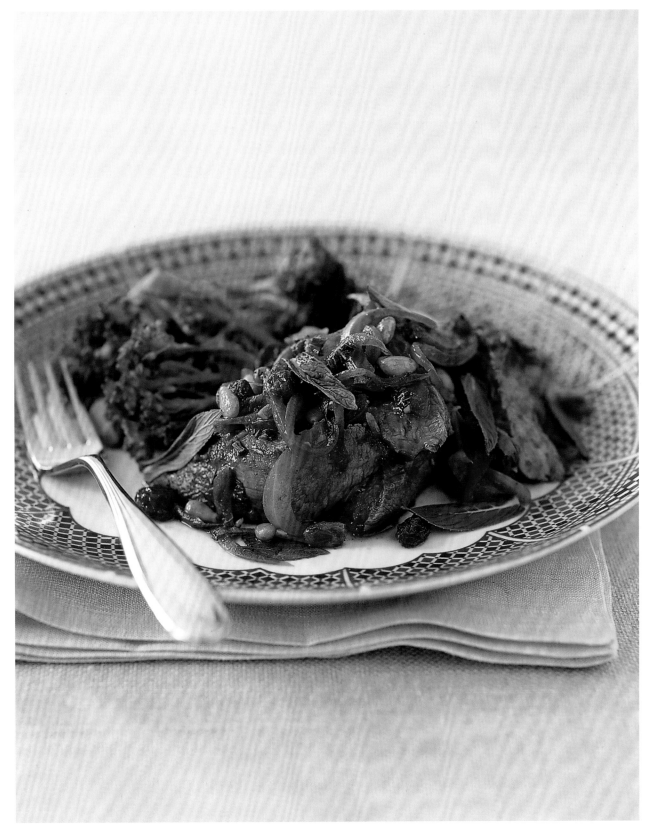

Braised Moroccan lamb

SERVES 4 PREP 15 mins COOK 1 hour 20 mins

1 tablespoon olive oil
800 g lean leg of lamb, trimmed
   of fat and cut into 3 cm chunks
1 onion, diced
2 cloves garlic, crushed
2 teaspoons ground cumin
1 teaspoon ground ginger
2 teaspoons sweet paprika
3 tablespoons roughly
   chopped coriander (cilantro)
1 × 400 g tin chopped tomatoes
2 tablespoons tomato paste (puree)
1 cup (250 ml) salt-reduced beef stock
1 tablespoon honey
8 green olives, chopped
small mint leaves, to garnish

Look for bright green Sicilian olives – their buttery flavour and soft texture work wonderfully in this braise.

1 Preheat the oven to 170°C.

2 Heat the olive oil in a flameproof casserole dish over high heat. Brown the lamb in batches, then remove from the dish.

3 Add the onion and garlic to the dish and cook for 2–3 minutes or until beginning to soften, then add the cumin, ginger and paprika and stir until fragrant. Return the lamb to the dish, along with the coriander, chopped tomatoes, tomato paste and stock.

4 Bring to a simmer, then cover and bake in the oven for 1 hour or until the lamb is tender. Just before serving, stir in the honey and garnish with a scattering of olives and mint leaves. Serve with couscous from your daily bread allowance and steamed green beans.

TIP Lamb meat is often sold packed and diced, which can cut down on preparation time. If you like, the diced lamb can be replaced with 4 × 200 g frenched lamb shanks.

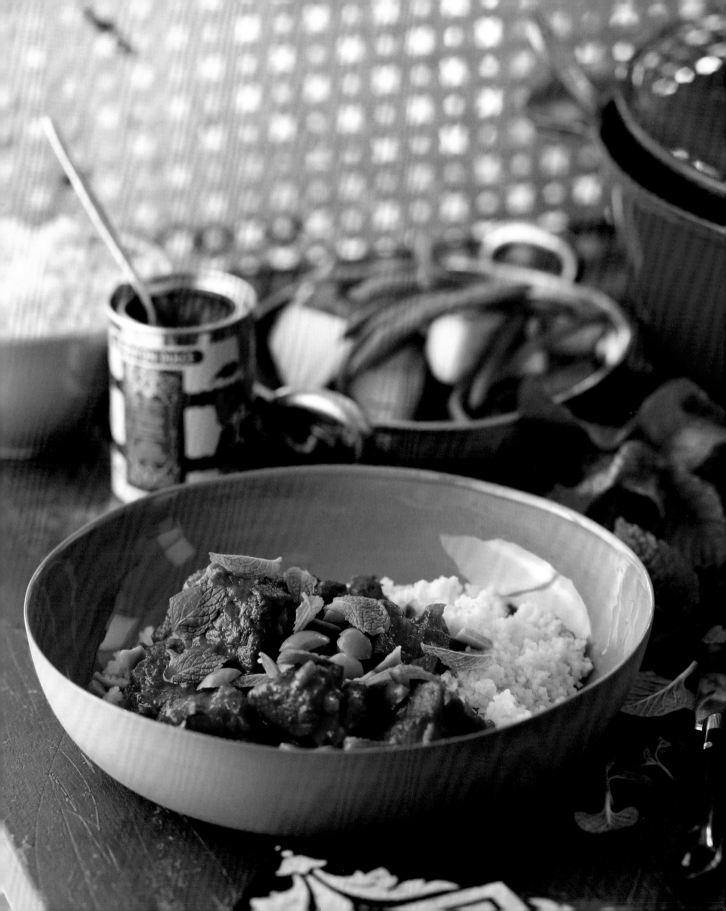

Lamb kofta curry

SERVES 4   PREP 25 mins   COOK 35 mins

The combination of spices in the kofta and sauce make this a very special dish. Double the quantities and store another meal for the family in the freezer.

700 g lean minced lamb
1 onion, finely chopped
2 cloves garlic, crushed
1 × 3 cm piece ginger,
    finely grated
½ teaspoon chilli powder
2 teaspoons ground coriander
4 tablespoons chopped
    coriander (cilantro)
2 eggs

SAUCE
1 tablespoon olive oil
1 onion, finely chopped
1 × 2 cm piece ginger,
    finely grated
2 cloves garlic, crushed
1 teaspoon ground cumin
1 teaspoon ground coriander
1 teaspoon sweet paprika
½–1 teaspoon chilli powder
    (or to taste)
1 cinnamon stick
1 × 400 g tin chopped tomatoes
1 teaspoon garam masala
1 tablespoon lemon juice
roughly chopped coriander
    (cilantro), to serve

1 Preheat the oven to 200°C and line a large baking tray with baking paper.

2 To prepare the koftas, place the minced lamb, onion, garlic, ginger, chilli powder, ground coriander, chopped coriander and eggs in a food processor and pulse until just combined. Form the mixture into small balls (this should make approximately 30 balls). Place on the prepared tray and bake for 15–20 minutes or until just cooked.

3 Meanwhile, to make the sauce, heat the olive oil in a large frying pan and cook the onion until browned.

4 Combine the ginger, garlic, cumin, coriander, paprika, chilli powder and 2 tablespoons water in a small bowl. Add to the pan with the cinnamon stick and cook until fragrant, then stir in the tomatoes and ½ cup (125 ml) water and simmer for 5 minutes. Add the meatballs in a single layer and simmer, covered, for 10–15 minutes or until the sauce has thickened.

5 Gently stir in the garam masala and lemon juice. Sprinkle with coriander and serve with steamed rice from your daily bread allowance and a green salad to the side.

TIP This dish can be frozen and stored for a later date. Either prepare the meatballs only and freeze, or complete the whole dish, without adding the coriander garnish, and freeze. Mince should always be as fresh as possible and kept refrigerated until you cook it.

Lamb kofta with roasted pumpkin, lemon and rocket salad

SERVES 4   PREP 30 mins   COOK 25 mins

800 g lean minced lamb
1 small onion, peeled and grated
¾ teaspoon ground allspice
2½ tablespoons finely chopped
  flat-leaf (Italian) parsley
1 tablespoon olive oil
400 g pumpkin (squash),
  peeled, seeded and cut
  into 1 cm thick slices
large handful rocket leaves
250 g yellow teardrop tomatoes,
  halved lengthways
½ cup (75 g) semi-dried tomatoes,
  well-drained
1 cup (250 ml) reduced-fat
  Greek-style yoghurt
2 teaspoons finely grated
  lemon zest
1½ tablespoons lemon juice

These kofta are made from minced lamb formed into a long, torpedo shape, which are quickly fried before being baked in the oven, then served with a hearty salad for dinner.

1 Preheat the oven to 180°C.

2 Combine the minced lamb, onion, allspice and parsley in a bowl and season to taste. Using your hands, knead the mixture for 4–5 minutes or until smooth. Take handfuls of the mixture and form into torpedo shapes about 9 cm long.

3 Heat the olive oil in a large ovenproof non-stick frying pan over medium heat. Add the kofta and cook, turning often, for 5 minutes or until cooked through. Transfer to a baking dish, place in the oven and bake for 20 minutes.

4 Meanwhile, place the pumpkin in the reserved frying pan, then transfer to the oven and bake for 20 minutes or until tender. Transfer the pumpkin to a large bowl, add the rocket, tomato and semi-dried tomatoes and combine well. Divide among plates, then place the kofta on top.

5 Combine the yoghurt, lemon zest and juice in a small bowl, then drizzle this dressing over the salad and kofta and serve immediately.

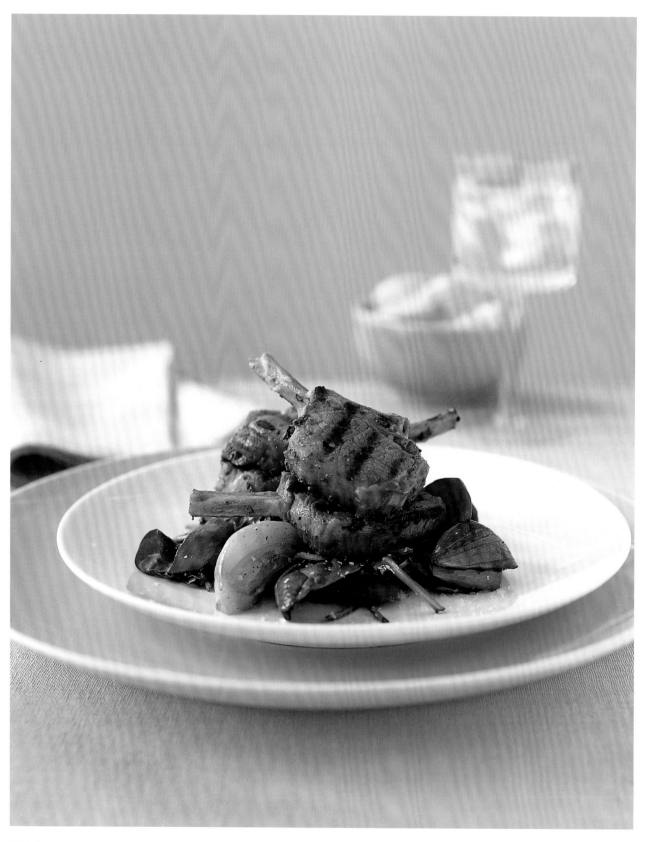

1 SERVE =
2 units protein
1 unit vegetables
2 units fats

Rosemary and lemon lamb cutlets with baked fennel and red onion

SERVES 4   PREP 15 mins + marinating time   COOK 20 mins

1.4 kg lamb cutlets (200 g meat
   per person), trimmed of fat
2 bulbs fennel, sliced
2 red (Spanish) onions,
   cut into wedges
1 tablespoon olive oil
100 g baby spinach leaves

MARINADE
2 tablespoons chopped rosemary
2 teaspoons chopped tarragon
2 teaspoons chopped flat-leaf
   (Italian) parsley
1 tablespoon olive oil
2 tablespoons lemon juice

1 Mix marinade ingredients and pour into a shallow dish. Add meat and turn to coat thoroughly. Cover and allow to marinate for 30 minutes.

2 Preheat oven to 180°C.

3 Place fennel and onion in a baking dish and drizzle with oil. Bake for 20 minutes.

4 Meanwhile, preheat grill plate or barbecue grill to hot. Add cutlets and cook for 1 minute each side, or until done to your liking. Set aside to rest.

5 Toss spinach leaves through hot vegetables and lightly season. Arrange on serving plates and top with cutlets.

1 SERVE =
2 units protein
2 units vegetables
1 unit fats

Lamb with turluturlu

SERVES 4   PREP 30 mins   COOK 50 mins

1 large eggplant (aubergine),
  trimmed and cut into 3 cm pieces
600 g pumpkin (squash), peeled,
  seeded and cut into 3 cm pieces
1 large red capsicum (pepper),
  trimmed, seeded and
  cut into 3 cm pieces
2 red (Spanish) onions,
  cut into large pieces
3 zucchini (courgettes),
  trimmed and thickly sliced
1 tablespoon olive oil
2 teaspoons ground coriander
1 teaspoon sweet paprika
1 teaspoon ground cumin
2 cups (500 ml) salt-reduced
  tomato passata
2 handfuls coriander (cilantro),
  chopped (optional)
olive oil spray
800 g lean lamb leg steaks,
  trimmed of fat

**Turluturlu is a Turkish-style ratatouille that goes beautifully
with lamb.**

1 Preheat the oven to 180°C. Place the vegetables in a large roasting tin,
  drizzle over the oil and toss to coat. Sprinkle with the ground spices,
  then season to taste. Bake for 40 minutes or until the vegetables are very
  tender. Remove the tin from the oven, pour over the passata and stir to
  combine, then sprinkle with coriander (if using) and bake for another
  10 minutes to heat through.

2 Meanwhile, heat a chargrill plate or large frying pan over medium heat.
  Once hot, spray with olive oil and cook the steaks for 2–3 minutes on
  each side for medium–rare or until cooked to your liking.

3 Thickly slice the steaks on the diagonal, then divide among warmed
  plates with the turluturlu.

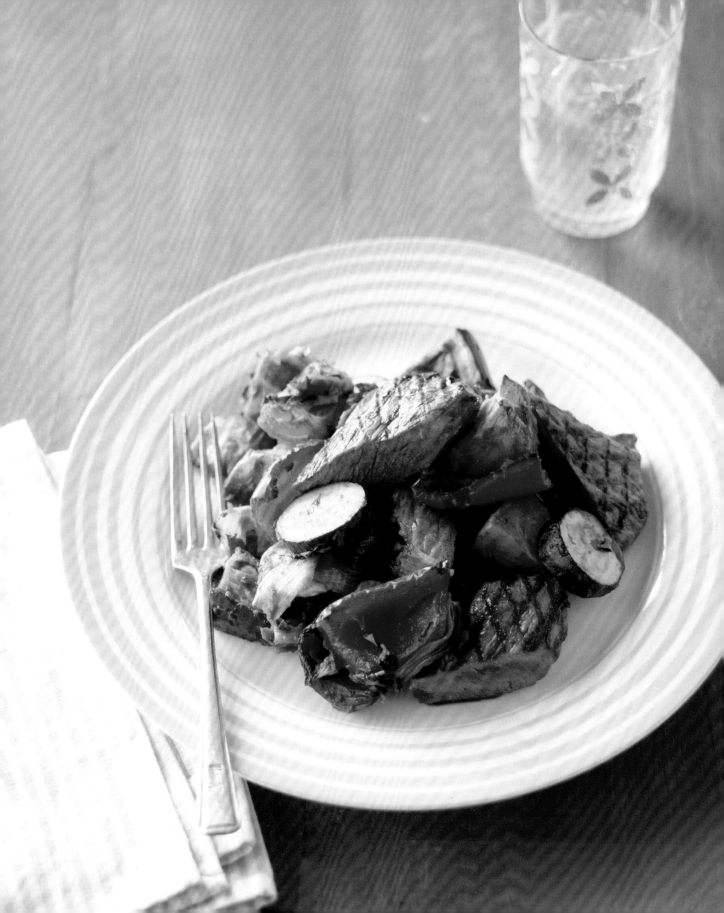

Roast leg of lamb with rosemary and garlic

SERVES 4   PREP 10 mins + resting time   COOK 1 hour

1 × 1.5 kg leg of lamb (200 g meat
   per person), trimmed of fat
1 tablespoon olive oil
2 sprigs rosemary
2 cloves garlic, skin on and halved
2 lemons, quartered
½ cup (125 ml) white wine

1 Preheat oven to 180°C.

2 Rub meat with oil and lightly season. Place rosemary, garlic and
   lemon in a baking dish and pour in wine. Place lamb on top and bake
   for 1 hour.

3 Remove from oven, cover loosely with foil and set aside to rest for
   10 minutes before carving. (This cooking time will produce pink
   lamb. If you prefer yours slightly more cooked, leave it in the oven
   for another 10–30 minutes.)

4 Serve with your favourite vegetables – either potato and pumpkin,
   peeled and added to the baking dish 1 hour before the end of
   cooking time; or fresh greens, such as peas or beans, steamed,
   boiled or blanched.

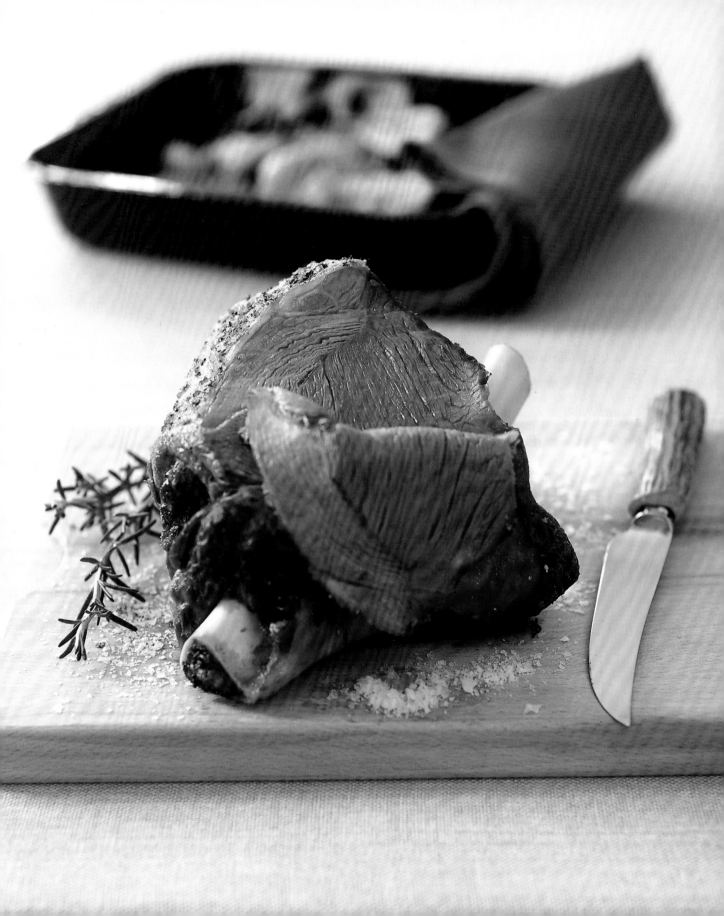

Indian lamb patties

SERVES 4   PREP 20 mins + refrigerating time   COOK 15 mins

750 g lean minced (ground) lamb
1 small onion, finely chopped
1 clove garlic, finely chopped
1 tablespoon garam masala
½ cup roughly chopped
   coriander (cilantro)
¼ cup roughly chopped mint
1 tablespoon spicy mango chutney
1 egg, lightly beaten
1 cup (280 g) reduced-fat
   natural yoghurt

1 Place all ingredients except yoghurt in a large bowl and mix well.
   Season lightly. Form mixture into 8 patties. Transfer to a plate, cover
   and refrigerate for 15 minutes.

2 Heat a grill plate or barbecue grill to high. Add patties and cook for
   6–8 minutes each side, or until cooked through. Serve with a dollop
   of yoghurt and steamed green vegetables or a salad.

1 SERVE =
2 units protein
1 unit fats

Garlic and herb butterflied leg of lamb

SERVES 4   PREP 10 mins + marinating time   COOK 35 mins

1 tablespoon olive oil
3 cloves garlic, crushed
juice of 2 lemons
2 tablespoons chopped rosemary
2 tablespoons chopped oregano
1 × 800 g leg of lamb, boned and
   butterflied (ask your butcher
   to do this)

Start this the night before, then let the oven do its magic while you enjoy the company of your guests.

1 Combine the olive oil, garlic, lemon juice, herbs, salt and pepper in a large shallow dish. Add the lamb and turn to coat well. Cover with plastic wrap and marinate in the refrigerator for up to 24 hours.

2 Preheat the oven to 200°C or the barbecue to medium–high.

3 If using the oven, heat a large frying pan over high heat. Add the lamb and cook each side for 5 minutes or until browned. Transfer to a roasting tin, then place in the oven and roast for 20–25 minutes or until cooked to your liking. If using the barbecue, grill the lamb for about 15 minutes each side or until cooked to your liking.

4 Regardless of which cooking method you choose, rest the lamb for 15–20 minutes. Serve drizzled with the pan juices, alongside the Greek and couscous salads (see pages 468 and 104).

TIP If you find yourself with leftover lamb, it makes a perfect addition to lunch the next day. Either serve it in a wholegrain sandwich with salad leaves and some seeded mustard, or shredded and tossed through a salad (see, for example, the warm lamb salad on page 118).

Lamb with minted zucchini salad and onion relish

SERVES 4   PREP 20 mins   COOK 30 mins

6 zucchini (courgettes), trimmed
 and sliced on the diagonal
olive oil spray
4 × 250 g lamb leg chops,
 trimmed of fat
½ cup (75 g) pitted kalamata olives
small handful mint leaves (optional)

ONION RELISH

2 teaspoons olive oil
2 large onions, very thinly sliced
1 cup (250 ml) red wine
1 cup (250 ml) salt-reduced
 chicken stock
2½ tablespoons red wine vinegar
2 teaspoons caster sugar or
 powdered sweetener

Lamb leg chops have a bone running through the middle and an edge of fat that needs trimming off, so accounting for this will take the average weight of a chop down to the requisite 200 g. They do vary in size, though, so be sure to weigh them after trimming.

1 To make the relish, heat the oil in a large non-stick saucepan over medium heat. Add the onion, then cover and cook, stirring occasionally, for 10 minutes or until very soft. Remove the lid, add the wine, stock, vinegar and sugar or sweetener, then cook, stirring frequently, for 15–20 minutes or until the liquid has reduced and the mixture is jammy.

2 Meanwhile, heat a chargrill plate or large heavy-based frying pan over medium heat. Spray the zucchini with olive oil, then, working in batches, cook for 3 minutes, turning once, or until cooked through. Transfer to a bowl and set aside.

3 Place the lamb on the chargrill plate or in the pan and cook for 3 minutes on each side for medium–rare or until cooked to your liking. Meanwhile, add the olives and mint (if using) to the bowl of zucchini and toss to combine well.

4 Divide the zucchini mixture among plates, add a lamb chop and spoon some of the onion relish over. Season with pepper and serve.

TIP Slow cooking makes the onions in the relish meltingly soft, so don't be tempted to rush the process. This relish keeps in the fridge for up to a week, so you could easily double the recipe and have plenty on hand to accompany grilled steak, poached chicken or lean roast pork.

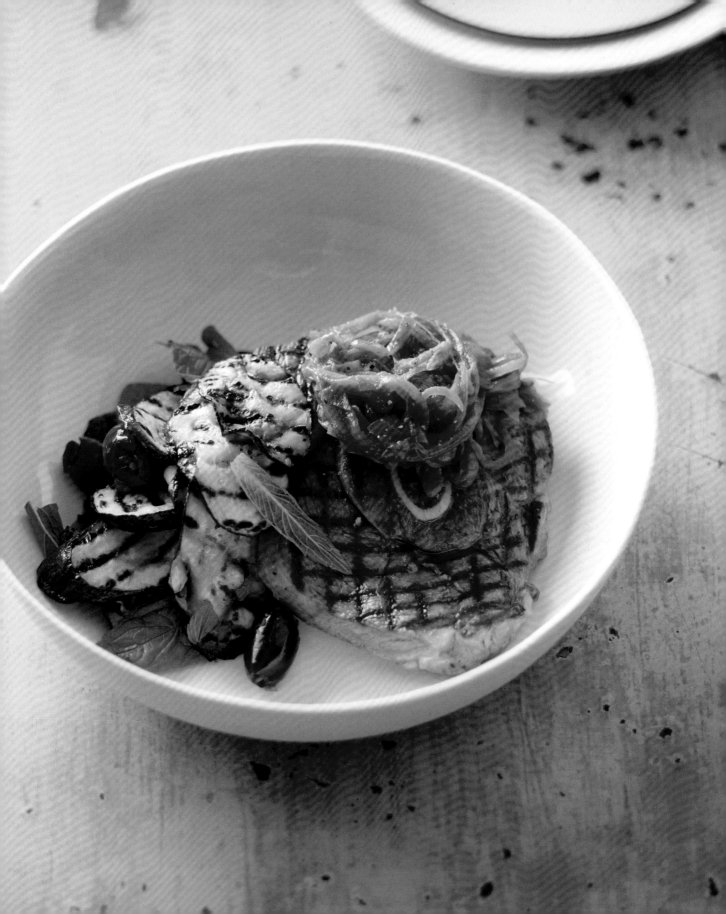

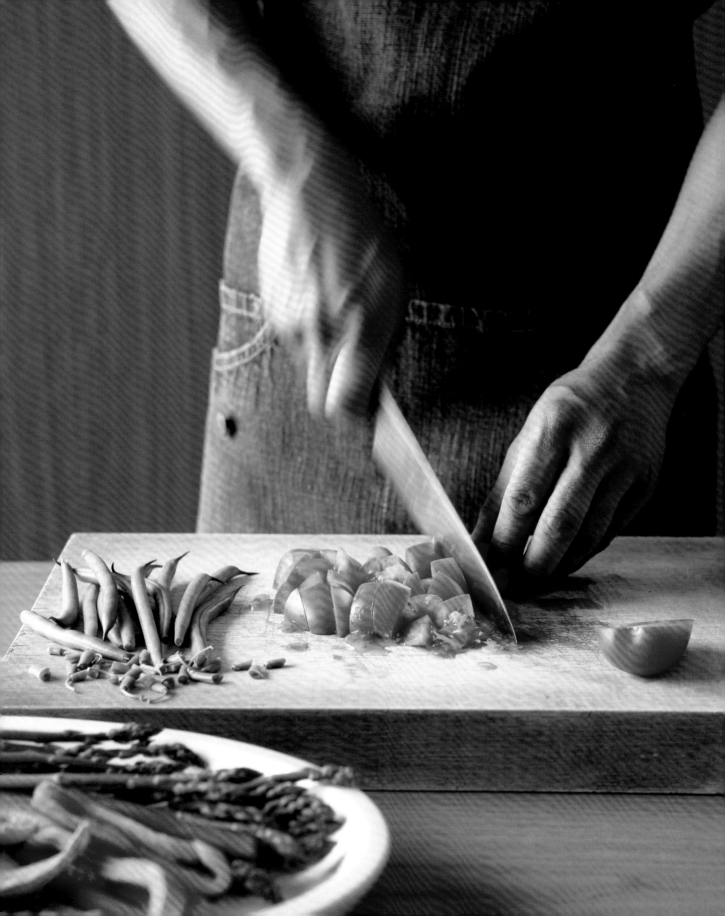

sides

Shaved cabbage and brussels sprout salad

SERVES 4   PREP 20 mins

200 g savoy cabbage, core
   and outer leaves removed
125 g brussels sprouts, trimmed
50 g finely shredded cos lettuce
½ red (Spanish) onion, thinly sliced
1½ tablespoons lemon juice
1½ tablespoons white wine vinegar
1 tablespoon extra virgin olive oil
50 g parmesan, finely grated
1 tablespoon balsamic vinegar

This crisp, refreshing salad makes a wonderful counterpoint to simply grilled chicken or barbecued meats.

1　Finely shred the cabbage and brussels sprouts with a mandolin or sharp knife. Combine in a large bowl with the cos lettuce and onion.

2　Whisk together the lemon juice, white wine vinegar and olive oil. Pour the dressing over the vegetables and gently toss. Sprinkle with parmesan and drizzle with balsamic vinegar just before serving.

1 SERVE =
1 unit vegetables
¼ unit fruit
2½ units fats

Spinach, pear and walnut salad

SERVES 4   PREP 10 mins   COOK 10 mins

40 g walnuts
1 tablespoon extra virgin olive oil
1 tablespoon balsamic vinegar
150 g baby spinach leaves
1 pear, thinly sliced

Use the freshest walnuts you can find for this dish. If stored for too long, they can become rancid.

1 Preheat the oven to 180°C and line a baking tray with baking paper. Spread out the walnuts on the prepared tray and toast them in the oven for 10 minutes or until golden brown and fragrant. Remove from the oven and allow to cool, then roughly chop.

2 Meanwhile, make a dressing by combining the olive oil and vinegar in a screw-top jar. Shake well to combine.

3 In a large bowl, gently toss together the spinach leaves, pear slices and dressing. Arrange on serving plates and scatter the walnuts over the top.

TIP You could serve this as a starter, side dish or, as the French do, following the main course of your dinner party. You can even serve this in place of the scallops with prosciutto and cauliflower puree (see page 199) if you want to keep your protein units down. 50 g shaved parmesan or reduced-fat goat's cheese would make a delicious addition to this salad, and would add ¼ unit dairy per serve.

Greek salad

SERVES 4   PREP 10 mins

1 cos (romaine) lettuce, torn
  into large pieces
2 Lebanese (short) cucumbers,
  roughly chopped
1 green capsicum (pepper),
  seeded and finely chopped
12 kalamata olives
4 Roma (plum) tomatoes, quartered
½ red (Spanish) onion, thinly sliced
2 tablespoons olive oil
1 tablespoon lemon juice
200 g reduced-fat feta

1 Put lettuce, cucumber, capsicum, olives, tomato and onion into a large
   salad bowl. Add oil and lemon juice and toss. Season to taste.

2 Crumble feta over top and serve.

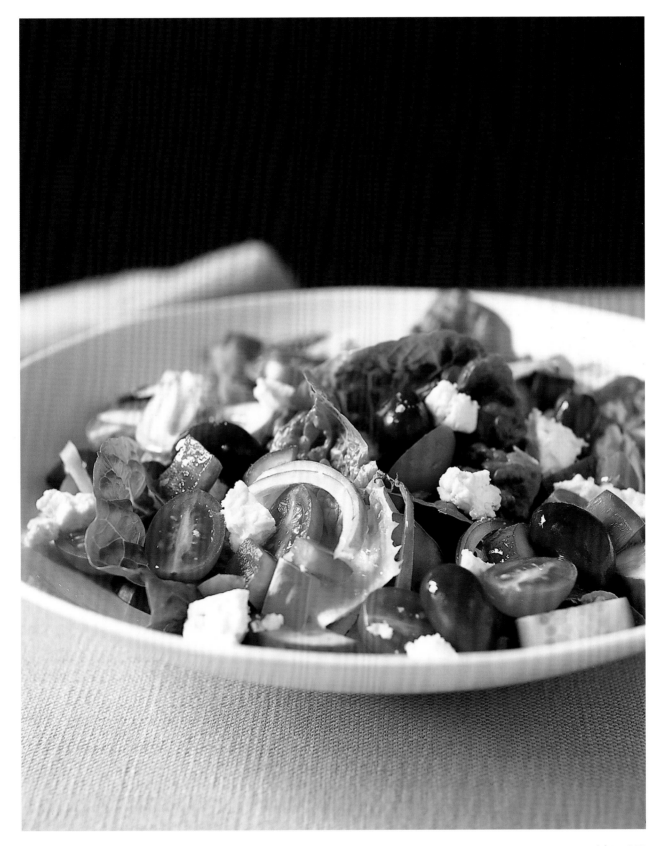

Potato, olive, mint and egg salad

SERVES 4   PREP 20 mins + cooling time   COOK 15 mins

2 red (Spanish) onions, peeled
   and cut into thin wedges
olive oil spray
600 g desiree potatoes,
   halved widthways
8 eggs, hard-boiled and peeled
100 g pitted kalamata olives
small handful mint leaves, torn
large handful rocket leaves

DRESSING
3 teaspoons seeded or Dijon mustard
2½ teaspoons red wine vinegar
¹/₃ cup (80 ml) extra virgin olive oil

Enjoy this for lunch – the sweetness of the charred red onion brings a special touch to this salad. If you like, halve the number of eggs and toss through 200 g flaked tuna or sliced cooked chicken.

1   Heat a chargrill plate over medium heat. Spray the onion wedges with olive oil, then cook, in batches if necessary, for 5–6 minutes on each side or until tender and lightly charred. Remove to a large bowl.

2   Meanwhile, cook the potato halves in a saucepan of boiling water for 15 minutes or until tender. Drain well and cool slightly, then slip off the skins and discard. Cut the potato into 1 cm pieces and add to the onion in the bowl. Cut the eggs into 1 cm pieces and add to the bowl along with the olives, mint and rocket leaves.

3   For the dressing, whisk the mustard and vinegar together in a small bowl, slowly adding the oil in a thin steady stream. Season to taste with salt and pepper, then pour over the salad. Toss gently to coat, then divide among plates or bowls and serve immediately.

1 SERVE =
1 unit vegetables
½ unit fats

Fennel and red onion salad

SERVES 4   PREP 10 mins

3 baby fennel bulbs, thinly sliced
   (preferably with a mandolin)
½ red (Spanish) onion, thinly sliced
handful of flat-leaf (Italian) parsley,
   shredded
2 teaspoons extra virgin olive oil
2 teaspoons lemon juice
2 teaspoons Dijon mustard

Fennel has a sweet fragrance and distinctive aniseed or licorice flavour. It is a good idea to remove the tough outer layers of the fennel bulbs and slice 1 cm off the base before preparing it for the salad.

1 Combine the fennel, onion and parsley in a large bowl.

2 Whisk together the remaining ingredients and pour over the vegetables. Season, then gently toss together.

Silverbeet cooked with anchovies, currants and vinegar

SERVES 4 **PREP** 15 mins **COOK** 18 mins

1 large bunch (about 1 kg) silverbeet (Swiss chard), stems trimmed and reserved, leaves washed and coarsely chopped
2 teaspoons olive oil
3 cloves garlic, thinly sliced
6 anchovy fillets, or to taste, drained of oil and chopped
¹/₃ cup (55 g) currants
¼ cup (60 ml) balsamic vinegar

The Italian-inspired, sweet and sour flavours of balsamic, anchovy and currants are the perfect way to transform an everyday vegetable into an interesting accompaniment.

1 Finely chop the silverbeet stems to give about 2 cups, then discard the remaining stems.

2 Heat the oil in a large saucepan over medium heat, then add the stems, garlic, anchovies and currants. Cover the pan, then cook, stirring often, for 8–10 minutes or until the stems are tender.

3 Add the leaves to the pan and cook, covered, for 5–6 minutes or until the leaves are tender. Add the vinegar, bring the mixture to the boil, then cook for 1–2 minutes to allow any excess liquid to evaporate.

4 Season to taste, then serve hot or at room temperature.

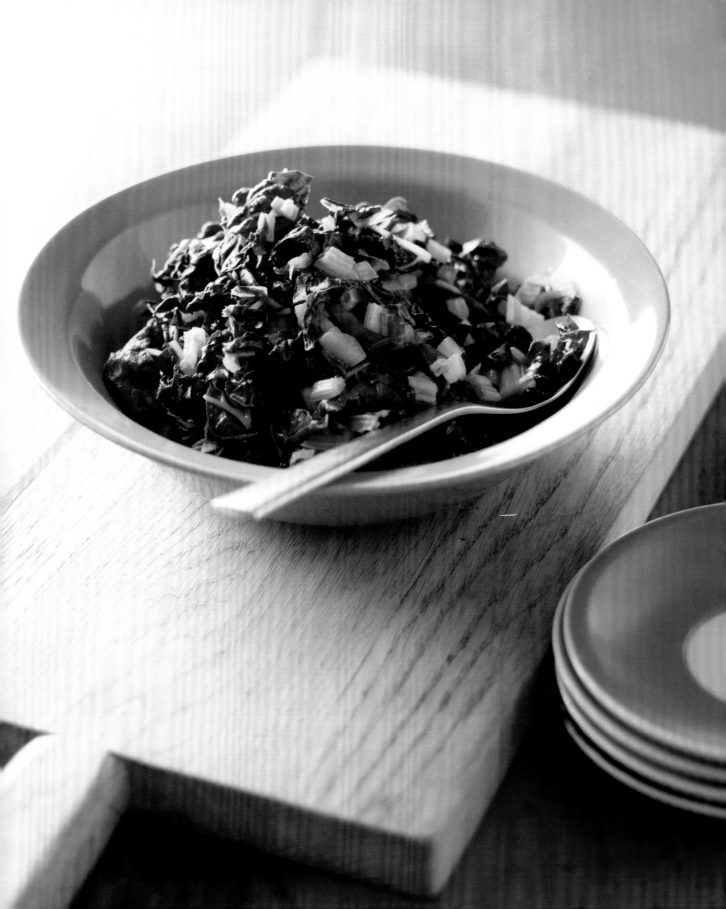

1 SERVE =
2 units vegetables
2 units fats

1 SERVE =
½ unit dairy
1 unit vegetables
1 unit fats

Pumpkin mash with cabbage and spring onions

SERVES 4   **PREP** 15 mins   **COOK** 20 mins

2 tablespoons olive oil
500 g cabbage, finely shredded
600 g butternut pumpkin, peeled
  and cut into large chunks
1 cup (250 ml) reduced-fat milk
4 spring onions (scallions),
  finely sliced

1 Heat olive oil in a large frying pan over medium heat. Add cabbage and saute for 5 minutes, or until soft. Remove from heat and set aside.

2 Fill a large saucepan with 2 cm lightly salted water and bring to a simmer. Add pumpkin, cover tightly, and cook for 15 minutes, or until tender. Drain well and return to pan. Add milk and mash pumpkin with a fork. To serve, season mash lightly and stir through cabbage and spring onions.

3 Goes well with beef or lamb.

Zucchini with spinach and goat's cheese

SERVES 4   **PREP** 10 mins   **COOK** 10 mins

3 zucchini (courgettes), finely
  sliced into rounds
150 g baby spinach
2 teaspoons finely grated lemon zest
1 tablespoon olive oil
50 g goat's cheese, crumbled
¼ cup torn basil

1 Bring a large saucepan of lightly salted water to a boil. Add zucchini and cook for 3 minutes. Drain zucchini in a colander and return to saucepan over low heat. Add spinach, lemon zest and olive oil and stir until spinach has wilted. Add goat's cheese and basil and season lightly.

2 Goes well with lamb or chicken.

1 SERVE =
1½ units dairy
1½ units vegetables

Cauliflower cheese

SERVES 4   PREP 15 mins   COOK 25 mins

1 small head cauliflower
   (about 800 g), trimmed
   and cut into florets
2½ cups (625 ml) reduced-fat milk
¼ cup (40 g) wholemeal flour
150 g reduced-fat cheddar, grated
large pinch cayenne pepper
   (optional)
large handful flat-leaf (Italian)
   parsley leaves, chopped (
   optional)

This reduced-fat version of everybody's favourite comfort food is also great served for lunch – just scatter over 70 g fresh breadcrumbs before baking, then serve with a green salad.

1 Preheat the oven to 180°C.

2 Bring a large saucepan of water to the boil, add the cauliflower and cook for 3–4 minutes or until almost tender. Drain well, then place in a baking dish.

3 Bring the milk to simmering point in a saucepan. Combine the flour and 4 tablespoons water in a small bowl and stir until smooth. Stirring constantly, add the flour mixture to the milk, bring to the boil, then cook for 1–2 minutes or until thickened.

4 Remove the milk mixture from the heat, stir in half the cheese, the cayenne (if using) and the parsley (if using) and season to taste. Pour the sauce over the cauliflower in the dish, then sprinkle over the remaining cheese. Bake for 20 minutes or until golden and bubbling.

TIP Try this tasty variation – reduce the amount of cheddar cheese to 100 g, and use 50 g grated parmesan and a large pinch of nutmeg instead of the cayenne.

Broad bean, pea and mint 'smash'

SERVES 4   PREP 10 mins   COOK 12 mins

400 g fresh podded or
   frozen broad beans
3 cups (360 g) fresh podded
   or frozen peas
small handful mint leaves, torn

A riot of green, this sweet and delicious side dish goes brilliantly with grilled lamb, beef or chicken.

1 Cook the broad beans in a saucepan of boiling water for 3–4 minutes or until tender. Drain well, reserving the cooking water, then plunge them into a bowl of cold water to cool. Drain again, then peel and set aside.

2 Return the reserved cooking water to the boil, then cook the peas for 3–4 minutes or until tender. Drain well, reserving about 100 ml of the cooking water. Return the peas to the pan with the broad beans and 2 tablespoons of the cooking water, then cover and place over low heat for 2–3 minutes to warm through.

3 Using a potato masher, coarsely mash the peas and beans, adding a little more cooking water if needed. Season to taste with salt and pepper, stir in the mint and serve immediately.

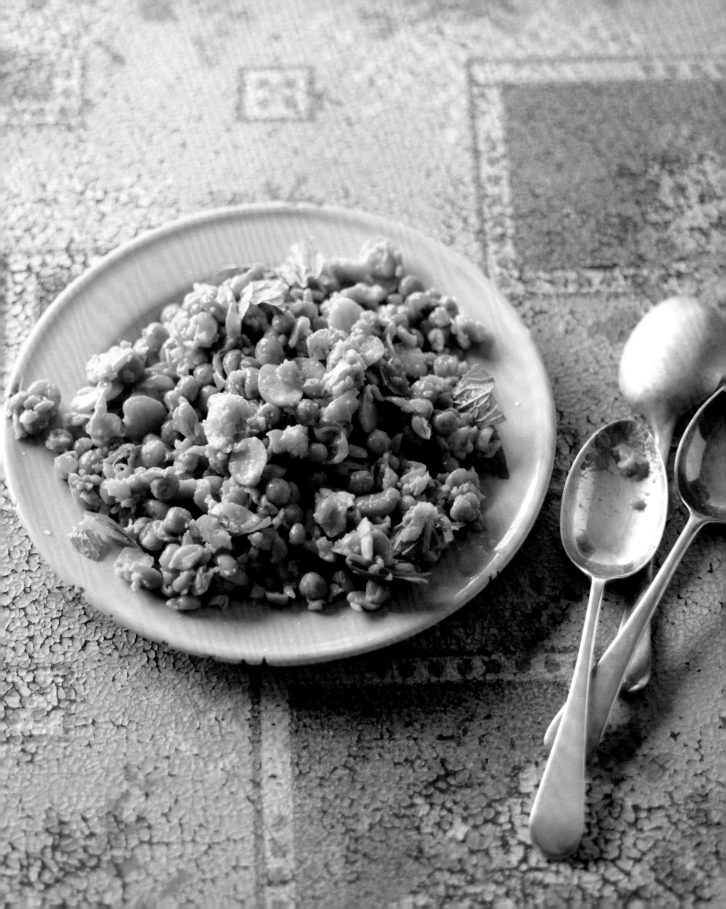

Warm eggplant salad

SERVES 8   PREP 20 mins   COOK 25 mins

4 medium eggplants (aubergines),
   peeled and diced
olive oil spray
2 tablespoons olive oil
2 red (Spanish) onions, chopped
2 teaspoons ground coriander
2 teaspoons ground cumin
2 teaspoons ground cinnamon
2 teaspoons sweet paprika
1–2 teaspoons chilli flakes
6 cloves garlic, crushed
2 × 400 g tins chopped tomatoes
1 teaspoon sugar
½ cup (25 g) chopped mint
½ cup (25 g) chopped coriander
   (cilantro)

Silky roast eggplant is combined with fragrant spices to create an extremely moreish side dish. This is particularly good with the lamb cutlets (see page 438).

1   Preheat the oven to 200°C and line a baking tray with baking paper.

2   Place the eggplants on the prepared tray and spray with olive oil. Roast for 25 minutes until tender.

3   Meanwhile, heat the olive oil in a pan over medium heat and cook the onion for 3–4 minutes or until it begins to soften. Add the ground spices and chilli flakes and stir until fragrant, then stir in the garlic, tomatoes and sugar and simmer for 5 minutes or until thickened.

4   Remove the pan from the heat. Stir in the eggplant, mint and coriander and serve.

> **TIP** If you prefer, the eggplants can be cooked whole on a chargrill or barbecue. Turn them frequently until the skins are blackened, then remove them from the heat and allow to cool. Peel, discarding the skins, then chop the flesh into cubes.

Zucchini, pumpkin and tomato gratin

SERVES 4   PREP 15 mins   COOK 45 mins

olive oil spray
500 g pumpkin (squash), peeled,
    seeded and thinly sliced
4 zucchini (courgettes), trimmed
    and thinly sliced lengthways
100 g finely grated parmesan
    or pecorino
2 roma (plum) tomatoes, thinly sliced
small handful basil or oregano leaves,
    torn (optional)
1 tablespoon balsamic vinegar

This easy gratin can be served hot, warm or at room temperature, and goes particularly well with roast or grilled lamb, beef or chicken.

1 Preheat the oven to 180°C.

2 Spray the base and sides of a 2 litre baking dish with olive oil spray. Place half the pumpkin slices over the base, overlapping slightly as necessary to cover the base. Season with salt and pepper, then use half the zucchini slices to cover the pumpkin in a single layer, overlapping as necessary. Sprinkle over half the cheese, then place the tomatoes in a layer on top and scatter over the basil or oregano leaves (if using). Use the remaining zucchini to form a layer, then season again and scatter over the remaining cheese. Finally, place the remaining pumpkin over the top in a neat layer.

3 Cover the dish with foil, then bake for 30 minutes. Remove the foil and bake for another 15 minutes or until the vegetables are tender.

TIP Omit the cheese if you like: it won't taste as rich, but will still be delicious.

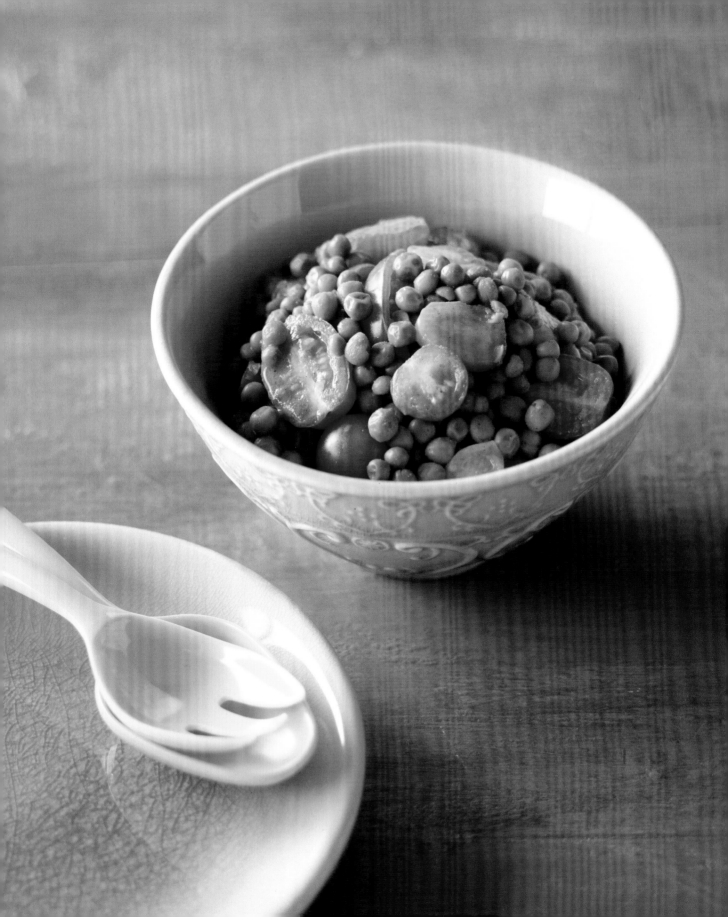

1 SERVE =
2 units vegetables
½ unit fats

Hot curried peas and tomatoes

SERVES 4   PREP 5 mins   COOK 10 mins

2 teaspoons vegetable oil
2½ teaspoons mild curry powder,
    or to taste
3 cups (360 g) frozen peas
250 g cherry tomatoes, halved
2 tablespoons lemon juice,
    or to taste

Serve this simple side dish with grilled red meat or chicken.

1 Heat the oil in a large saucepan over medium heat, then sprinkle in
   the curry powder and cook, stirring, for 1 minute or until fragrant.
   Add the peas, cover with the lid and cook, stirring occasionally,
   for 3–4 minutes or until the peas have softened slightly.

2 Add the tomato and ½ cup (125 ml) water, then cook, covered for
   5 minutes, stirring occasionally, until the tomato has softened and
   the peas are tender. Add a little more water if necessary.

3 Season to taste with salt and pepper, add the lemon juice, then serve.

Sweet potato and ginger mash

SERVES 4   PREP 15 mins   **COOK** 20 mins

2 teaspoons vegetable oil
1 × 2.5 cm piece ginger,
   peeled and finely chopped
1 teaspoon ground ginger
2 large sweet potatoes,
   peeled and chopped

This is a hearty, spicy side that goes well with grilled fish or meats.

1   Heat the oil in a medium-sized saucepan, add the ginger then cook, stirring, over medium heat for 1–2 minutes or until fragrant. Add the ground ginger, sweet potato and enough water to just cover, then bring to the boil. Reduce the heat to low–medium, then cover and cook for 20 minutes or until the sweet potato is tender.

2   Drain well, reserving the cooking liquid, then mash with a vegetable masher, adding enough of the reserved cooking liquid as is necessary to form a soft mash.

3   Season to taste with salt and pepper and serve immediately.

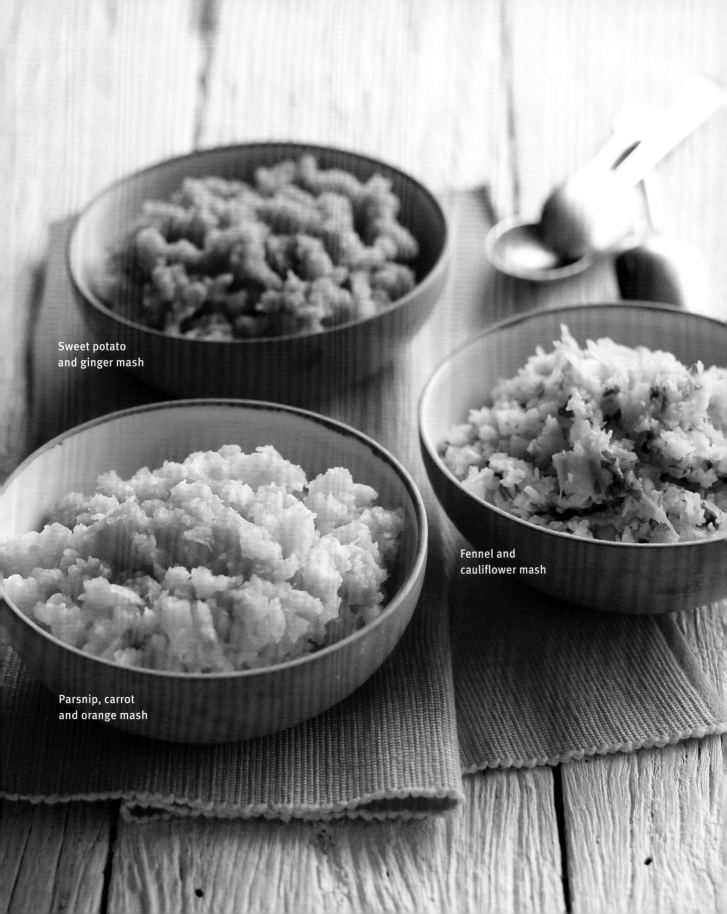

Sweet potato
and ginger mash

Fennel and
cauliflower mash

Parsnip, carrot
and orange mash

Fennel and cauliflower mash

SERVES 4   PREP 12 mins   COOK 25 mins

½ large head cauliflower, trimmed
 and coarsely chopped
2 bulbs fennel, trimmed and
 coarsely chopped
approximately 1 litre reduced-fat milk
small handful flat-leaf (Italian)
 parsley leaves, finely chopped
 (optional)

This mash has a subtle flavour and a lovely soft texture. Try it with fish or chicken.

1   Place the vegetables and milk in a saucepan, adding more milk or water to just cover the vegetables. Bring to simmering point, then cover and cook over low–medium heat for 25 minutes or until the vegetables are very tender.

2   Drain, reserving the cooking liquid. Mash the vegetables with a vegetable masher, adding enough of the reserved cooking liquid as is necessary to form a soft mash.

3   Season to taste with salt and pepper and return the mash to the saucepan. Place over low heat, cover and cook for 2–3 minutes, stirring often, to heat through. Stir through the parsley (if using) and serve.

1 SERVE =
½ unit fruit
1½ units vegetables

Parsnip, carrot and orange mash

SERVES 4 PREP 10 mins COOK 20 mins

2 parsnips, peeled and chopped
4 carrots, chopped
¾ cup (180 ml) orange juice
2 teaspoons finely grated orange zest

Lighter than ordinary mash, with the added zestiness of orange, this goes beautifully with any pork or chicken dish.

1 Combine the parsnip and carrot in a saucepan, cover with cold water, then bring to the boil. Cook over medium heat for 20 minutes or until the vegetables are tender, then drain well.

2 Add the orange juice and zest, then mash well with a vegetable masher.

> **TIP** Use a stick blender to puree the vegetables for a smoother texture if you like.

Spiced red lentils with green beans and mint

SERVES 4   PREP 15 mins   COOK 45 mins

1 tablespoon olive oil
1 onion, chopped
2 cloves garlic, crushed
1 tablespoon grated ginger
½ teaspoon fennel seeds
2 teaspoons turmeric
1 tablespoon garam masala
½ teaspoon cardamom seeds
1 green chilli, seeded and
    finely chopped
1 × 400 g tin diced tomatoes
400 g red lentils, rinsed
200 g pumpkin, peeled
    and cut into 2 cm dice
1 cup (250 ml) water
150 g green beans
2 tablespoons shredded mint
$^1/_3$ cup (95 g) reduced-fat
    natural yoghurt, to serve

1 Heat oil in a large saucepan over medium heat.
   Add onion, garlic and ginger and cook, stirring, for
   5 minutes, or until onion is golden. Add spices and
   chilli and cook, stirring constantly, for 1 minute. Add
   tomato, lentils, pumpkin and water (the vegetables
   should be covered – if not, just add a little more
   water), and bring to a boil. Reduce heat and
   simmer for 30 minutes, or until lentils are soft.

2 Add beans and cook for a further 3 minutes. Gently
   stir mint through and lightly season. Serve with
   a dollop of yoghurt and rice from your daily bread
   allowance, if desired.

Carrot and dill bake

SERVES 4   PREP 15 mins   COOK 30 mins

**This is a lovely, warming side dish that goes
well with fish or chicken.**

650 g carrots, grated
2 tablespoons plain flour
4 egg whites
small handful dill, chopped
olive oil spray

1 Preheat the oven to 180°C.

2 Combine the grated carrot and flour in a large bowl,
   season to taste with salt and pepper, then toss to
   combine well. Using electric beaters, whisk the egg
   whites until soft peaks form, then stir into the carrot
   mixture along with the dill.

3 Spray a large baking dish with olive oil, then pour the
   carrot mixture in, smoothing the top evenly. Bake for
   40 minutes or until the surface is deep golden and
   crisp and the carrot is tender. Serve hot.

1 SERVE =
1½ units vegetables
1 unit fats

Grilled vegetable salad with basil and black olives

SERVES 8 PREP 20 mins COOK 10 mins

Grilling vegetables seems to enhance and condense their flavour, adding a smokiness that makes them hard to resist. The olives add a salty contrast.

16 baby roma (plum) tomatoes, halved
2 zucchini (courgettes), thinly sliced
2 red capsicums (peppers), seeded and cut into strips
16 spears asparagus, trimmed
olive oil spray
200 g baby salad leaves
16 black olives, pitted
1 cup (50 g) shredded basil

VINAIGRETTE
2 cloves garlic, crushed
2 tablespoons extra virgin olive oil
¼ cup (60 ml) verjuice or white wine vinegar

1 Combine the vinaigrette ingredients in a screw-top jar and shake well to combine.

2 Heat a barbecue or chargrill to hot. Spray the tomato, zucchini, capsicum and asparagus with olive oil, then grill for 2–3 minutes each side, or until cooked through.

3 Place the salad leaves on a platter and top with the grilled vegetables, olives and basil. Pour the dressing over the top and serve.

TIP Try introducing other vegetables into this salad, such as diced eggplant, sliced fennel, sliced onion, or mushrooms.

Roasted herb and allspice onions

SERVES 4   PREP 8 mins   COOK 45 mins

2 teaspoons olive oil
1 clove garlic, crushed
1 tablespoon finely chopped
   flat-leaf (Italian) parsley
2 teaspoons finely chopped rosemary
3 teaspoons finely chopped
   thyme leaves
½ teaspoon ground allspice
pinch ground cloves
6 onions, unpeeled and
   halved lengthways

These sweet spiced onions will be a real hit. Serve with your favourite grilled or lean roast meats – these go especially well with beef and lamb.

1 Preheat the oven to 180°C.

2 Place the olive oil, garlic, herbs and spices in a bowl and toss to combine well.

3 Place the onion halves in a roasting dish, cut-side up, then spoon the herb mixture over. Roast for 25–30 minutes or until golden, then cover the dish with foil and roast for another 15 minutes or until the onion halves are tender.

TIP Peel the onions first if you like, but take care to leave the root end intact or they will fall apart as they cook.

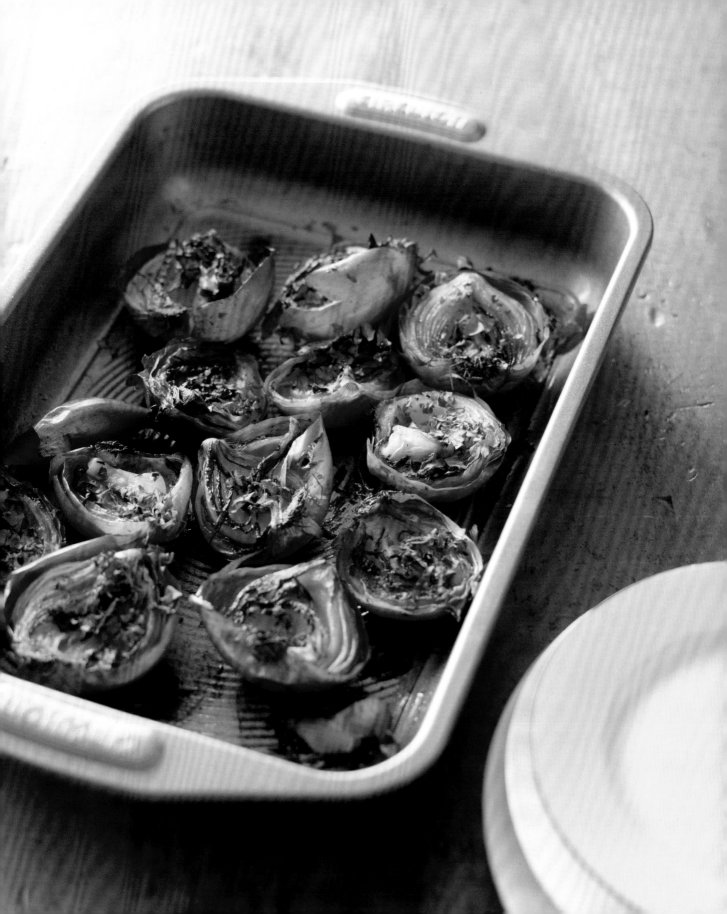

Roasted cherry tomatoes and asparagus with lemon thyme

SERVES 4   **PREP** 10 mins   **COOK** 10 mins

2 punnets cherry tomatoes
24 spears asparagus, cut into
  6 cm pieces
1 tablespoon olive oil
1 tablespoon picked lemon
  thyme leaves
100 g rocket (arugula)

1 Preheat oven to 200°C.

2 Place tomatoes, asparagus, oil and thyme in a large bowl and mix well. Lightly season. Transfer to an ovenproof dish and bake for 10 minutes, or until tomatoes start to split. Remove from oven and toss vegetables through rocket. Serve immediately.

3 Goes well with lamb, pork, chicken or fish.

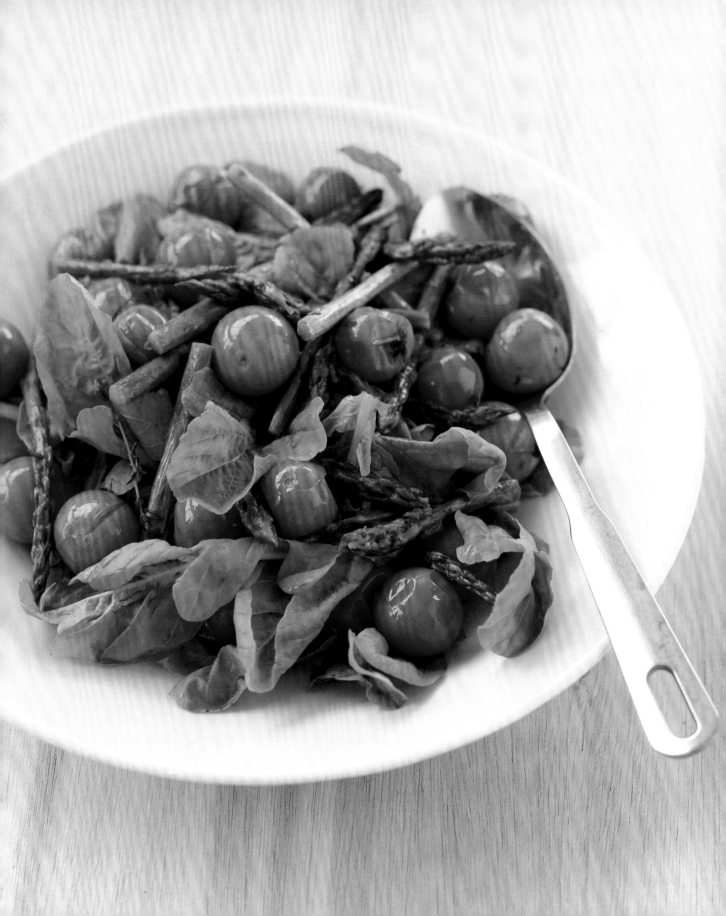

Green beans and asparagus with garlic breadcrumbs

SERVES 4   PREP 10 mins   COOK 10 mins

2 slices wholegrain bread
150 g green beans, trimmed
12 spears asparagus, trimmed
1 tablespoon olive oil
2 cloves garlic, crushed

The crunchy breadcrumbs in this dish transform the steamed greens into something special.

1   Pulse the bread in a food processor to form fine breadcrumbs.

2   Steam or microwave the green beans and asparagus for 4–5 minutes or until tender and just cooked.

3   Heat the olive oil in a small frying pan over medium heat, add the breadcrumbs and garlic and cook, stirring, for 5 minutes or until the crumbs are golden and crunchy.

4   Serve the beans and asparagus topped with the garlic breadcrumbs.

North African vegetable stew

SERVES 4   PREP 25 mins   COOK 25 mins

2 teaspoons olive oil

2 tablespoons Moroccan spice mix

3 carrots, thinly sliced

½ head cauliflower, cut into florets

1 large red capsicum (pepper),
trimmed, seeded and cut
into large pieces

¾ cup (180 ml) salt-reduced
chicken stock

500 g pumpkin (squash), peeled,
seeded and cut into 2 cm pieces

3 tomatoes, cut into 2 cm pieces

handful mint leaves, chopped
(optional)

This rustic stew is lovely served with couscous (see page 518) for lunch, or enjoy it for dinner served with your favourite grilled meat or fish and a green salad alongside.

1   Heat the oil in a large non-stick saucepan over low–medium heat, then add the spice mix and cook, stirring, for 1–2 minutes or until fragrant. Add the carrot, cauliflower, capsicum and stock and stir to combine well. Bring to a simmer, then cover and cook for 5 minutes.

2   Add the pumpkin, and a little extra water if necessary to just cover the pumpkin, then cover with the lid and cook for 12 minutes or until all the vegetables are tender. Add the tomato, season to taste with salt and pepper, then cover and cook for 5 minutes or until the tomato is heated through. Stir through the mint (if using) and serve.

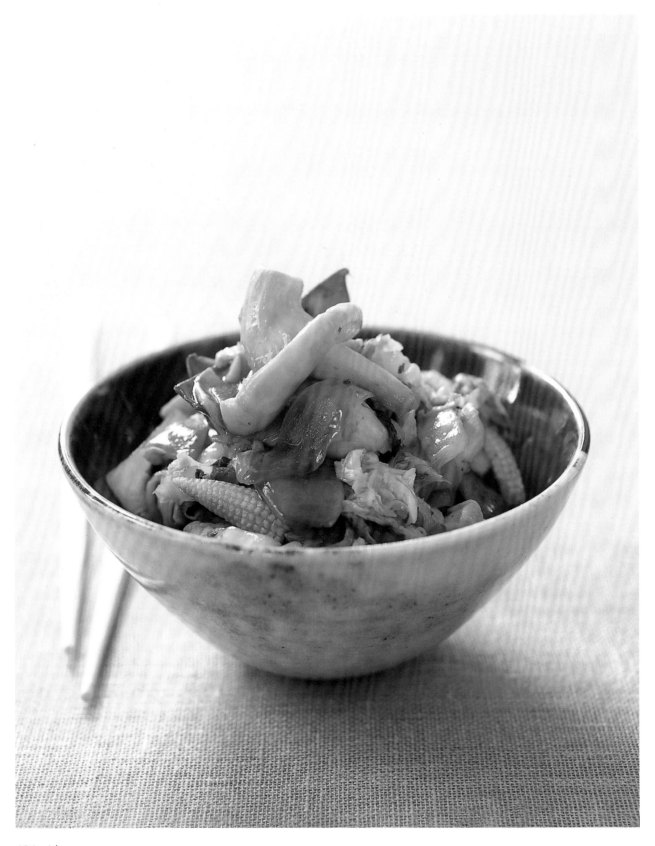

Stir-fried baby corn
with snowpeas

SERVES 4   PREP 10 mins   COOK 10 mins

1 tablespoon peanut oil
1 clove garlic
1 teaspoon grated ginger
1 onion, sliced
150 g snowpeas (mange-tout)
150 g oyster mushrooms
350 g Chinese cabbage, shredded
100 g baby corn
2 tablespoons oyster sauce
1 tablespoon light soy sauce
2 tablespoons coriander
   (cilantro) leaves

1   Heat a wok or large frying pan over high heat. Add oil and, when smoking, add garlic, ginger and onion and stir-fry for 2–3 minutes, or until onion begins to soften. Add snowpeas, mushrooms, cabbage and corn and stir-fry for 5 minutes, or until almost cooked. Add oyster sauce, soy sauce and coriander and cook for 1 minute. Serve immediately.

Italian broccoli

SERVES 4   PREP 20 mins   COOK 45 mins

800 g broccoli (about 2 heads)

4 anchovy fillets, drained of oil
    and finely chopped

6 cloves garlic, finely chopped

¹/₃ cup (80 ml) lemon juice

¼ cup (50 g) drained
    capers (optional)

300 ml salt-reduced chicken
    or vegetable stock

handful flat-leaf (Italian) parsley
    leaves, chopped

dried chilli flakes, to taste (optional)

This chunky 'sauce' can be served for lunch with pasta or on bruschetta or pizza, or with grilled meat or fish for dinner. It's easy and quick to prepare and needs barely any attention once it's cooking. Don't be alarmed by the amount of garlic – the long cooking renders it sweet and mild and not at all overpowering.

1   Using a large, sharp knife, trim 1 cm from the end of the broccoli stems, then finely chop the broccoli, including the stems.

2   Combine all the ingredients except the parsley and chilli flakes in a saucepan. Bring the mixture to simmering point, cover the pan and cook over medium heat for 35 minutes or until the broccoli is very tender and most of the liquid has evaporated. Remove the lid and cook for 5–10 minutes to allow the excess liquid to evaporate.

3   Season with salt and pepper, stir in the parsley and chilli flakes to taste (if using), then serve hot or at room temperature.

TIP This freezes well, so when broccoli is in season you can easily double the recipe to have some leftover to freeze.

Sesame tofu with Asian mushrooms

SERVES 4   **PREP** 10 mins   **COOK** 20 mins

2 teaspoons sesame seeds
400 g firm tofu
2 tablespoons olive oil
1 cup shiitake mushrooms
1 cup enoki mushrooms
1 cup oyster mushrooms
1 clove garlic, finely sliced
¼ cup (60 ml) light soy sauce
¼ cup (60 ml) vegetable stock
½ cup finely sliced spring
   onion (scallion)
1 teaspoon cornflour (cornstarch)
1 tablespoon cold water
1 tablespoon chopped coriander
   (cilantro) leaves

1   Preheat oven to 150°C.

2   Heat a small non-stick frying pan over medium heat. Add sesame seeds and toss for 5 minutes, or until lightly toasted. Set aside.

3   Cut tofu into 1.5 cm slices and dab with paper towel to absorb as much water as possible. Heat half the oil in a large non-stick frying pan over high heat. Add tofu and cook for 3 minutes each side, or until golden. Transfer tofu to a serving plate and keep warm in the oven.

4   Reduce heat to medium and add remaining oil to pan. Add mushrooms and garlic and saute for 5 minutes, or until mushrooms are soft and golden. Add soy sauce and stock and bring to a boil. Add spring onion. Mix cornflour with water, then pour into liquid in pan and stir over heat until sauce has thickened. Add coriander. Arrange tofu on serving plates, spoon mushroom mixture over and sprinkle with toasted sesame seeds.

1 SERVE =
2½ units vegetables
2 units fats

Chunky ratatouille bake

SERVES 4   PREP 15 mins   COOK 45 mins

1 red (Spanish) onion, peeled leaving
   root end intact and cut into wedges
1 red capsicum (pepper), trimmed,
   seeded and cut into large pieces
1 green capsicum (pepper), trimmed,
   seeded and cut into large pieces
1 eggplant (aubergine), trimmed
   and cut into 3 cm pieces
3 zucchini (courgettes), trimmed
   and cut into large pieces
3 tomatoes, cut into chunks
   or wedges
1 tablespoon olive oil
¼ cup (60 ml) balsamic or
   red wine vinegar
¾ cup (120 g) pitted kalamata olives
1 tablespoon fresh thyme leaves or
   1½ teaspoons dried thyme

These flavours go well with almost any type of meat or fish.

1 Preheat the oven to 180°C. Combine all the vegetables in one or
   two roasting dishes (make sure the vegetables are not too crowded).
   Drizzle over the oil and vinegar and toss to coat, then scatter over
   the olives and thyme.

2 Bake for 45 minutes or until the vegetables are tender, then season
   to taste with salt and pepper and serve.

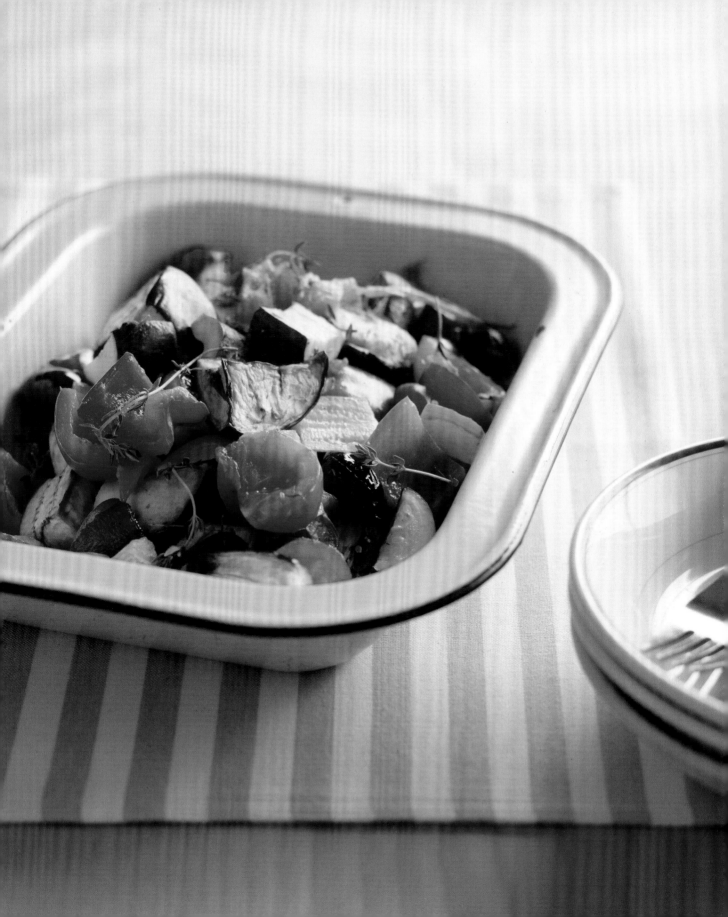

Cos lettuce with buttermilk dressing

SERVES 4   PREP 10 mins

4 baby cos lettuce, tough outer
   leaves removed, lettuce
   halved lengthways

BUTTERMILK DRESSING
¾ cup (180 ml) reduced-fat buttermilk
1 tablespoon lemon juice
2½ teaspoons Dijon mustard
2½ teaspoons horseradish cream
1 bunch dill, chopped

A simple, elegant side dish that goes with just about everything. Break up the cos lettuce and pour the dressing over if you want a tossed salad.

1   For the dressing, place all the ingredients in a bowl and whisk until smooth and well combined.

2   Divide the lettuce among plates, then drizzle over the dressing and serve immediately.

TIP Use iceberg or your favourite lettuce instead of cos.

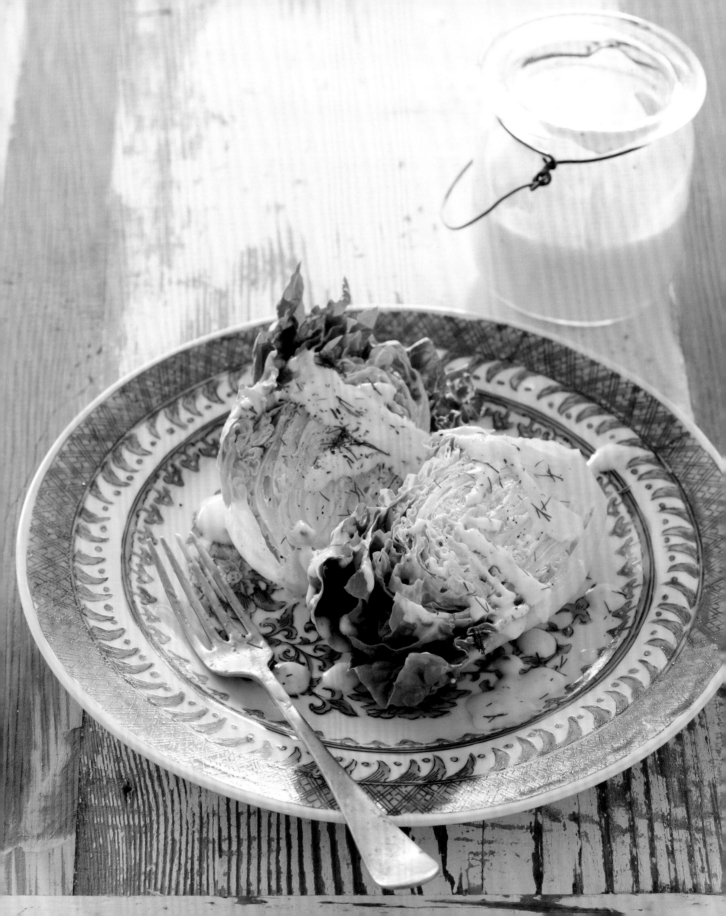

1 SERVE =
¼ unit fruit
2 units vegetables
½ unit fats

Mixed cabbage and pear coleslaw

SERVES 4   **PREP** 15 mins

about ¼ small red cabbage,
  finely shredded (you'll need
  2½ cups shredded cabbage)
about ¼ small green cabbage,
  finely shredded (you'll need
  2½ cups shredded cabbage)
250 g kohlrabi, trimmed, peeled
  and cut into fine matchsticks
1 firm ripe pear, halved, cored
  and thinly sliced
large handful flat-leaf (Italian)
  parsley leaves
½ cup (125 ml) reduced-fat
  mayonnaise
¼ cup (60 ml) lemon juice

A sweet and colourful version of classic coleslaw. If you can't find kohlrabi at the greengrocers, use celeriac or celery instead.

1   Place all the ingredients in a large bowl and gently toss to combine
    well. Serve immediately.

Stir-fried beans, mushrooms and asparagus

SERVES 4   PREP 10 mins   COOK 5 mins

1 tablespoon olive oil

250 g green beans or snake beans, trimmed and cut into 5 cm lengths

150 g mushrooms, halved if large

1 bunch asparagus, trimmed and halved

2 cloves garlic, crushed

1 tablespoon grated ginger

4 spring onions, sliced

1 tablespoon oyster sauce

2 tablespoons soy sauce

¼ cup (60 ml) salt-reduced chicken stock or water

coriander (cilantro) leaves, to serve (optional)

This is a delicious combination, but the ingredients given below are just suggestions – vary the vegetables according to what you have to hand, and where possible use a mixture of mushrooms for added interest.

1 Heat the olive oil in a wok or frying pan over high heat. Add the beans, mushrooms and asparagus and stir-fry for 3 minutes or until the vegetables are just starting to colour (you may need to do this in two batches to maintain the heat).

2 Add the garlic, ginger and spring onion and cook for 30 seconds until fragrant. Pour in the oyster sauce, soy sauce and stock or water and toss until heated through. Serve immediately, garnished with coriander leaves (if using), with protein from your daily allowance.

Lemon-thyme braised leeks and radishes

SERVES 4   PREP 10 mins   COOK 45 mins

4 leeks, trimmed leaving the root
    end intact, and washed
2 bunches radishes, washed,
    trimmed and halved
1 bay leaf, bruised
2 sprigs thyme
1½ cups (375 ml) salt-reduced
    chicken stock
¼ cup (60 ml) lemon juice
zest of 1 lemon, removed in strips
    with a vegetable peeler and cut
    into fine matchsticks

**Serve this warm or at room temperature. This works equally
well with parsley or chives if you don't have thyme.**

1   Preheat the oven to 180°C and place the leeks and radishes in a baking
    dish or roasting tin.

2   Combine the remaining ingredients in a saucepan and bring to the
    boil. Pour this mixture over the vegetables in the dish, then season to
    taste with salt and pepper. Cover the dish tightly with foil and braise
    in the oven for 45 minutes or until the vegetables are very tender.

3   Serve hot, warm or at room temperature.

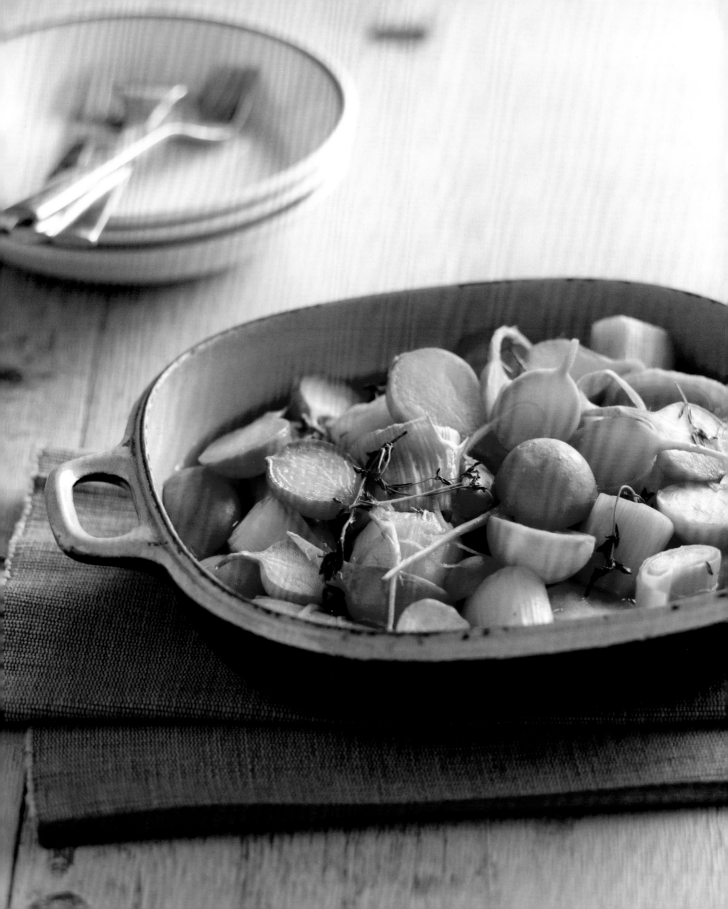

Spicy roasted cauliflower

SERVES 4   PREP 5 mins   COOK 30 mins

1 small or ½ large cauliflower,
   cut into florets
1 tablespoon extra virgin olive oil
1 tablespoon Cajun spice mix
reduced-fat natural yoghurt,
   to serve (optional)

This simple recipe makes a delicious accompaniment for grilled chicken, lamb or fish. If you don't have any Cajun spice mix in the pantry, use Moroccan spice mix or curry powder instead.

1 Preheat the oven to 200°C and line a baking tray with baking paper.

2 Combine the cauliflower, olive oil and spice mix in a bowl and toss to coat. Place the cauliflower on the tray in a single layer and roast for 30 minutes or until well coloured, turning once or twice.

3 Serve with a dollop of yoghurt, if desired, and protein from your daily allowance.

Grilled eggplant with tomatoes and balsamic vinegar

SERVES 4   **PREP** 15 mins   **COOK** 15 mins

3 eggplants (aubergines),
   sliced into rounds
2 tablespoons olive oil
2 red (Spanish) onions, diced
2 cloves garlic, crushed
800 g tomatoes, diced
¼ cup roughly chopped mint
¼ cup roughly torn basil
2 tablespoons balsamic vinegar
1 tablespoon capers, chopped

1   Preheat a grill plate or barbecue grill to high. Lightly brush eggplant slices with half the oil, and season lightly. Grill for 2 minutes each side, or until browned. Transfer to a large mixing bowl and set aside.

2   Heat remaining oil in a large saucepan over high heat. Add onions and garlic and cook for 5 minutes, or until onions begin to soften. Add tomatoes and cook for a further 2 minutes. Season to taste. Pour tomato mixture over eggplant and add herbs, balsamic vinegar and capers. Carefully toss, and serve warm or cold.

3   Goes well with chicken or fish.

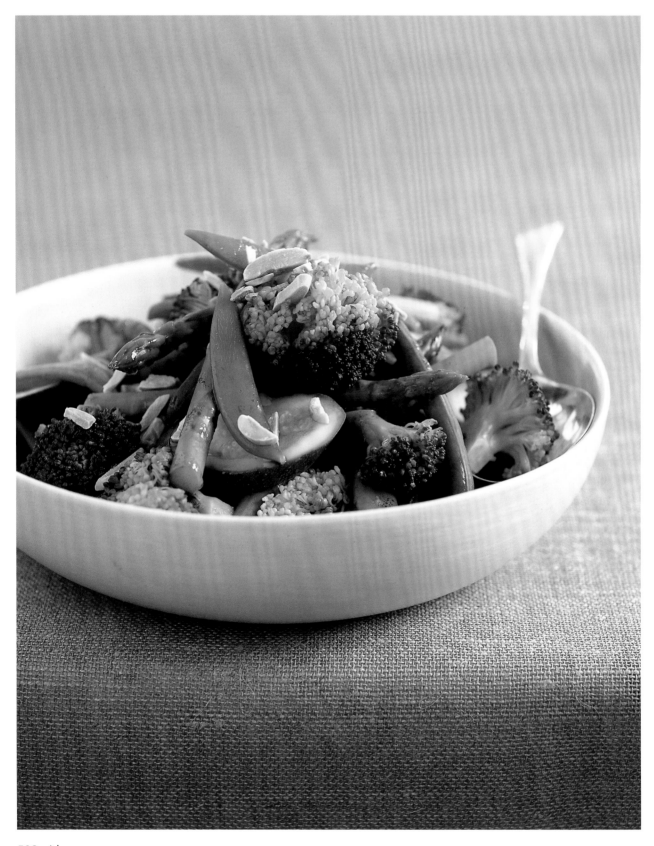

Steamed greens with toasted almonds

SERVES 4   **PREP** 5 mins   **COOK** 15 mins

2 tablespoons flaked almonds

12 spears asparagus

250 g broccoli, broken into florets

2 zucchini (courgette), chopped
into 4 cm lengths

150 g baby beans

100 g sugar snap peas

2 teaspoons olive oil

1 teaspoon balsamic vinegar

1 Heat a small non-stick frying pan over medium heat. Add almonds and toss for 5 minutes, or until lightly toasted. Set aside.

2 Place asparagus in a steamer and steam for 3 minutes. Add broccoli, zucchini, beans and peas and steam for a further 5 minutes, or until all vegetables are tender. Transfer to a bowl and toss gently with oil and balsamic vinegar. Scatter with almonds and serve immediately.

Green salad

SERVES 4   PREP 10 mins

1 butter lettuce, tough outer
  leaves discarded
1 head radicchio, tough outer leaves
  discarded *or* 1 bunch curly endive
  (frisee), trimmed
large handful rocket leaves
2 baby cos lettuces, tough
  outer leaves discarded
¼ cup (60 ml) balsamic vinegar,
  or to taste

Consider using a variety of three or four different types of leaves for added flavour and texture when making a salad. A bitter leaf, such as radicchio or curly endive, can make a nice contrast to the softer, sweeter leaves, such as butter lettuce or oak leaf lettuce. Cos lettuce is wonderful for adding crispness, as is witlof (not a lettuce at all, but a member of the endive family and lovely eaten raw in salads). A peppery leaf, such as rocket or watercress, is another excellent flavour to introduce.

To avoid dipping into your fats allowance, use lemon juice, red wine vinegar, balsamic vinegar, lime or orange juice to dress the salad. Add the dressing at the very last minute to avoid the leaves turning soggy.

1   Remove the leaves from the lettuces and gently wash them by submerging them in a large bowl or sink of cold water. Shake off excess water, then, working in batches, spin the leaves dry in a salad spinner and transfer to a large bowl.

2   Drizzle over the vinegar and toss to combine well. Season to taste with salt and pepper, then serve.

TIP If you're short of time, make a salad using a bag of pre-mixed leaves available from the supermarket. Allow about 2 cups of leaves per person.

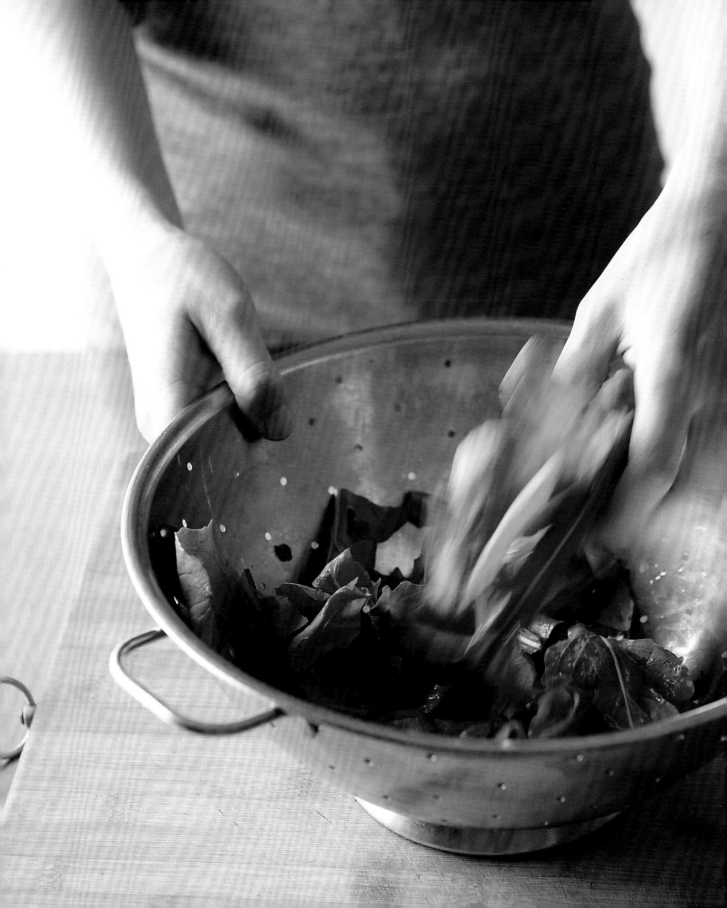

1 SERVE =
2 units protein
1 unit vegetables
1 unit fats

Steamed tofu with Asian greens

SERVES 4   PREP 10 mins   COOK 15 mins

800 g silken tofu, drained
2 teaspoons sesame oil
2 teaspoons vegetable oil
100 ml light soy sauce
2 teaspoons oyster sauce
1 red chilli, seeded and
    finely chopped
4 spring onions, finely sliced
handful of coriander (cilantro) leaves
8 baby bok choy or other Asian
    greens, steamed or blanched

This light and delicate dish works really well as a balanced meat-free option for lunch or dinner.

1   Pour water into the base of a steamer or a wok with a steamer basket and bring to the boil. Place the tofu on a plate which will fit in the steamer and cut it into 4 cm pieces but do not break apart. Cover and steam for about 10 minutes, then drain the liquid from the steamed tofu.

2   Meanwhile, heat the oils, soy sauce and oyster sauce in a small saucepan. Stir in the chilli and spring onion, then remove from the heat.

3   Pour the sauce over the tofu and sprinkle with coriander leaves. Serve with the Asian greens and rice from your daily bread allowance.

TIP   To save time and to increase the vegetable content of the meal, steam an assortment of chopped vegetables with the tofu.

1 SERVE =
1½ units vegetables
½ unit fats

Asparagus, snowpea and mushroom stir-fry

SERVES 4 **PREP** 15 mins **COOK** 6 mins

2 teaspoons vegetable oil

2 cloves garlic, crushed

1 × 2.5 cm piece ginger, finely chopped

300 g button mushrooms, thinly sliced

2 bunches asparagus, trimmed, spears halved lengthways, then chopped into 5 cm pieces

300 g snowpeas (mange-tout), trimmed

¼ cup (60 ml) mirin

2 tablespoons rice wine vinegar

1 tablespoon salt-reduced light soy sauce

1½ teaspoons cornflour

A fresh and crunchy accompaniment that's so easy to make.

1 Heat the oil in a wok over high heat. Add the garlic, ginger, mushrooms, asparagus and snowpeas and stir-fry for 3–4 minutes or until the vegetables have softened.

2 Add the mirin, rice wine vinegar and soy sauce and stir-fry, tossing the wok often, for 1 minute or until the liquid boils. Meanwhile, combine the cornflour with 1 tablespoon water to form a paste, then add to the wok and cook for 1 minute or until the liquid has thickened and the vegetables are tender. Serve immediately.

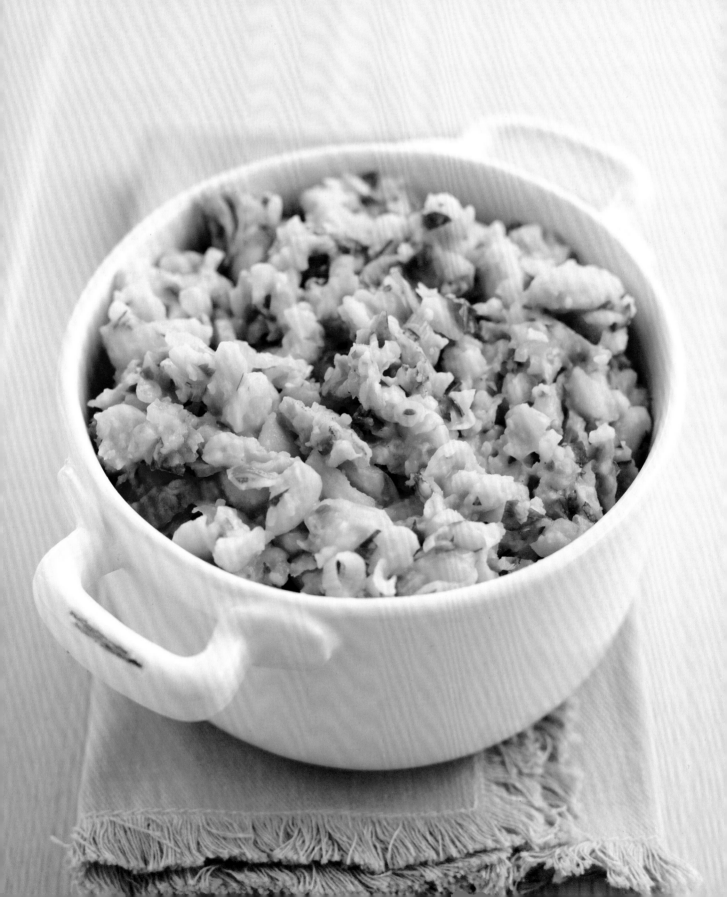

1 SERVE =
1 unit bread
1 unit fats

White beans with spring onions and fresh herbs

SERVES 4 **PREP** 10 mins **COOK** 10 mins

1 tablespoon olive oil
4 spring onions (scallions),
   finely sliced
1 clove garlic, finely chopped
½ green chilli, finely chopped
4 slices prosciutto, finely chopped
1 × 400 g tin cannellini beans,
   drained and rinsed
½ cup (125 ml) chicken stock
1 tablespoon chopped flat-leaf
   (Italian) parsley
1 tablespoon chopped oregano

1 Heat oil in a large heavy-based saucepan over high heat. Add spring onions, garlic and chilli and cook for 30 seconds. Add prosciutto and cook for a further minute. Add beans and stir well, then add stock and bring to a boil. Reduce heat and simmer for 5 minutes. Lightly crush beans with a fork, then stir through the herbs.

2 Goes well with pork or chicken.

Stir-fried vegetables

SERVES 4   PREP 10 mins   COOK 7 mins

2 teaspoons sesame oil
1 bunch Chinese broccoli (gai lan), trimmed, stems thinly sliced
1 bunch choy sum, trimmed, stems thinly sliced
3 cloves garlic, crushed
1 × 3 cm piece ginger, peeled and cut into fine matchsticks
4 baby bok choy, trimmed and quartered lengthways
¼ cup (60 ml) hoisin sauce
¼ cup (60 ml) salt-reduced chicken stock
2 tablespoons Chinese shaohsing rice wine or dry sherry

Stir-fried vegetables make for a crispy, crunchy and delicious side dish. A wide variety of Asian vegetables is readily available: try Chinese cabbage, bok choy, choy sum, tat soy and mustard leaves. Don't waste the hard stalks you trim away – thinly slice them and cook them for 3–4 minutes to soften them, before adding the leaves, either whole or sliced. Thinly sliced onion, celery, carrot and mushrooms are also great in stir-fries, as are beans, peas, asparagus, snowpeas, sugar snap peas and spinach. Thick vegetables, such as beans and asparagus, should be sliced or chopped for stir-frying. Flavourings can include chopped chilli, galangal or lemongrass, and you can use fish, oyster or black bean sauce instead of hoisin sauce.

1 Heat a wok over medium–high heat. Once hot, add the oil, Chinese broccoli stems, choy sum stems, garlic, ginger and bok choy, then stir-fry for about 4 minutes or until the stems have softened.

2 Add the remaining ingredients, including the Chinese broccoli and choy sum leaves, then toss to combine well. Stir-fry, tossing the wok often, for 3 minutes or until the vegetables are tender and the liquid has reduced and thickened. Serve immediately.

TIP If your wok is small, then cook the vegetables in batches. Start with those that take the longest, then remove them from the wok and cook the quick-cooking veg. Return them all to the wok to toss through just before serving.

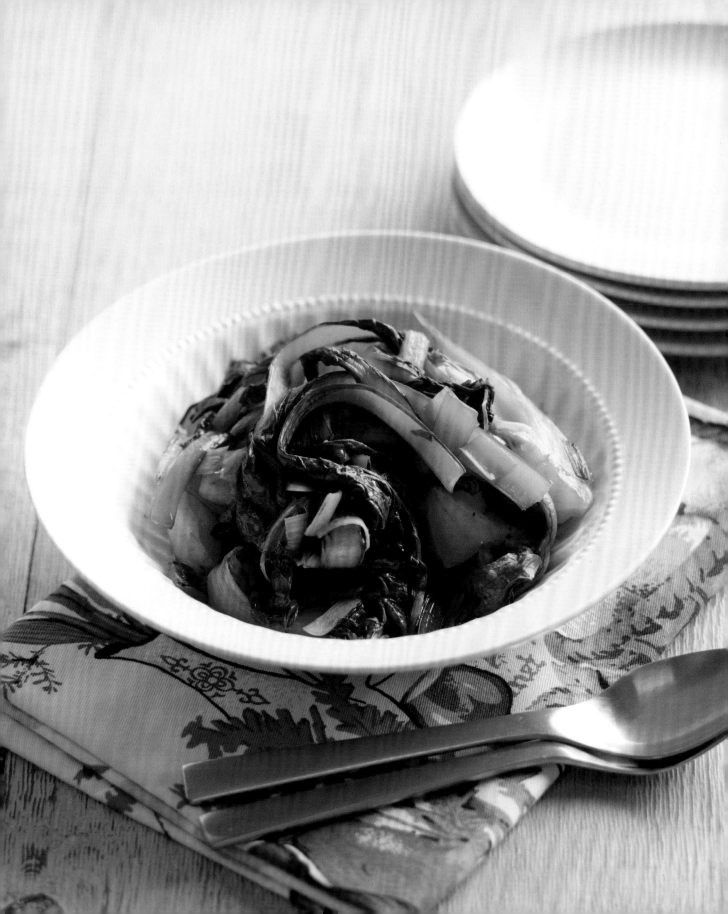

Couscous

SERVES 4   PREP 5 mins + standing time

Couscous is such a versatile staple – so quick and easy to prepare and a great base to add all kinds of flavourings to.

½ cup (100 g) couscous
½ cup (125 ml) boiling water

1 Place the couscous in a heatproof bowl. Pour over the boiling water, then cover the bowl with plastic wrap. Leave the couscous to stand for 5 minutes, or until the liquid has been absorbed and the grains are softened.

2 Fluff the couscous with a fork, separating the grains. Add your desired flavourings, then season to taste and serve.

VARIATIONS

Substitute hot orange juice for the water. Before serving, stir through 60 g currants and 1 teaspoon finely grated orange zest (this will add ½ unit fruit). Peel and finely chop 1 × 1 cm piece ginger and add to the couscous with 1 teaspoon finely grated lemon zest before adding the water. Before serving, stir in a small handful of chopped coriander leaves. Add 80 g chopped pistachios, 60 g chopped dried apricots and a pinch of saffron threads to the couscous before adding the water. Stir in a small handful of chopped mint before serving (this will add ½ unit fruit and 1 unit fats).

Steamed rice

SERVES 4   COOK 12 mins + standing time

Cook rice in salt-reduced chicken stock instead of water for a richer flavour.

²/₃ cup (130 g) long-grain rice
1¹/₃ cups (330 ml) cold water

1 Combine the rice and water in a small saucepan, then cover and bring slowly to simmering point over medium heat. Reduce the heat to very low and cook the rice for about 12 minutes or until all the liquid has been absorbed.

2 Remove from the heat and leave to stand, covered, for 5 minutes before serving.

VARIATIONS

Replace half the water with tomato juice and add 1 finely chopped tomato to the rice at the start of cooking. Add a large handful of chopped spinach leaves, a small handful of chopped flat-leaf (Italian) parsley leaves and some chopped coriander to the rice at the start of cooking. For spice-scented rice, add half a cinnamon stick, a star anise and 2–3 slices of fresh ginger to the rice at the start of cooking.

Oven-steamed vegetables

SERVES 4   PREP 15 mins   COOK 15 mins

1 cup (250 ml) salt-reduced
    chicken stock
½ small head cauliflower, trimmed
    and cut into large florets
300 g brussels sprouts, trimmed
    and halved lengthways
1 head broccoli (about 400 g),
    trimmed and cut into large florets
1 large green capsicum (pepper),
    trimmed, seeded and cut into
    2 cm pieces
finely grated zest and juice
    of 1 large lemon
3 sprigs thyme
1 bay leaf
handful flat-leaf (Italian)
    parsley leaves, chopped
    (optional)

Although these vegetables are cooked in the oven, they actually steam rather than bake due to the amount of liquid in the roasting tin. Not only is this a great alternative to cooking in a steamer, but you can also add all sorts of herbs and aromatics to the steaming liquid to add flavour to your vegetables.

Many types of vegetables can be steamed in this way, including carrots, snowpeas, beans, asparagus, peas, broad beans, leeks, silverbeet, spinach, bok choy and other Asian greens, corn and zucchini. Just make sure the vegetables are all cut into roughly the same-sized pieces, and take care not to overcrowd the roasting tin.

1 Preheat the oven to 200°C. Bring the chicken stock to the boil in a small saucepan.

2 Combine all the vegetables in a large roasting tin. Season to taste with salt and pepper, then sprinkle over the lemon zest and juice. Scatter over the thyme and bay leaf, then pour over the hot stock.

3 Cover the tin tightly with foil and bake for 15 minutes or until the vegetables are tender. Sprinkle over the parsley (if using), then serve immediately.

VARIATIONS

Peel and finely chop 1 × 2 cm piece ginger. Use orange juice as the steaming liquid and add the ginger and 2 teaspoons grated orange zest to it. Once the vegetables are cooked, strain off the steaming liquid into a saucepan, boil it for 2–3 minutes over high heat to reduce, then serve it poured over the vegetables.

Use white wine as the steaming liquid and add to it 2 teaspoons chopped tarragon and 1 clove chopped garlic. Once the vegetables are cooked, strain off the steaming liquid into a saucepan, boil it over high heat for 2–3 minutes to reduce, then serve it poured over the vegetables.

1 SERVE =
1 unit bread
2 units vegetables
1 unit fats

Roasted vegetables

SERVES 4   PREP 15 mins   COOK 45 mins

4 carrots, halved lengthways
1 large sweet potato, peeled
    and cut into thick rounds
3 turnips, peeled and halved
2 red (Spanish) onions, peeled,
    leaving root end intact, then
    cut into thick wedges
400 g pumpkin (squash),
    peeled, seeded and cut
    into thick wedges
1 tablespoon olive oil

Get the maximum flavour from vegetables by roasting; they will be golden and crisp on the outside, and soft and fluffy inside. A dash of oil is needed in order to achieve a nice crispness. For extra flavour, add 1 tablespoon coarsely chopped rosemary or thyme leaves in with the oil.

1   Preheat the oven to 180°C.

2   Combine all the vegetables in a single layer in a large roasting tin, drizzle with the oil then toss to coat. Season to taste with salt and pepper, then roast for 45 minutes, turning once, or until golden and tender.

VARIATIONS

Replace turnips with one large or two small red capsicums (peppers), trimmed, seeded and cut into large pieces. Add ½ cup (75 g) finely chopped pitted kalamata olives 30 minutes before the end of the cooking time, then scatter over some torn basil or mint leaves (or both) and drizzle with balsamic vinegar to taste.

Combine 2 bunches trimmed asparagus with 400 g large button mushrooms and 1 tablespoon chopped oregano in a roasting tin, drizzle over 1 tablespoon olive oil and season to taste. Roast at 180°C for 30 minutes, turning once, or until tender.

Trim ½ large head cauliflower and 2 heads broccoli and cut into florets. Place in a roasting tin, drizzle with 1 tablespoon olive oil, then season to taste and add a teaspoon caraway seeds or 2–3 teaspoons poppy seeds if desired. Roast at 180°C for 40 minutes or until golden and tender.

To roast beetroots, trim off their stems and scrub to clean. Dry the beetroots, then wrap each one tightly in foil. Place in a roasting tin and roast at 180°C for 1½ hours (depending on size) or until tender when pierced with a skewer. When

cool enough to handle, remove skins. Cut into wedges to serve – a tablespoon of reduced-fat natural yoghurt and a sprinkling of dill or chives for each serving is a nice accompaniment.

To roast tomatoes, cut firm, ripe medium-sized tomatoes in half, then cut each half into three wedges. Place in a roasting tin and drizzle with 1 tablespoon each of olive oil and balsamic vinegar. Season to taste, then roast in a 150°C oven for 2–2½ hours or until the tomatoes have shrivelled slightly and are nicely browned around the edges.

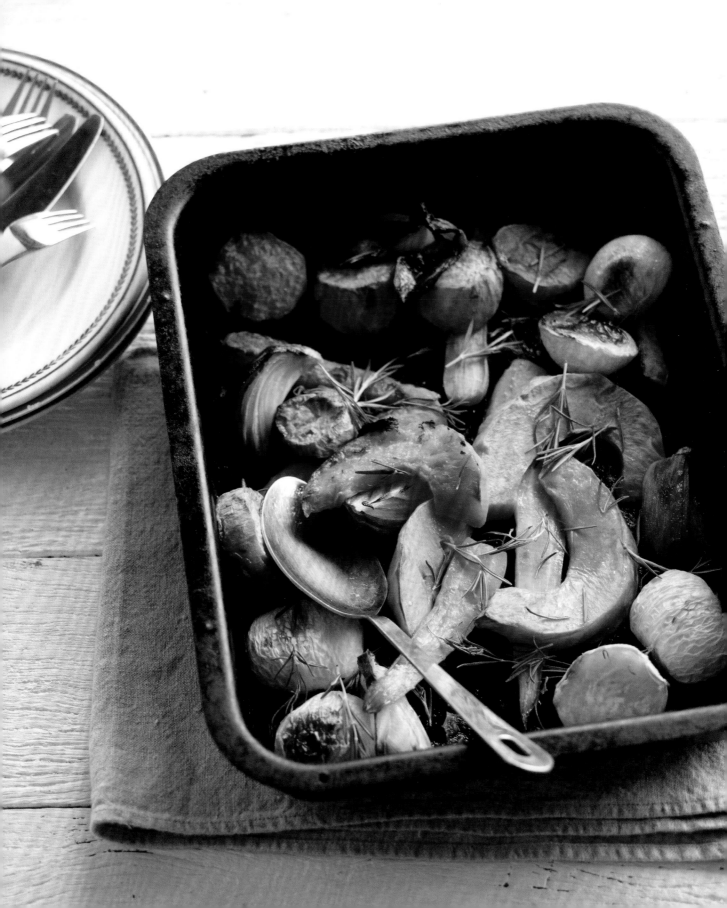

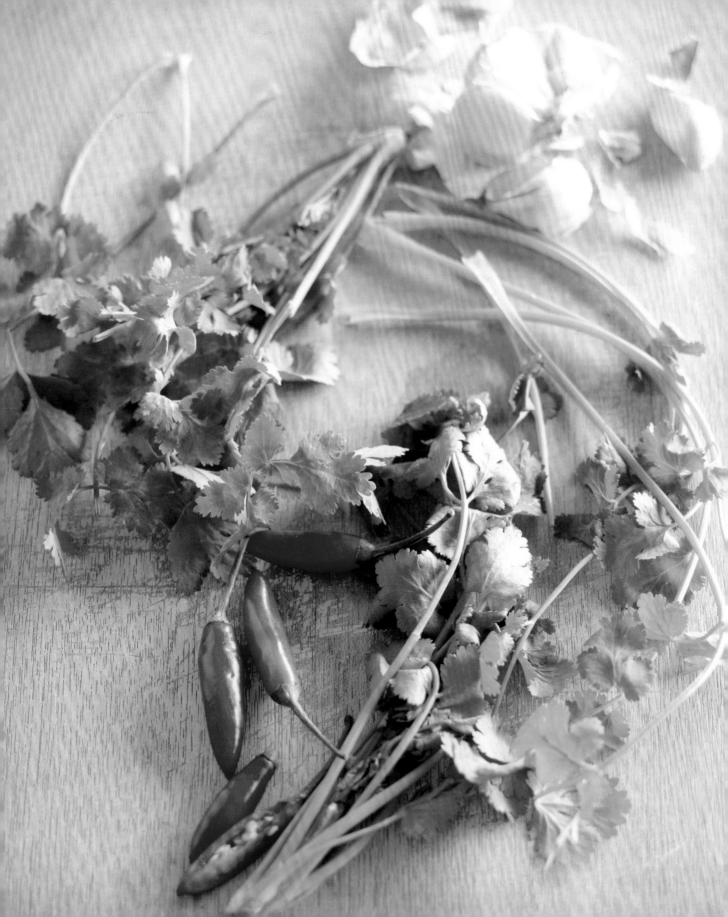

basics

Marinades

Marinades can be used to tenderise or flavour meat or fish. Active agents, such as vinegar and lemon juice, tenderise meat, and work well on tougher cuts. Oil- or water-based marinades are primarily used to enhance flavour.

The following marinades are sufficient for 800 g red meat, chicken or fish. To prepare each marinade, simply mix all ingredients in a small bowl. Place the meat in a shallow dish and pour over the marinade. Turn the meat to coat it thoroughly, then cover and refrigerate for up to 24 hours. Remove the meat from the marinade and cook as desired.

It is important not to use any leftover marinade as a sauce, unless it has been cooked in some way (for example tandoori sauce basted onto baking meat). After it has come into contact with raw meat or fish, there has been a transfer of bacteria that can be harmful to humans.

Chilli and lime

1 teaspoon sugar
$^1/_3$ cup (80 ml) light soy sauce
juice of 2 limes
1 teaspoon fish sauce
½ red chilli, finely sliced
1 teaspoon sesame oil
1 clove garlic, crushed
1 × 2 cm piece ginger, shredded
3 spring onions (scallions),
   finely sliced

Beef or lamb

½ cup (125 ml) red wine
1 tablespoon balsamic vinegar
1 tablespoon olive oil
sprigs of thyme
sprigs of rosemary
1 clove of garlic, crushed
2 bay leaves
2 spring onions (scallions),
   roughly chopped

Ginger soy

¼ cup (60 ml) soy sauce
1 teaspoon grated ginger
2 teaspoons honey
1 tablespoon lemon juice

Seafood

1 tablespoon olive oil
2 tablespoons white wine vinegar
2 teaspoons ground fennel
½ clove garlic, finely chopped

Greek-style

¼ cup (60 ml) lemon juice
2 teaspoons lemon zest
1 tablespoon chopped flat-leaf
   (Italian) parsley
1 tablespoon chopped basil
1 clove garlic, finely chopped
2 tablespoons olive oil
2 teaspoons oregano

Tandoori

$^1/_3$ cup (100 g) tandoori paste
1 teaspoon ground cumin
1 tablespoon lemon juice
250 g reduced-fat natural yoghurt
1 clove garlic, crushed

Five-spice chinese

2 tablespoons oyster sauce
1 tablespoon hoi sin sauce
1 tablespoon dry sherry
½ clove garlic, crushed
1 teaspoon five-spice powder

Thai-style

¼ cup (60 ml) lime juice
2 tablespoons fish sauce
1 small red chilli, finely chopped
1 teaspoon brown sugar
¼ cup coriander (cilantro) leaves

Rubs

Rubs are perhaps the quickest and easiest way to jazz up a piece of meat or fish. There is no secret trick to rubs: just choose your favourite herbs and spices and sprinkle or rub them with a little oil onto raw meat. Work the rub into the meat with your fingers to ensure the entire surface is covered. Rubs work best when the meat is then char-grilled: be sure to oil the meat, not the hotplate, or the meat will fry rather than grill.

Most of the following recipes can be mixed by hand in a small bowl. Those with larger ingredients, such as bay leaves, may require blending in a food processor or with a hand-held processor. Using a mortar and pestle is also an excellent way to blend herbs without losing any of their freshness. Just add enough oil to moisten the rub – it shouldn't be too wet, otherwise the meat won't char-grill effectively.

Rubs do not keep: make them as you need them.

Lemon pepper

lemon pepper
thyme

Zesty

mint
lemon zest
paprika

Mexican-style

lemon zest
ground cumin
ground coriander
jalapeno chilli (or cayenne pepper)

Fish rub

sliced spring onions (scallions)
finely chopped garlic
caraway seeds
ground coriander

Italian-style

oregano
thyme
basil
chopped chives
finely chopped garlic

Chicken rub

bay leaf
rosemary
lemon zest and juice
freshly ground black pepper

Lamb rub

paprika
ground cumin
ground coriander
finely chopped garlic

Capsicum, tomato and orange puree

MAKES ABOUT 3 CUPS (750 ML)   PREP 10 mins   COOK 20 mins

1 tablespoon olive oil

3 large red capsicums (peppers), trimmed, seeded and coarsely chopped

2 cloves garlic, crushed

$^1/_3$ cup (50 g) semi-dried tomatoes, drained

½ cup (125 ml) orange juice

1 teaspoon finely grated orange zest

small handful chopped basil (optional)

This can be used as a sauce to go with steamed or boiled vegetables or grilled meats, or is delicious as a dip. It will keep for up to 3 days stored in an airtight container in the fridge.

1   Heat the olive oil in a saucepan over medium heat. Add the capsicum and garlic and stir to combine, then cover the pan and cook, stirring often, for about 15 minutes or until the capsicum is very soft.

2   Stir in the tomatoes, orange juice and zest, cover and cook for another 5 minutes, then remove from the heat and puree with a stick blender.

3   Season to taste, then leave to cool to room temperature. Stir in the basil, if using, then serve.

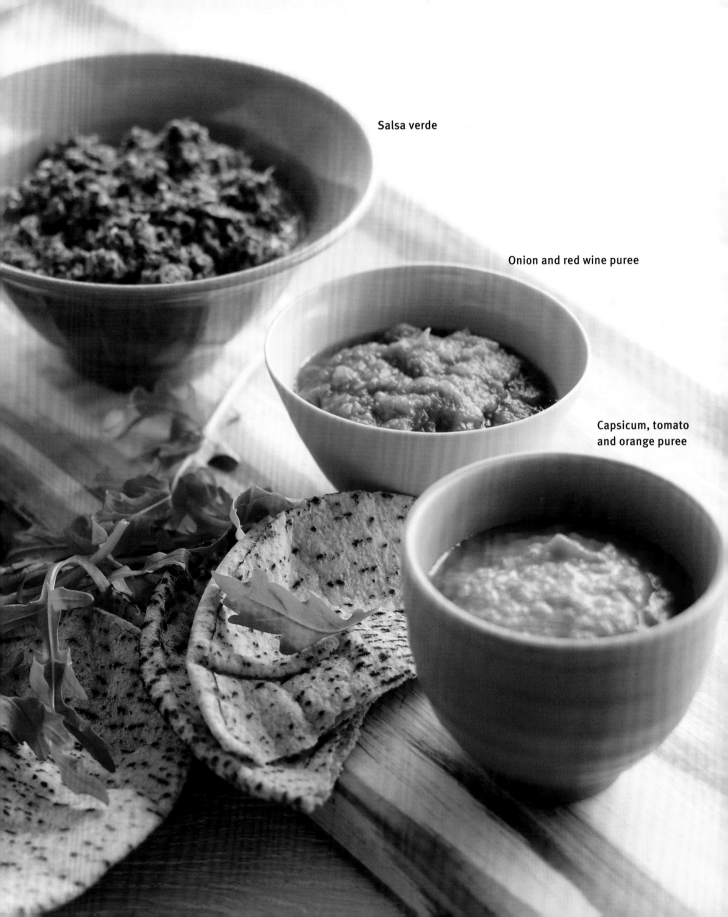

Salsa verde

Onion and red wine puree

Capsicum, tomato
and orange puree

Salsa verde

MAKES ABOUT 3 CUPS (750 ML)   **PREP** 15 mins   **COOK** 7 mins

1 egg
1 bunch curly-leaf parsley,
 leaves picked
1 bunch mint, leaves picked
2 tablespoons drained capers
2½ tablespoons chopped gherkins
4 anchovy fillets, drained of oil
 and coarsely chopped
2½ tablespoons lemon juice
2 teaspoons Dijon mustard
1 tablespoon olive oil
approximately 150 ml salt-reduced
 vegetable stock

This piquant sauce is loaded with herbs and is excellent with lamb, steak, poached chicken or grilled, poached or steamed fish. Stored in an airtight container and kept in the fridge, salsa verde will keep for up to 4 days.

1 Hard-boil the egg in a small saucepan of simmering water for 7–8 minutes, then drain well and cool in cold water. Peel and set aside.

2 Place the remaining ingredients in a food processor. Chop the egg and add to the mixture, then process until a coarse paste forms, adding more stock or water if necessary. Season to taste, then serve.

TIP Make this a day in advance, then cover closely with plastic wrap and refrigerate overnight to allow the flavours to mellow. Bring to room temperature before serving.

Onion and red wine puree

MAKES ABOUT 3 CUPS (750 ML)   PREP 10 mins   COOK 45 mins

1 tablespoon olive oil
4 sprigs thyme
750 g onions (about 4), thinly sliced
1½ tablespoons red wine vinegar
½ cup (125 ml) red wine
1 cup (250 ml) salt-reduced chicken
　or vegetable stock

The perfect accompaniment to grilled or roast meats, especially pork, beef or lamb, or you could serve it as one of a series of dips for crudites when entertaining.

1　Heat the oil in a saucepan over medium heat, then add the thyme and onion. Reduce the heat to low–medium, then cover and cook, stirring often, for 20 minutes or until the onion is very tender.

2　Add the remaining ingredients and stir to combine, then bring to simmering point. Cook over low heat, stirring occasionally, for about 20 minutes or until the liquid has reduced. Remove the thyme and discard.

3　Transfer the mixture to a food processor then process until smooth. Return to the saucepan and cook, stirring, over medium heat for 3–4 minutes to reheat, then serve.

TIP　This sauce is best served warm, so if stored in the fridge, reheat before serving.

1 SERVE =
½ unit protein
1½ units fats

1 SERVE =
1 unit bread
¼ unit dairy
¼ unit vegetables

Hummus

SERVES 4 **PREP** 10 mins

Taste this as you go and add more lemon juice or chilli to suit your palate. Include any leftover dip in a salad sandwich or wrap the next day.

1 × 400 g tin chickpeas,
   rinsed and drained
2 cloves garlic, crushed
3 tablespoons lemon juice
2 tablespoons tahini
½ teaspoon chilli powder (optional)

1 Process all the ingredients in a food processor until smooth, adding a little water if it's too thick. Season to taste, then serve with vegetables cut into sticks or wholemeal pita bread from your daily bread allowance.

> **TIP** Hailing from the Middle East, tahini is a smooth, thick paste made from hulled and ground sesame seeds. It is available from most supermarkets and health-food shops.

Beetroot dip with pita chips

SERVES 4 **PREP** 10 mins **COOK** 10 mins

A delicious dip with a fabulous colour. And the good thing about making it yourself is that you know exactly what went into it.

4 wholemeal pita breads
olive oil spray
1 × 450 g tin baby beetroot, drained
200 g reduced-fat natural yoghurt
1 clove garlic, crushed
2 tablespoons lemon juice
1 teaspoon ground cumin

1 Preheat the oven to 180°C. Split the pita breads in half and cut them into pieces. Spray with olive oil and place on a baking tray in a single layer. Bake for 10 minutes or until crisp.

2 Place the remaining ingredients in a food processor and process until smooth. Serve the beetroot dip with the pita chips.

1 SERVE =
¼ unit vegetables
1 unit fats

Grilled eggplant dip

SERVES 4   PREP 10 mins   COOK 20 mins

1 large eggplant (aubergine)
olive oil spray
1 tablespoon extra virgin olive oil
1 onion, finely chopped
2 cloves garlic, crushed
½ teaspoon ground cumin
2 tablespoons lemon juice

Roasting the eggplant until the skin is black and blistered may look alarming, but this is what gives the dip its unique smoky flavour.

1 Heat a chargrill or barbecue to medium–hot.

2 Spray the eggplant with olive oil and grill, turning, for 15 minutes or until the skin is blackened all over. Cool slightly then peel away the blackened skin. Discard the skin and mash the flesh with a fork in a bowl.

3 Heat the olive oil in a medium saucepan over medium heat and cook the onion until soft. Add the garlic and cumin and cook for a minute longer. Add the onion mixture and lemon juice to the mashed eggplant and mix well. Season to taste and serve with vegetables cut into sticks or wholemeal pita bread from your daily bread allowance.

TIP If you prefer, you can also cook the eggplant under a grill or roast it in a preheated 200°C oven for 50 minutes.

1 SERVE =
1 unit protein
½ unit dairy
* 1 unit vegetables with serving
suggestion

Tuna, ricotta and red onion spread

SERVES 4   PREP 10 mins

1 × 425 g tin tuna, drained
100 g reduced-fat ricotta
1 clove garlic, crushed
½ small red (Spanish) onion,
   finely chopped
1 tablespoon lemon juice
1 teaspoon Worcestershire sauce

This versatile spread can be served simply with wholemeal bread, or offered as a dip with sliced vegetables and grilled pita bread.

1 Combine all the ingredients in a food processor and process until smooth. Season to taste.

2 Serve with crispbread or bread from your daily allowance, as a dip with vegetable sticks, or use as a sandwich filling with salad.

Baked ricotta with chilli and olives

SERVES 4   **PREP** 15 mins + standing time   **COOK** 30 mins

450 g fresh reduced-fat ricotta
olive oil spray
3 tablespoons chopped mixed herbs
   (such as parsley, basil or oregano)
2 cloves garlic, crushed
1 teaspoon dried chilli flakes
12 black olives, pitted

Enjoy this creamy ricotta spread on grilled wholemeal pita bread or toasted wholegrain bread, sprinkled with your favourite fresh herbs.

1 Place the ricotta in a sieve over a bowl and set aside in the refrigerator for at least a couple of hours to drain any excess liquid.

2 Preheat the oven to 180°C. Spray four ¾ cup (185 ml) baking dishes or Texas muffin tins with olive oil and line the base with baking paper.

3 Combine the ricotta, chopped herbs, garlic and chilli flakes in a bowl and season with salt and pepper. Spoon the ricotta mixture into the baking dishes and smooth the surface. Divide the olives among the dishes and gently press into the mixture. Spray lightly with olive oil, then bake for 30 minutes or until risen and firm. Serve hot or cold with wholegrain bread from your daily bread allowance.

Sauces

How long is a piece of string? The number of sauces in cooking is just about infinite, and everyone has their particular favourite. Here are a number of commonly used sauces that are delicious and well within the parameters of the Total Wellbeing Diet.

1 SERVE (1 TABLESPOON) =
1 unit fats

1 SERVE (1 TABLESPOON) =
1 unit fats

Olive gremolata

MAKES ABOUT 1½ CUPS

1 bunch flat-leaf (Italian) parsley
grated zest of 1 lemon
juice of ½ lemon
2 cloves garlic
100 g pitted green olives
¼ cup (60 ml) olive oil
freshly ground black pepper

1 Place all ingredients except the oil and pepper in a food processor. Lightly process, then, with the motor still running, add enough oil to form a thick paste. Season to taste with pepper. Serve on top of baked fish or chicken.

Parsley relish

MAKES ABOUT 1½ CUPS

1 bunch flat-leaf (Italian) parsley
6 anchovy fillets
2 tablespoons baby capers
grated zest of 2 lemons
½ cup (125 ml) lemon juice
¼ cup (60 ml) olive oil
freshly ground black pepper

1 Place all ingredients except oil and pepper in a food processor. Lightly process, then, with the motor still running, add enough oil to form a thick paste. Season to taste with pepper. Serve cooked lamb or beef with a dollop of relish on top.

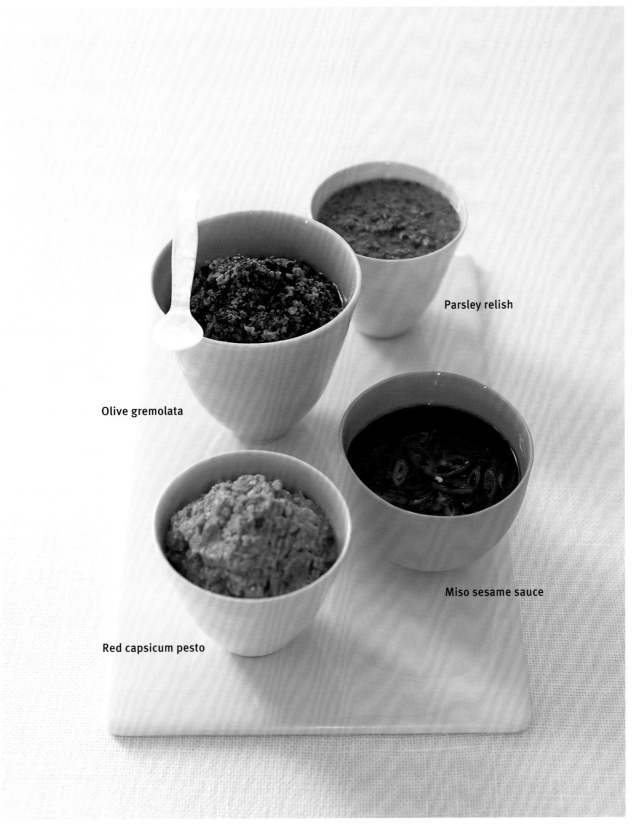

Parsley relish

Olive gremolata

Miso sesame sauce

Red capsicum pesto

Yoghurt sauce

MAKES ABOUT 1 CUP (250 ML)

1 cup (280 ml) reduced-fat natural yoghurt
1 tablespoon chopped mint
½ clove garlic, finely chopped
2 teaspoons lemon juice
½ teaspoon ground cumin

1 Place all ingredients in a bowl and mix well. Season to taste. Cover and refrigerate for 10 minutes before using. If the sauce is too thick, add a little water to thin it out.

2 Serve with grilled lamb or chicken.

Miso sesame sauce

MAKES ABOUT 1 CUP (250 ML)

2 tablespoons sesame seeds
1 tablespoon red miso paste
1 teaspoon brown sugar
1 teaspoon grated ginger
1 tablespoon lemon juice
½ cup (125 ml) chicken stock

1 Fry sesame seeds in a dry non-stick frying pan over medium heat for 5 minutes, or until golden.

2 Place all ingredients in a bowl and mix well. Serve drizzled over fish, chicken or vegetables.

Red capsicum pesto

MAKES ABOUT 1½ CUPS (375 ML)

2 red capsicums (peppers),
  halved and seeded
2 tablespoons olive oil
2 cloves garlic
50 g parmesan
2 tablespoons pine nuts

1 Preheat oven to 180°C.

2 Place capsicums in a shallow baking dish skin-side
up and drizzle with half the oil. Roast for 25 minutes.
Remove from oven, cover with foil and allow to cool
slightly. Peel off and discard skin.

3 Place all ingredients in a food processor and blend
to a smooth paste. Season to taste.

4 Serve with grilled lamb, beef or chicken, or use
to coat lamb fillets before barbecuing them.

Tomato and chilli sauce

MAKES ABOUT 2½ CUPS (625 ML)

1 teaspoon olive oil
½ onion, finely chopped
1 clove garlic, finely chopped
6 tomatoes, chopped
1 red chilli, finely chopped
1 teaspoon raw sugar
½ cup (125 ml) water
1 tablespoon finely chopped
  flat-leaf (Italian) parsley
1 tablespoon finely chopped
  coriander (cilantro) leaves

1 Heat oil in a medium-sized saucepan over low heat.
Add onion and garlic and cook for 5 minutes, or until
soft. Add tomato, chilli, sugar and water. Increase
heat to medium, then coverand cook for 10 minutes.

2 Uncover and simmer for a further 10 minutes, or
until thick.

3 Stir through herbs and season well. Pour sauce into
a sterilised bottle or jar and store, refrigerated, for up
to 2 weeks.

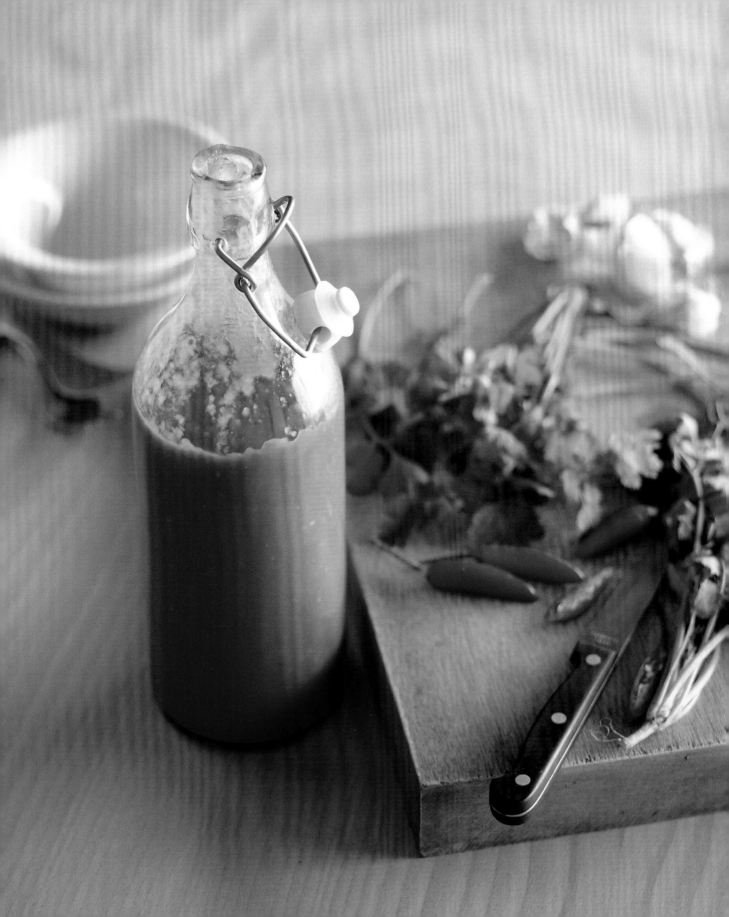

Tomato sauce

MAKES ABOUT 1.25 LITRES   PREP 15 mins   COOK 30 mins

1 tablespoon olive oil
1 large onion, very finely chopped
3 cloves garlic, crushed
2 tablespoons tomato paste (puree)
½ cup (125 ml) red wine
2 × 400 g tins chopped tomato
2 tablespoons red wine vinegar
1 tablespoon Worcestershire sauce,
   or to taste
2½ tablespoons caster sugar or
   powdered sweetener

A great all-purpose tomato sauce. Make a batch of this every now and then and you'll always have some on hand. Just a spoonful will lift grilled meat, chicken or fish to new heights.

1 Heat the olive oil in a medium-sized saucepan over medium heat. Add the onion and garlic and cook, stirring often, for 5 minutes or until the onion has softened. Add the tomato paste and cook, stirring, for 2 minutes. Add the red wine, stir to combine, then cook, stirring, for 3 minutes or until the liquid has boiled and reduced a little.

2 Add the remaining ingredients, then bring to simmering point. Reduce the heat to low and cook for 15–20 minutes or until the sauce has thickened slightly.

3 Use a stick blender to process the sauce until smooth. Leave to cool to room temperature, then transfer to airtight containers and store in the refrigerator.

TIP Stored in an airtight container, this sauce will keep in the fridge for up to 1 week, and in the freezer for up to 10 weeks.

Tomato sauce

VARIATIONS

Lemongrass tomato sauce Add two bruised, knotted stalks of lemongrass with the onion, and use $1/3$ cup (80 ml) fish sauce instead of the vinegar. Omit the Worcestershire sauce and add 2 tablespoons lemon juice, or to taste, instead. Add the finely grated zest of a lemon at the end, removing the lemongrass stalks before using.

Italian tomato sauce Add 3 tablespoons chopped drained capers and 6–8 drained and chopped anchovy fillets (or to taste) in with the onion, and use balsamic vinegar instead of the red wine vinegar. Add a small handful of chopped basil at the end.

Ginger and sherry tomato sauce Use sweet sherry (or orange juice) instead of the red wine, and add 1 × 4 cm piece of ginger, peeled and chopped, in with the onion. Use sherry vinegar instead of the red wine vinegar, and omit the Worcestershire. Add the finely grated zest of an orange at the end, too, if you like.

Thai green curry paste

MAKES ½ CUP (150 G)   PREP 15 mins   COOK 10 mins

1 tablespoon shrimp paste
8–12 small green chillies,
   roughly chopped
1 teaspoon freshly ground
   black pepper
8 cloves garlic
2 teaspoons grated ginger
1 red (Spanish) onion,
   roughly chopped
2 tablespoons coriander
   (cilantro) roots and stems
2 stalks lemongrass, white part
   only, roughly chopped
2 teaspoons ground coriander
1 teaspoon ground cumin
4 kaffir lime leaves, chopped

**It's much healthier to make your own curry paste as the
supermarket varieties are often laden with unnecessary
amounts of fats and sugars. This homemade paste can be
used in the green roast chicken curry on page 277, or in
the Thai fishcakes on page 62.**

1   Preheat the oven to 180°C

2   Wrap the shrimp paste in foil and roast for 5–10 minutes or until
    warmed through.

3   Pound the roasted shrimp paste with the remaining ingredients
    in a mortar and pestle, or blend together in a food processor to
    make a thick paste.

4   Divide into portions, then place in an airtight container and freeze
    for a later date. It will keep for a month or so.

TIP Shrimp paste (or belachan) is sold in Asian supermarkets and some
mainstream supermarkets – try looking in the international food section.
Don't be put off by the smell – it adds a delicious flavour to your curry.
Roasting it helps mellow the flavour. Kaffir lime leaves are available from
supermarkets and greengrocers. Freeze any leftovers in a zip-lock bag
for future use.

GREEN CURRY

Fry 2–3 tablespoons curry paste in 1 tablespoon vegetable oil until
fragrant, then add 1–2 cups (250–500 ml) fish or chicken stock and
½ cup (125 ml) reduced-fat coconut milk. Add 2 cups (320 g) trimmed
and diced fish or chicken and 1–2 cups (100–200 g) sliced and diced
mixed vegetables and simmer for 5–10 minutes or until cooked through.
Serve with lemon wedges, fresh coriander or mint and rice from your
daily bread allowance.

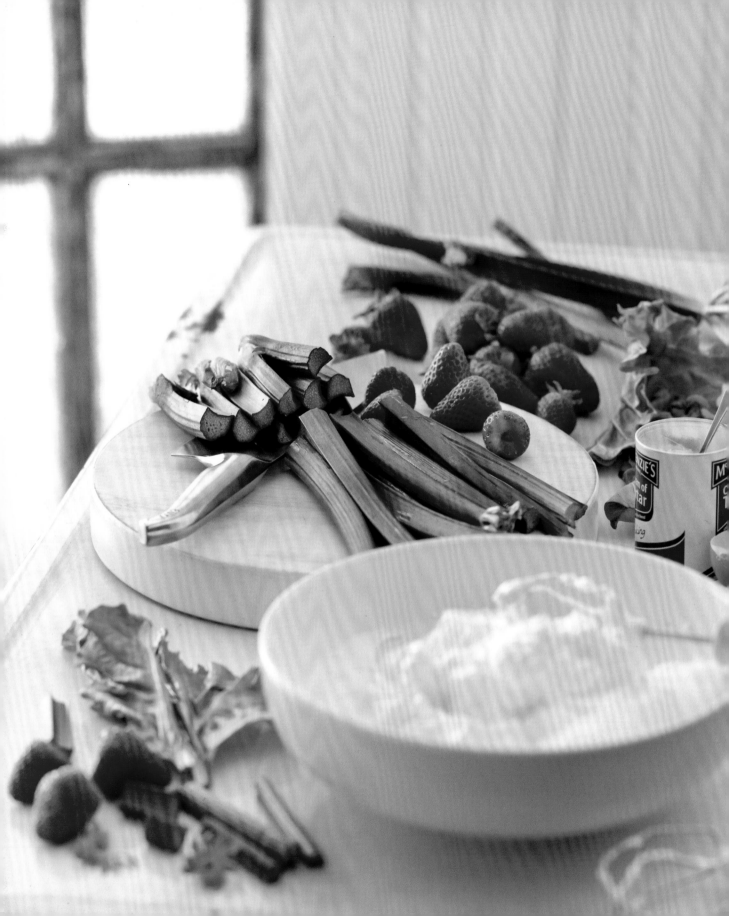

desserts

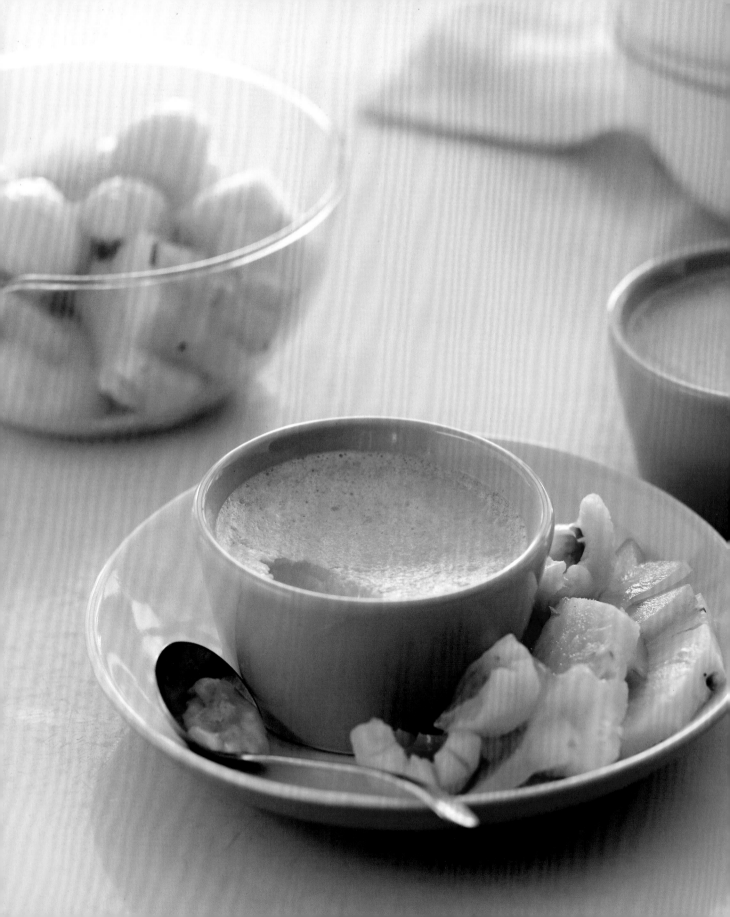

1 SERVE =
½ unit protein
½ unit dairy

Coconut custard

SERVES 4   PREP 10 mins   COOK 30 mins

4 eggs
1½ cups (375 ml) reduced-fat
   coconut-flavoured evaporated milk
½ cup (125 ml) reduced-fat milk
¹/₃ cup (75 g) powdered sweetener

This custard pudding is a summery delight, and can be served with any seasonal fruit.

1 Preheat the oven to 160°C.

2 Whisk together all the ingredients until well combined. Strain and pour into four 200 ml ramekins or ovenproof dishes. Place the ramekins in a roasting tin and pour enough hot water into the tin to come halfway up the sides of the ramekins.

3 Bake for 30 minutes or until just set (the centre should still be wobbly). Remove the custards from the roasting tin and allow to cool. If not eating within an hour of cooling, refrigerate until ready to serve. Serve with your choice of fruit.

TIP This can also be made with unflavoured evaporated milk and served with mixed berries and/or oranges. For a winning tropical fruit combination, serve the custard with a mix of pineapple, kiwi fruit, star fruit and lychees.

Layered espresso and milk jellies

SERVES 4   PREP 15 mins + refrigerating time   COOK 8 mins

5 teaspoons powdered gelatine
2 cups (500 ml) freshly
    brewed espresso
¼ cup (55 g) powdered sweetener
1 cup (250 ml) reduced-fat
    evaporated milk

This is ideal for coffee lovers, and a great dessert to make when entertaining, as it can be prepared in advance and refrigerated until you are ready to serve.

1   Place 3 tablespoons cold water in a heatproof cup or small bowl, then sprinkle in 3½ teaspoons of the gelatine and leave to stand for 5 minutes or until softened. Place the cup or bowl in a small saucepan containing enough hot water to come halfway up the sides of the cup or bowl. Place over low heat for 3–4 minutes or until the gelatine has dissolved.

2   Stir the gelatine mixture into the warm coffee with 2 tablespoons of the sweetener, then leave to stand, stirring occasionally, until it has cooled to room temperature and the sugar has dissolved. Divide among four 1 cup (250 ml) capacity glasses, then chill for 1 hour or until set.

3   Place 2 tablespoons water in a heatproof cup or small bowl and sprinkle in the remaining gelatine. Leave to stand for 5 minutes, then place the cup or bowl in a small saucepan containing enough hot water to come halfway up the sides of the cup or bowl. Place over low heat for 3–4 minutes or until the gelatine has dissolved.

4   Meanwhile, warm the milk over low heat until just heated through. Combine the gelatine with the remaining sweetener and the warm milk in a bowl. Cool to room temperature, then divide among the espresso jellies. Refrigerate for 1 hour or until set, then serve.

TIP Using sweetener in this delicious dessert makes it equivalent to just 130 calories.

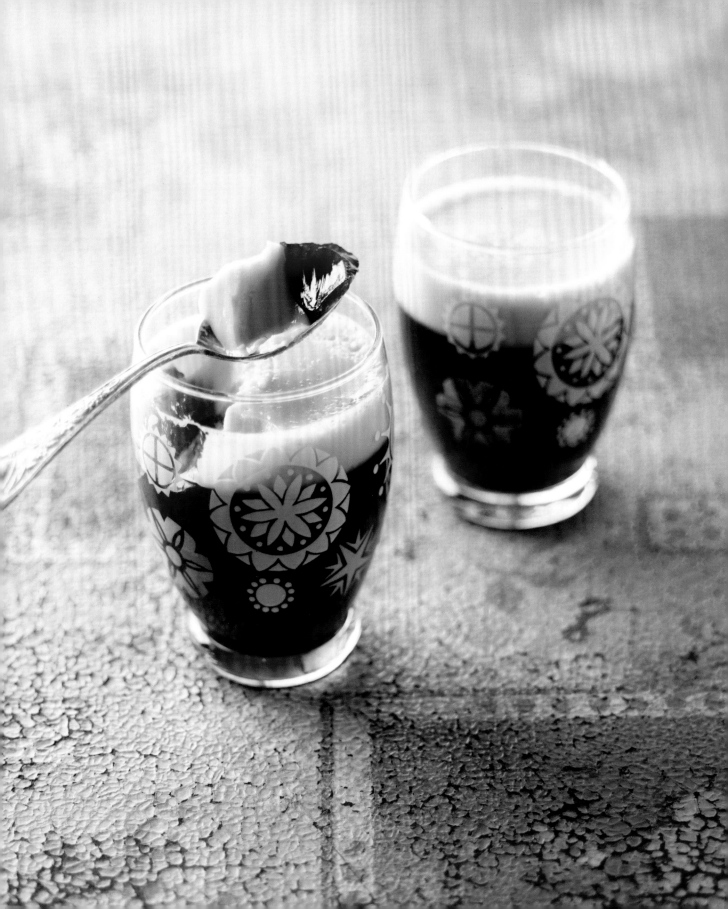

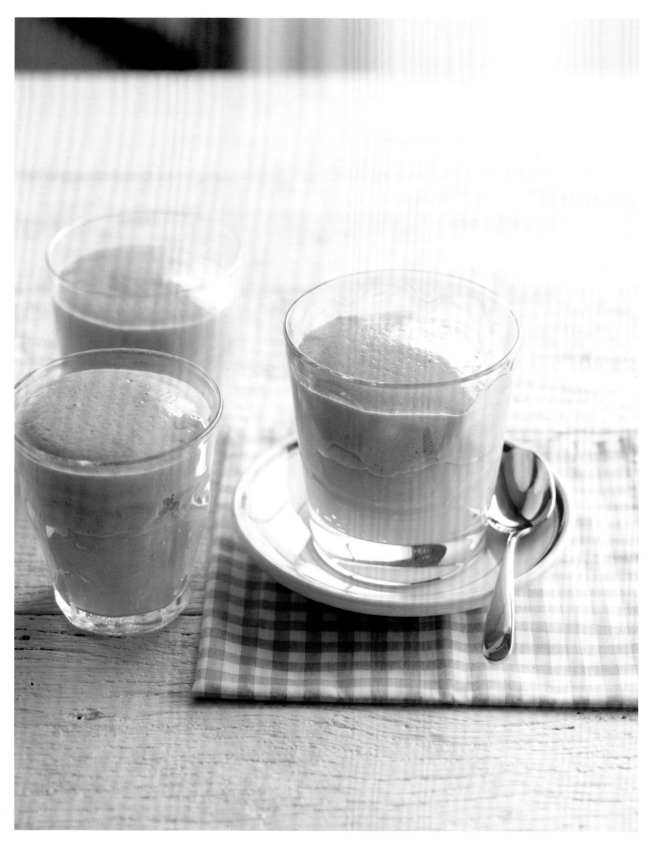

Apple and red wine zabaglione parfait

SERVES 4   PREP 10 mins   COOK 20 mins

4 granny smith apples, cut
   into small chunks
2 tablespoons powdered sweetener

RED WINE ZABAGLIONE
4 egg yolks
1 cup (250 ml) red wine
2 tablespoons powdered sweetener
2 tablespoons caster sugar

This silky smooth dessert tastes rich and decadent and is perfect to serve at a dinner party.

1 Place the apples in a saucepan with ½ cup (125 ml) water, then cover and bring to simmering point. Reduce the heat to low, then cook for 10 minutes or until the apples are tender. Remove the lid, then cook for 6–7 minutes or until all the excess liquid has evaporated. Remove from the heat, stir to break down the apples into a puree, then stir in the sweetener and set aside to cool.

2 Meanwhile, to make the zabaglione, half-fill a medium-sized saucepan with water and bring to simmering point. Choose a bowl large enough to fit over the pan without touching the water. Away from the heat, combine the egg yolks, red wine, sweetener and caster sugar in the bowl, then, using hand-held electric beaters, whisk to combine well. Place the bowl over the boiling water and whisk continually for 10–12 minutes or until the mixture is very thick and pale and has increased in volume.

3 Remove the bowl from the heat and continue to whisk until the zabaglione has cooled to room temperature. Divide the apple mixture among large serving glasses, then spoon the zabaglione over and serve immediately.

1 SERVE =
½ unit dairy
½ unit fruit

Mango pudding

SERVES 4   PREP 10 mins + refrigerating time

2 medium mangoes, peeled
    and stones removed
200 ml reduced-fat evaporated milk
$^1/_3$ cup (75 g) powdered sweetener
1½ tablespoons powdered gelatine
fresh berries, to serve (optional)

For mango lovers everywhere, this creamy dessert is sure to be a hit.

1   Puree the mangoes in a food processor or blender. Transfer to a bowl and mix in the milk and sweetener.

2   Stir the gelatine into 200 ml hot water until dissolved. Add to the mango mixture and stir well to combine.

3   Pour the mixture into four glasses or bowls and refrigerate for 2 hours or until set. Serve with fresh berries, if liked.

TIP You can use 400 g tinned or thawed frozen mango flesh if fresh mangoes aren't in season. This is the perfect dessert to follow a spicy Asian meal. Try serving it with a squeeze of lime juice.

Baked banana with flaked almonds and grand marnier

SERVES 6   PREP 10 mins   COOK 20 mins

½ teaspoon ground cardamom
juice and finely grated zest of 1 lemon
juice and finely grated zest of 1 orange
1 tablespoon Equal or other
  powdered sweetener
1 tablespoon maple syrup
¼ cup (80 g) low-joule apricot jam
120 ml Grand Marnier
4 large bananas
2 tablespoons flaked almonds,
  toasted
500 g reduced-fat natural yoghurt

1 Preheat oven to 190°C. Lightly grease a medium-sized ovenproof dish.

2 Place cardamom, lemon juice and zest, orange juice and zest, Equal, maple syrup, apricot jam and Grand Marnier in a small saucepan. Bring to a simmer, then remove from heat and set aside.

3 Cut bananas into 3 cm pieces and place in prepared ovenproof dish. Pour warm syrup over bananas. Bake for 15 minutes, or until bananas are soft. Serve bananas sprinkled with almonds, and with yoghurt alongside.

1 SERVE =
1 unit dairy
1 unit fruit

Cherry soup with cream-cheese float

SERVES 4 PREP 5 mins + cooling time COOK 12 mins

3 cups (600 g) fresh pitted
   or frozen cherries
1½ cups (375 ml) red wine
1 cinnamon stick
2½ tablespoons caster sugar
   or powdered sweetener
200 g reduced-fat cream cheese
ground cinnamon, to serve

A decadent-tasting dessert combining cherries with cinnamon.

1 Combine the cherries, wine, cinnamon stick and the sugar or sweetener with 1 cup (250 ml) water in a saucepan. Bring to simmering point, then cover and cook over low–medium heat for 5–6 minutes or until the cherries are just soft. Set aside to cool.

2 Discard the cinnamon stick, then divide the cherry soup among bowls. Place a dollop of cream cheese on top, sprinkle with ground cinnamon and serve immediately.

TIP Use orange juice instead of wine if you like, but remember to include it in your fruit allowance.

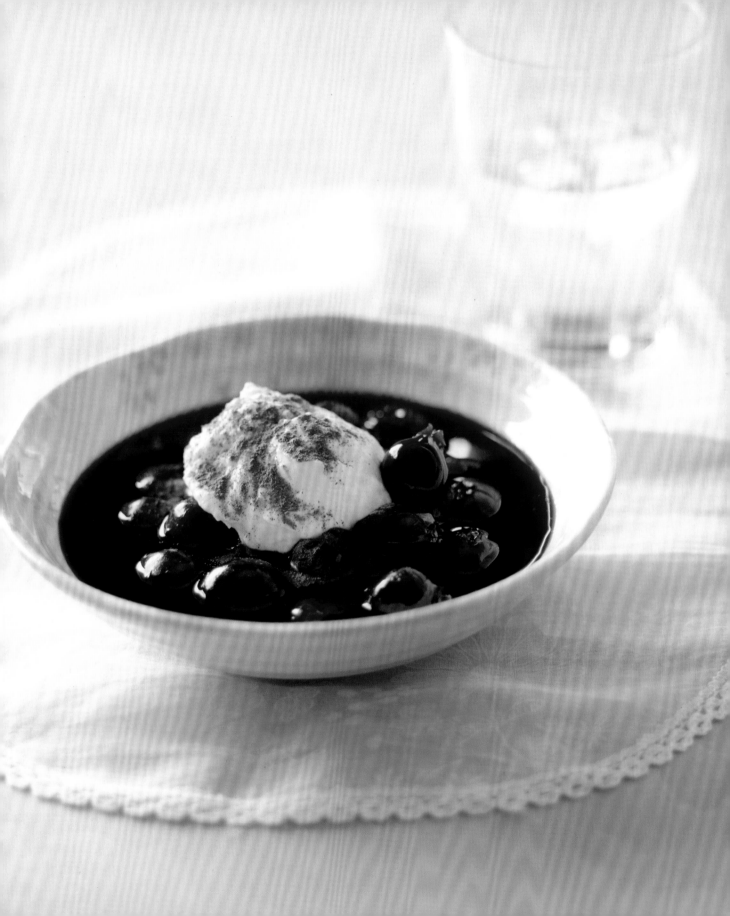

Watermelon sorbet

SERVES 4   PREP 25 mins   CHILL 5 hours

700 g seedless watermelon,
    roughly diced and chilled
2 tablespoons lime juice
2 tablespoons sugar or
    powdered sweetener

For a cooling treat on a hot summer's day, indulge in this lovely dessert.

1   Combine all the ingredients in a food processor and process until smooth.

2   If you have an ice-cream maker, churn the ice-cream according to the manufacturer's instructions.

3   If you don't have an ice-cream maker, freeze the watermelon mixture in a shallow container for 2–3 hours or until just set. Pulse in a food processor or blender until smooth, then return to the freezer for a further hour or until frozen. Once again, pulse in a food processor or blender until smooth, then return to the freezer and allow the sorbet to freeze until solid. Remove from the freezer 20 minutes before serving.

TIP Depending on what is in season, use other fruits, such as rockmelon or peach, in place of the watermelon.

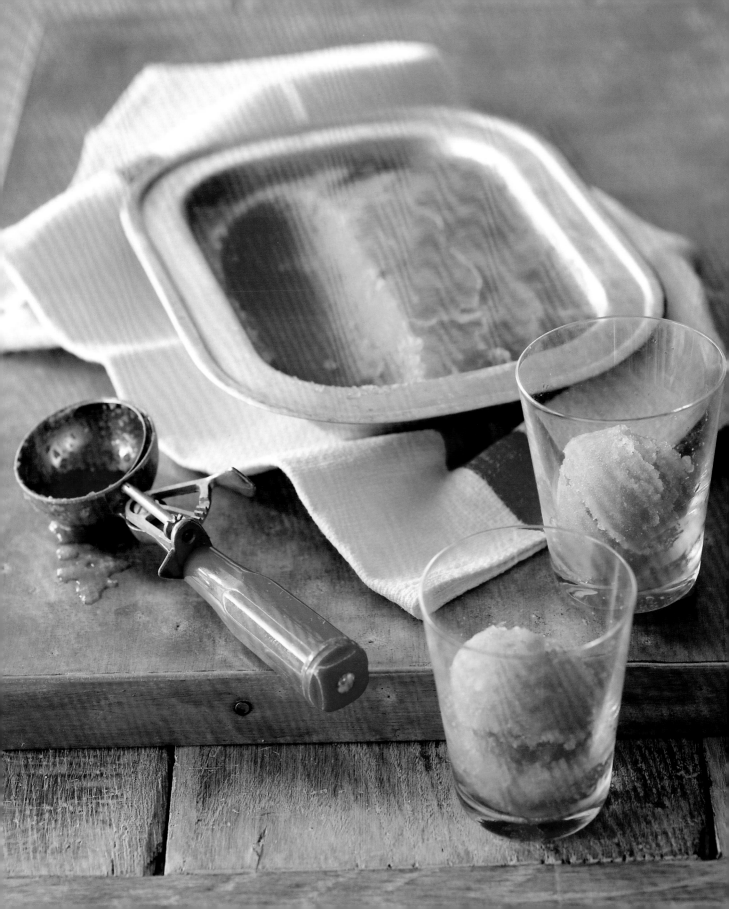

Grilled pineapple with lychee and ginger salad

SERVES 4   **PREP** 15 mins + standing time   **COOK** 6 mins

½ ripe pineapple, peeled
¼ cup (60 ml) white rum
vegetable oil spray
16 fresh lychees, peeled,
   seeded and quartered
1 × 1.5 cm piece ginger,
   or to taste, peeled and
   cut into very fine strips
small handful mint leaves

If fresh lychees are not in season just grill a little extra pineapple and scatter with the ginger and mint; the dish will still be delicious.

1   Cut the pineapple in half lengthways then cut out the hard core. Cut each half into slices about 5 mm thick. Place in a shallow dish, pour over the rum, then cover and leave to stand for 1 hour. Drain well, reserving any liquid.

2   Heat a chargrill plate or large heavy-based frying pan over medium heat. Once hot, spray with vegetable spray. Working in batches, cook the pineapple slices for 2–3 minutes on each side or until golden.

3   Meanwhile, combine the lychees, ginger and the reserved soaking liquid in a bowl and toss to combine well.

4   Divide the pineapple slices among plates, scatter over the lychee mixture and the mint leaves, drizzle with juices and serve.

Grape and fennel-seed clafoutis

SERVES 4   PREP 15 mins   **COOK** 30 mins

2 eggs, lightly beaten
1 egg yolk
50 g caster sugar or
   powdered sweetener
¼ cup (40 g) plain wholemeal flour
200 ml reduced-fat milk
1 teaspoon fennel seeds
olive oil spray
400 g green or red seedless grapes
icing sugar, to serve

The addition of fennel seeds to the batter adds a unique, aniseed-like flavour to this easy dessert.

1   Preheat the oven to 190°C, then place in a 1.25 litre capacity baking dish.

2   Whisk the eggs, egg yolk, sugar or sweetener and flour together until smooth, then gradually add the milk, whisking constantly to prevent lumps forming. Stir in the fennel seeds.

3   Remove the preheated dish from the oven and spray with olive oil. Place in the grapes and pour the batter over, then bake for 30 minutes or until the batter is deep-golden and set. Dust with icing sugar and serve immediately.

TIP   The same batter can be used with pitted cherries or sliced, pitted plums instead of grapes.

Almond jelly with orange segments

SERVES 6   PREP 15 mins + refrigerating time

450 ml boiling water
7 teaspoons powdered gelatine
375 ml light evaporated milk
1 teaspoon almond essence
2 teaspoons Equal or other
**   powdered sweetener**
6 oranges, segmented
¼ cup mint leaves

1   Pour water into a jug, add gelatine and whisk with a fork to dissolve.
    Add evaporated milk, almond essence and Equal, and mix well. Pour
    into 6 small ramekins, or other moulds, and refrigerate for 2 hours,
    or until set.

2   Before serving, toss orange segments with mint. Serve jellies either in
    the ramekins or turned out onto plates, and with orange segments.

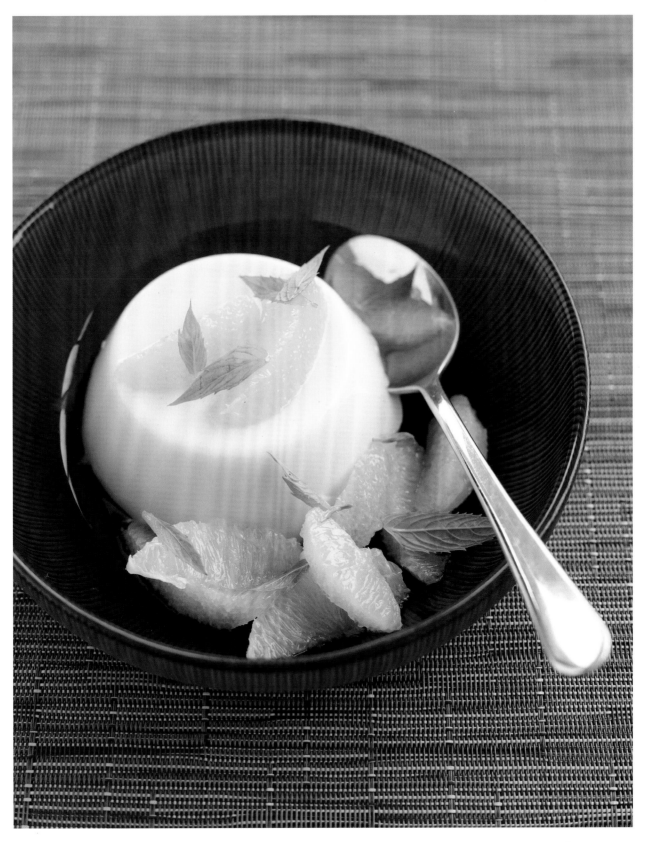

1 SERVE =
½ unit protein
2½ units dairy
1 unit fruit
½ unit fats

Lemon-ricotta cheesecake with blueberries

SERVES 10   **PREP** 15 mins   **COOK** 50 mins

1 kg fresh reduced-fat ricotta
1 tablespoon finely grated lemon zest
2½ tablespoons lemon juice
½ cup (110 g) powdered sweetener
5 eggs
¼ cup (35 g) plain flour
½ cup (40 g) flaked almonds (optional)
300 g blueberries
icing sugar (optional), to serve

Quick and very easy to make, this crustless cheesecake is perfect for when you have a crowd to feed. It keeps well in the fridge for several days too so any leftovers can be enjoyed long after your guests have gone.

1   Preheat the oven to 180°C.

2   Lightly grease, then flour a 24 cm springform cake tin. Line the base with baking paper. Place the ricotta, lemon zest and juice, sweetener and eggs in a food processor. Process the mixture until very smooth, stopping to scrape the mixture down with a flexible spatula as necessary. Add the flour, then pulse just until the flour is combined.

3   Transfer the ricotta mixture to the prepared tin, smoothing the top so it is even. Sprinkle over the flaked almonds, if using, then bake for 50 minutes or until light golden and just set in the middle. Turn off the oven, then leave the cheesecake to cool in the oven with the door ajar.

4   Serve the cheesecake in wedges, with blueberries scattered over and dusted with icing sugar (if using).

> **TIP** Use orange, or even lime, zest and juice for a totally different flavour.

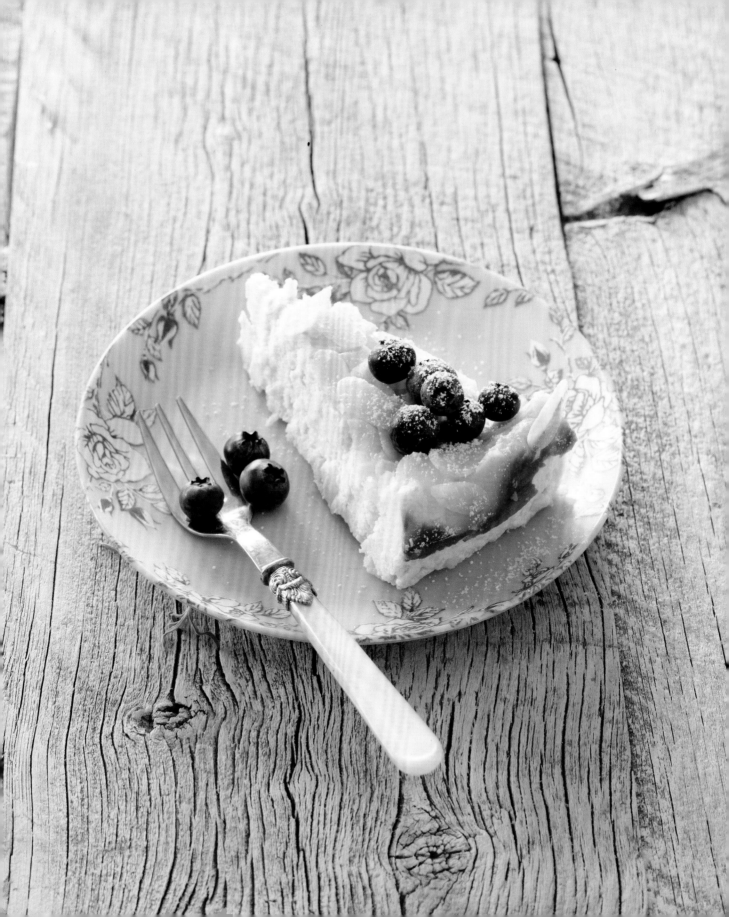

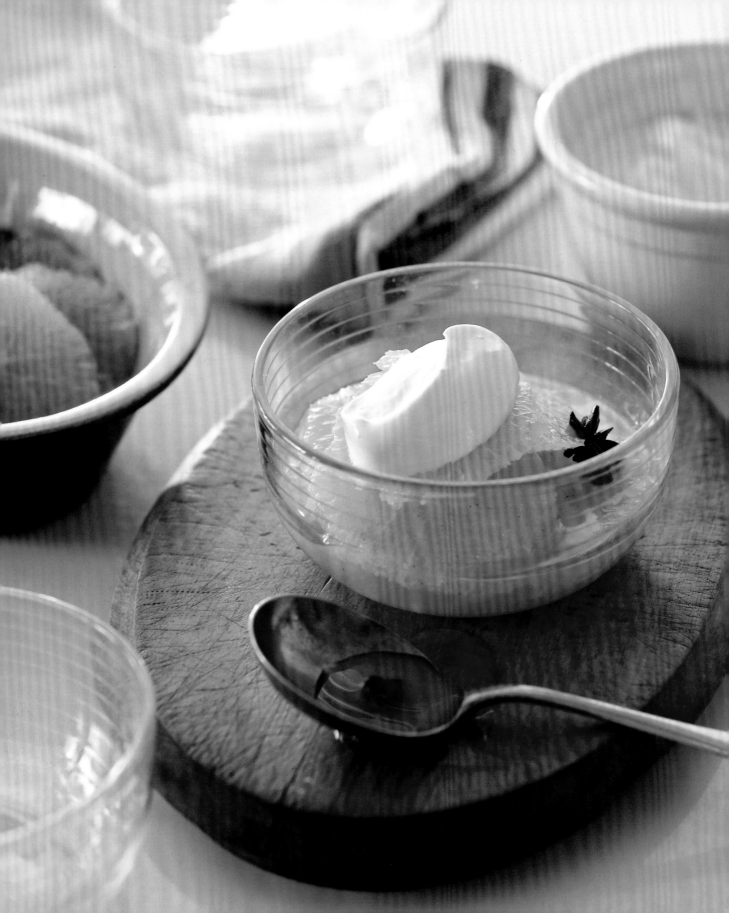

Cinnamon oranges with spiced yoghurt

SERVES 4 PREP 10 mins + refrigerating time COOK 10 mins

2 tablespoons sugar
1 cinnamon stick
2 cloves
1 star anise
4 oranges, peeled and sliced,
    reserving the peel from 1 orange
½ teaspoon vanilla bean paste

SPICED YOGHURT
400 g reduced-fat vanilla yoghurt
1 tablespoon honey
¼ teaspoon ground cinnamon,
    plus extra to serve (optional)

This simple recipe lets the spices do the talking. The creamy spiced yoghurt brings it all together beautifully.

1 Combine the sugar and 1 cup (250 ml) water in a small saucepan over medium heat and bring to the boil, stirring until the sugar has dissolved. Add the cinnamon, cloves, star anise and reserved orange peel. Simmer for 5 minutes, then remove from the heat and set aside to cool.

2 Stir the vanilla paste through the spice syrup, then strain, discarding the solids. Place the orange slices in a large bowl and pour the strained syrup evenly over the top. Cover with plastic wrap and refrigerate for at least 2 hours or overnight.

3 To make the spiced yoghurt, combine all the ingredients in a bowl.

4 Divide the orange slices among four bowls and top with a dollop of spiced yoghurt. Garnish with star anise or sprinkle with a little extra cinnamon, if desired, and serve.

TIP Vanilla bean paste is a convenient substitute for vanilla beans, and is available in the baking section at your local supermarket. Unlike vanilla essence or extract, it contains vanilla seeds. You can substitute vanilla extract if vanilla bean paste is not available. This dessert looks gorgeous if you use blood oranges when in season, or a mixture of both regular and blood oranges.

1 SERVE =
½ unit bread
½ unit dairy
1 unit fruit
1 unit fats

Apple crumble with custard

SERVES 4   PREP 10 mins   COOK 35 mins

1 × 800 g tin apple pie fruit
$^1/_3$ cup (50 g) plain wholemeal flour
$^1/_3$ cup (30 g) rolled oats
2 tablespoons brown sugar
½ teaspoon ground cinnamon
2 tablespoons light margarine
400 g reduced-fat custard

This crumble is a warming end to any meal, and can be made with many different fruit combinations so you will never tire of it.

1 Preheat the oven to 180°C.

2 Spread the apple in the base of an 18 cm × 18 cm ovenproof dish.

3 Combine the flour, oats, sugar and cinnamon in a medium bowl. Using your fingers, rub the margarine into the dry ingredients until the mixture resembles coarse breadcrumbs. Sprinkle the crumble mix over the apple.

4 Bake for 35 minutes, then serve hot with a splash of reduced-fat custard.

TIP Spraying the top lightly with olive oil halfway through cooking will result in a darker golden crumble topping. Using different fruit in your crumble can produce equally delicious results – try tinned pears, mangoes or apricots, or stewed rhubarb and strawberry.

1 SERVE =
½ unit dairy
½ unit fruit
1 unit fats

Apricot and almond yoghurt pops

SERVES 4 PREP 10 mins **CHILL** overnight

20 g flaked almonds
30 g sultanas
400 g reduced-fat apricot yoghurt
1 tablespoon sesame seeds

Kids and adults alike will enjoy cooling down with these icy pops. You can vary the fruit and nut combinations according to taste – the options are endless!

1 Finely chop the almonds and sultanas or pulse in a food processor. Combine with the yoghurt and sesame seeds in a large bowl, then divide among four 100 ml icy-pole moulds. Place in the freezer overnight.

2 To serve, dip the moulds in hot water to loosen.

TIP These can be made with other fruit-flavoured reduced-fat yoghurts: try mango, strawberry or blueberry – whatever takes your fancy.

Stewed rhubarb

SERVES 4　PREP　10 mins + cooling and refrigerating time　COOK　8 mins

12 stalks rhubarb (or 600 g other
　fruit), chopped into 2 cm pieces
juice and finely grated zest of 1 lemon
1 tablespoon Equal
1 teaspoon vanilla essence
1 teaspoon ground cinnamon
2 tablespoons orange juice
a little slivered orange zest

1　Place all ingredients in a deep stainless-steel frying pan. Cook over low heat for 8 minutes, or until soft. Allow to cool until just warm. Refrigerate until needed. Serve with reduced-fat natural yoghurt.

2　Try stewing other fruits, varying the other ingredients to taste.

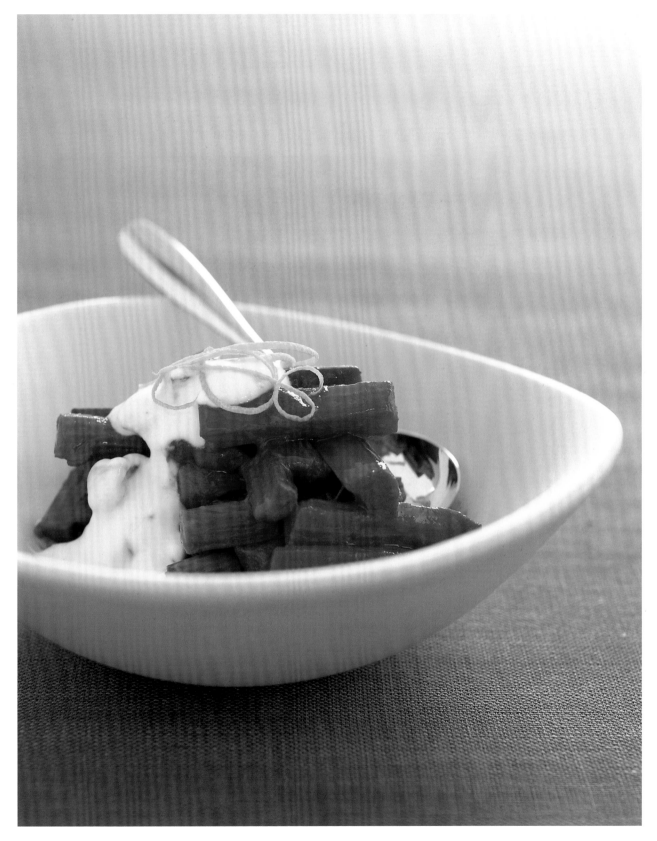

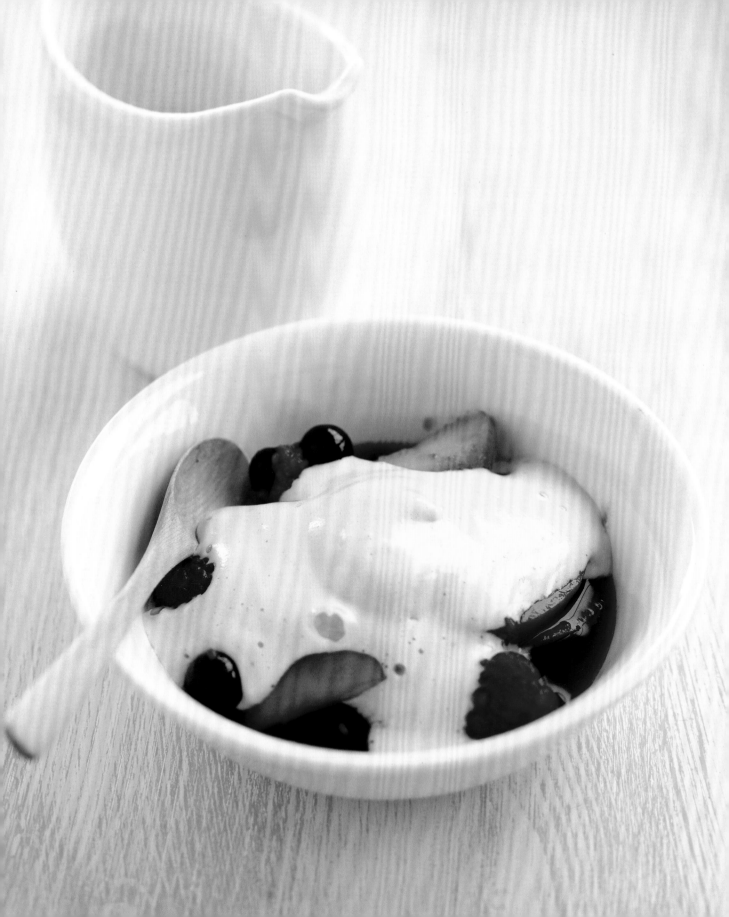

1 SERVE =
1 unit protein
1 unit fruit

Zabaglione

SERVES 4 PREP 5 mins **COOK** 10 mins

8 egg yolks
²/₃ cup Equal or other
   powdered sweetener
1 teaspoon finely grated
   lemon zest
1 teaspoon vanilla essence
¹/₃ cup marsala
650 g stewed fruit

1 Half-fill a saucepan with water and bring to a boil, then reduce heat to a simmer. Place egg yolks and Equal in a heatproof bowl that will fit neatly on top of the saucepan, without touching the water. Using a hand-held electric mixer, lightly beat yolks. Position bowl on top of saucepan and continue to beat until yolks are pale and frothy. Add lemon zest and vanilla essence, and continue to beat while adding marsala a couple of drops at a time. When the mixture begins to resemble a soft, frothy cream, remove from heat.

2 To serve, pour zabaglione over stewed fruit.

Berry banana freeze

SERVES 4   PREP 5 mins   CHILL 2–3 hours

3 bananas
200 g frozen mixed berries

Another icy treat for a warm day. It takes just a few minutes to whip this up, and the results are sensational.

1 Peel and roughly chop the bananas and place in a freezer bag. Freeze for 2–3 hours or until solid.

2 Puree the banana and berries in a food processor until smooth. Serve immediately or scoop into an airtight container and return to the freezer until ready to serve.

TIP You could use this mixture to make icy poles for the kids. Just scoop into six 100 ml icy-pole moulds and return to the freezer for 1–2 hours until solid.

Passionfruit meringues with mango

SERVES 6 **PREP** 15 mins + cooling time **COOK** 45 mins

6 egg whites
1 cup (160 g) **Equal or other powdered sweetener**
2 passionfruit
1 teaspoon vanilla essence
1 teaspoon finely grated lemon zest
250 ml reduced-fat passionfruit yoghurt
500 g fresh mango, sliced

1 Preheat oven to 150°C. Line a baking tray with baking paper.

2 Place egg whites in a clean, dry bowl and, using a hand-held electric mixer, beat until soft peaks form. Gradually beat in Equal until mixture becomes stiff. Spoon mixture onto prepared baking tray in 6 equal-sized blobs and bake for 45 minutes, or until firm. Remove from oven and turn out onto a wire rack to cool.

3 Meanwhile, scoop passionfruit pulp into a bowl and stir in vanilla essence, lemon zest and yoghurt. Place meringues on serving plates, top with a dollop of passionfruit yoghurt and serve with fresh mango slices.

1 SERVE =
½ unit cereal
½ unit dairy
½ unit fruit

Yoghurt Atholl Brose
with raspberries

SERVES 4   **PREP** 10 mins   **COOK** 10 mins

80 g quick-cook rolled oats
2 teaspoons caster sugar or
    powdered sweetener
2 teaspoons honey
¼ cup (60 ml) whisky
400 g reduced-fat Greek-style
    yoghurt
300 g raspberries

Based on a traditional Scottish dessert, this version uses yoghurt instead of the original cream. You could use any type of fruit for this: try seedless grapes cut in half, strawberries hulled and halved, or chopped ripe stone fruits such as apricots or peaches.

1 Preheat the oven to 180°C. Place the oats on a baking tray and bake for 8–10 minutes or until they are light golden, taking the tray out and shaking it occasionally. Remove from the oven and set aside to cool.

2 Place the sugar or sweetener, honey and whisky in a bowl and stir to combine well. Add the oats and yoghurt and combine.

3 Divide among four 1 cup (250 ml) capacity glasses, top with raspberries and serve immediately.

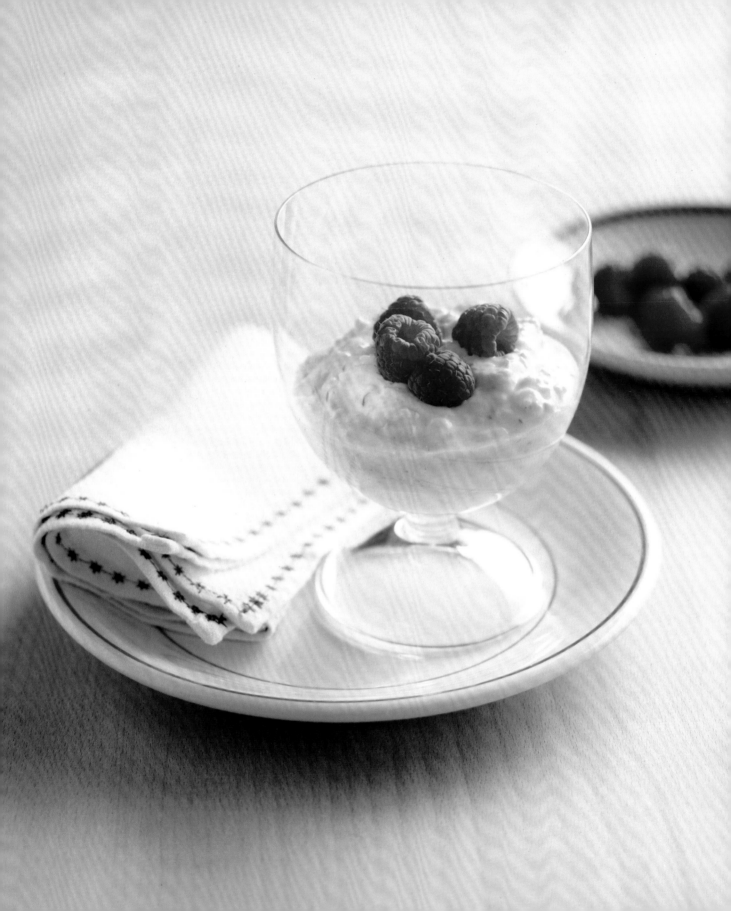

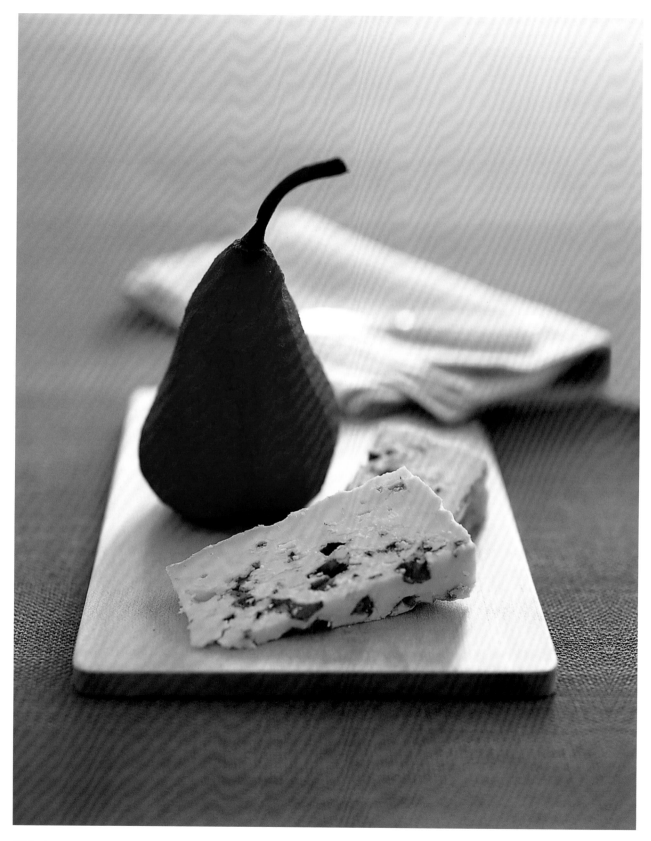

Poached pears with blue cheese

SERVES 4   **PREP** 10 mins + standing time   **COOK** 20 mins

4 firm pears, peeled
2 cinnamon sticks
2 cloves
1 teaspoon allspice
1 teaspoon black peppercorns
1 bay leaf
2 cups (500 ml) red wine
300 ml water
100 g blue cheese
1 teaspoon Equal

1   Place all ingredients except cheese and Equal into a saucepan and bring to a boil. Reduce heat and simmer for 20 minutes. Remove from heat and allow to cool slightly. Add Equal and mix well. Set aside for 4 hours.

2   Drain pears and serve with 25 g cheese per person.

1 SERVE =
½ unit dairy
1 unit fruit

Spiced strawberries with ricotta cream

SERVES 4   PREP 10 mins + cooling time   COOK 10 mins

500 g strawberries, washed
  and hulled
1 cup (250 ml) unsweetened
  orange juice
2 tablespoons sugar
1 cinnamon stick
4 star anise
2 teaspoons Grand Marnier (optional)

RICOTTA CREAM
100 g reduced-fat ricotta
200 g reduced-fat vanilla yoghurt
1 teaspoon caster sugar or
  powdered sweetener

The perfect ending to a friendly barbecue get-together or a sweet treat for any time of the week.

1 Place the strawberries in a large bowl and set aside.

2 Combine the orange juice, sugar, cinnamon and star anise in a medium saucepan over medium heat, stirring until the sugar has dissolved. Bring to the boil, then reduce the heat and simmer for 5 minutes or until slightly reduced. Stir in the Grand Marnier (if using), then cool to room temperature. Pour the syrup over the strawberries and set aside for 30 minutes to develop the flavours.

3 Meanwhile, to make the ricotta cream, combine all the ingredients in a food processor until smooth.

4 To serve, remove the cinnamon and star anise from the strawberry mix and spoon the strawberries into four bowls or serving glasses. Drizzle with a little of the syrup and serve with the ricotta cream.

TIP Other berries may be used in this recipe (raspberries, blackberries or mixed) or try a combination of strawberry and mango. As always, buy what's fresh and in season. Vary the liqueur if you like – try framboise. Leave it out altogether if serving children or replace it with ½ teaspoon vanilla extract.

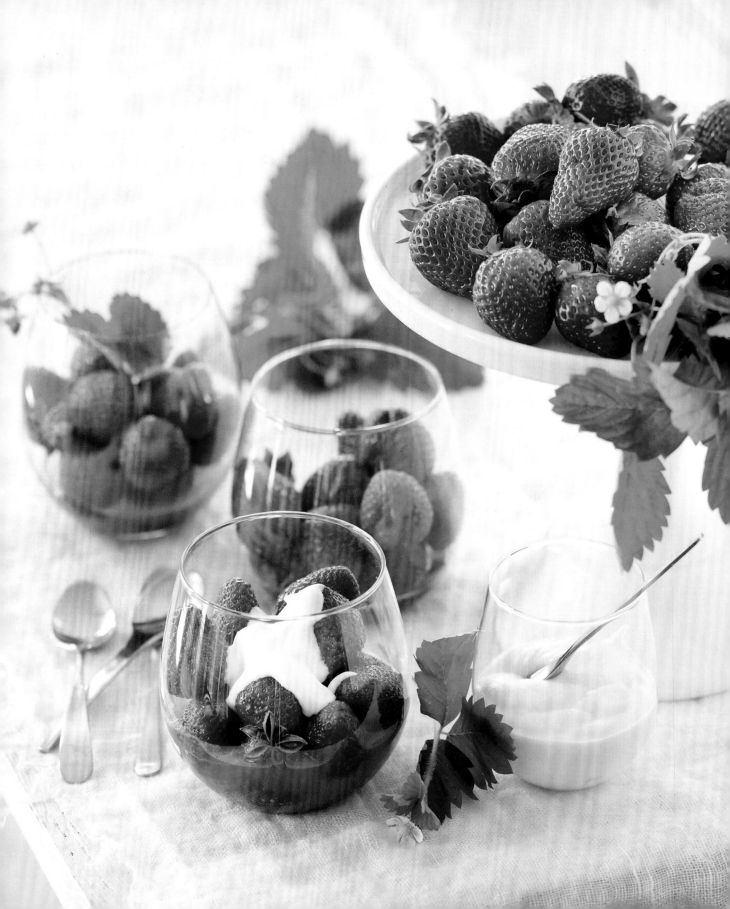

Mango, orange and pawpaw in lime syrup

SERVES 4 PREP 15 mins

¹/₃ cup (80 ml) lime juice
2 teaspoons finely grated lime zest
¼ cup (55 g) powdered sweetener
2 oranges, peeled and all
    white pith removed
1 small mango, peeled and
    stone removed, flesh sliced
½ small pawpaw, peeled and
    stone removed, flesh sliced

This is as simple as can be, and the zesty combination of flavours makes a great finish to the evening meal.

1 Combine the lime juice, zest, sweetener and 2½ tablespoons water in a bowl and stir to combine well. Using a small sharp knife, remove the segments from the oranges, holding the oranges over the lime syrup to collect any juices.

2 Combine the orange segments in a bowl with the remaining ingredients and toss gently to combine. Divide among bowls, drizzle over the syrup and serve.

1 SERVE =
¼ unit dairy
1½ units fruit
¼ unit fats

Roasted summer fruits with rosewater yoghurt and pistachios

SERVES 4   **PREP** 10 mins   **COOK** 15 mins

3 apricots, halved and pitted
3 plums, halved and pitted
1 nectarine, halved and pitted
1 peach, halved and pitted
1 tablespoon honey
1 tablespoon chopped pistachios

ROSEWATER YOGHURT
100 g reduced-fat Greek-style yoghurt
½ teaspoon rosewater, or to taste

You can use any in-season fruit for this dessert – it should be ripe but still firm. In winter, apples and pears work well, although you'll need to extend the roasting time to about 25–30 minutes for these.

1   Preheat the oven to 180°C.

2   Place the fruit halves in a baking dish, then drizzle the honey over and roast for 15 minutes or until the fruit is soft and golden around the edges. Cool slightly.

3   Meanwhile, to make the rosewater yoghurt, combine the yoghurt and the rosewater and stir to combine well.

4   Serve the fruit warm or at room temperature sprinkled with pistachios, with the yoghurt alongside.

TIP Try to get freestone stone fruit if you can, as they pull apart much more easily.

Apricot bread pudding

SERVES 4   PREP 10 mins   COOK 25 mins

olive oil spray
4 slices day-old wholemeal bread,
   crusts discarded, chopped into
   small pieces
1 × 400 g tin apricots in juice,
   drained well, quartered
400 ml reduced-fat milk
4 eggs, lightly beaten
2 tablespoons caster sugar
   or powdered sweetener
1 teaspoon vanilla extract
icing sugar, to serve

Comfort food at its best. Use fresh apricots when they are in season.

1 Preheat the oven to 180°C. Spray the base and sides of four 300 ml capacity baking or ovenproof dishes with olive oil spray and place in a roasting tin.

2 Divide half the chopped bread among the dishes, add the apricot pieces, then place the remaining bread on top.

3 Combine the milk, eggs, sugar or sweetener and vanilla in a bowl and whisk to combine well, then divide this mixture among the dishes. Pour enough boiling water into the tin to come halfway up the sides of the dishes, then bake for 25 minutes or until just set in the middle. Cool slightly, then serve warm dusted with icing sugar.

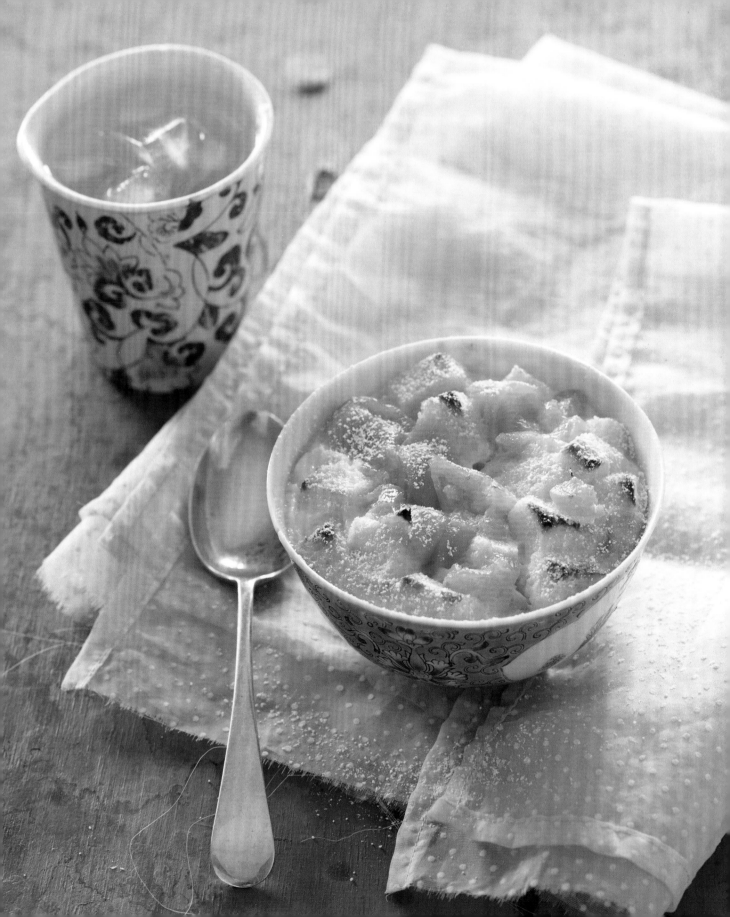

Spiced rhubarb and apple pie

SERVES 4   **PREP** 25 mins + resting time   **COOK** 45 mins

1 teaspoon finely grated lemon zest
1 tablespoon lemon juice
¼ cup (40 g) Equal or other
   powdered sweetener
2 teaspoons vanilla essence
½ teaspoon mixed spice
6 green apples, peeled,
   cored and quartered
1 cup apple juice
1 bunch rhubarb, cut
   into 4 cm pieces
1 quantity olive oil pastry
   (see page 54)
reduced-fat milk, for brushing

1 Preheat oven to 200°C.

2 Place lemon zest, lemon juice, Equal, vanilla essence, mixed spice, apples and apple juice into a large saucepan and bring to a boil. Reduce heat and simmer for 10 minutes, or until apple is soft but still holding its shape. Add rhubarb and cook for 2 minutes, or until rhubarb softens slightly. Remove from heat and pour into a shallow pie dish.

3 Roll out pastry to 5 mm thickness and the size of the pie dish. Brush rim of dish with a little milk, then drape pastry over, pressing the edges firmly onto the rim of the dish. Trim away excess pastry. Brush pastry lid with a little more milk and bake for 30 minutes, or until golden.

4 Serve warm with low-fat ice-cream or yoghurt, if desired.

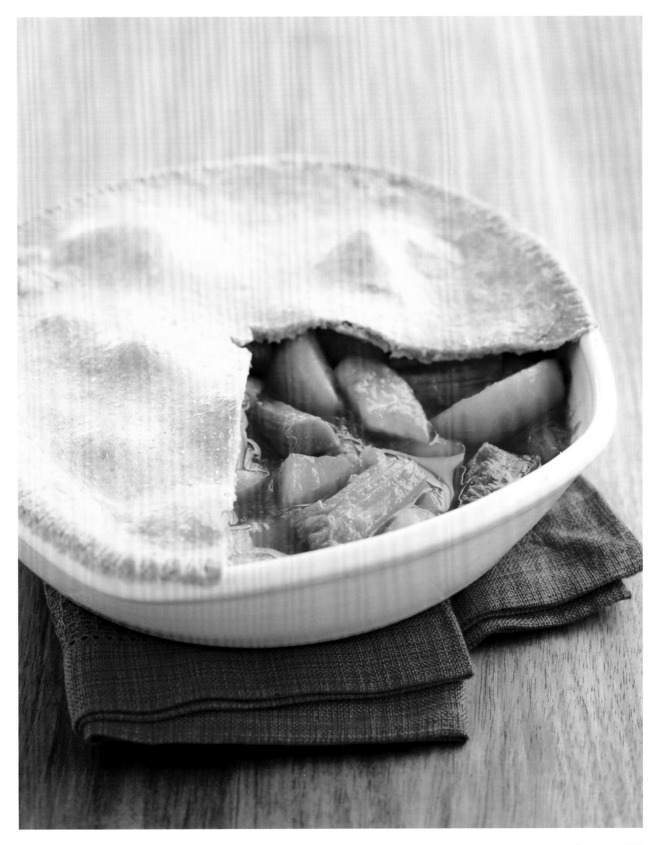

Grilled peaches with raspberry coulis

SERVES 4   PREP 5 mins   COOK 5 mins

4 peaches, peeled, halved
    and stones removed
olive oil spray

RASPBERRY COULIS
300 g frozen raspberries, thawed
1 tablespoon sugar or
    powdered sweetener
¼ cup (60 ml) orange juice

This dessert can also be made with other seasonal fruits, such as mangoes, apricots, pineapple or nectarines.

1 To prepare the raspberry coulis, combine the raspberries, sugar or powdered sweetener and orange juice in a food processor and blend until smooth. Strain and set aside.

2 Heat a chargrill or heavy-based frying pan over medium heat. Spray the peaches with olive oil and grill for 2–3 minutes each side or until golden.

3 Divide the grilled peaches among four plates, drizzle with the raspberry coulis and serve with a small scoop of reduced-fat, sugar-free ice-cream or dairy dessert from your daily dairy allowance, if liked.

TIP The peaches can easily be grilled on the barbecue for a sweet end to a weekend get-together. If liked, the raspberry coulis may be heated and served as a hot syrup. It also makes an excellent topping to a scoop of reduced-fat ice-cream for a quick and easy dessert.

Plum pie with olive oil and rosemary pastry

SERVES 4   PREP 15 mins + resting time   COOK 50 mins

600 g plums, halved and pitted,
   then quartered
1 cinnamon stick
1½ tablespoons caster sugar
   or powdered sweetener
icing sugar, to serve

OLIVE OIL AND ROSEMARY PASTRY
100 g wholemeal flour, plus
   extra for dusting
1 tablespoon caster sugar or
   powdered sweetener
2 teaspoons finely chopped rosemary
1 egg, beaten
1½ tablespoons extra virgin olive oil
ice-cold water, to mix

If plums are not in season, use tinned plums instead. Choose ones that are tinned in juice, not syrup, then drain them well and remove the stones.

1 Place the plums and cinnamon stick in a saucepan. Cover tightly with a lid, then cook over low–medium heat for 15 minutes or until the plums are soft. Stir in the sugar or sweetener, then remove the pan from the heat and leave to cool to room temperature. Discard the cinnamon stick.

2 Meanwhile, for the pastry, combine the flour, sugar or sweetener and rosemary in a bowl and make a well in the centre. Add the egg, olive oil and 1 tablespoon of ice-cold water to the well, then gradually incorporate the dry ingredients with the wet ingredients, adding a little more water as necessary to form a firm dough. Transfer the mixture to a clean, floured benchtop and knead lightly to bring it together. Form the pastry into a disc, cover with plastic wrap and refrigerate for 20 minutes.

3 Preheat the oven to 180°C.

4 Place the plum mixture in a 1 litre capacity baking dish. On a clean, floured benchtop, roll out the pastry into a piece 1–2 cms larger than the surface of the baking dish. Carefully transfer the pastry to the dish to cover the plums. Trim the edges, then bake for 35 minutes or until the pastry is golden and cooked through.

5 Serve the pie hot, warm or at room temperature, dusted with icing sugar.

TIP Always rest pastry in the fridge before rolling it out. You can make it a day in advance if you like and refrigerate it until ready to bake.

Buttermilk puddings with fresh berries

SERVES 6   PREP 10 mins + cooling and refrigerating time   **COOK** 5 mins

1 vanilla bean, split
600 ml buttermilk
7 teaspoons powdered gelatine
¼ cup (40 g) Equal or other
    powdered sweetener
250 ml reduced-fat vanilla yoghurt
600 g fresh seasonal berries
    (strawberries, raspberries,
    blueberries, etc.)

1 Place vanilla bean and half the buttermilk in a small saucepan and bring to a simmer. Remove from heat and add gelatine, stirring well to dissolve. Allow to cool slightly, stir in Equal, then strain through a fine-mesh sieve.

2 Place yoghurt and remaining buttermilk in a bowl and add buttermilk-gelatine mixture. Stir gently, then pour into 6 small ramekins or glasses. Refrigerate for 2 hours, or until set.

3 Serve puddings either in the ramekins or turned out onto plates, and with fresh berries.

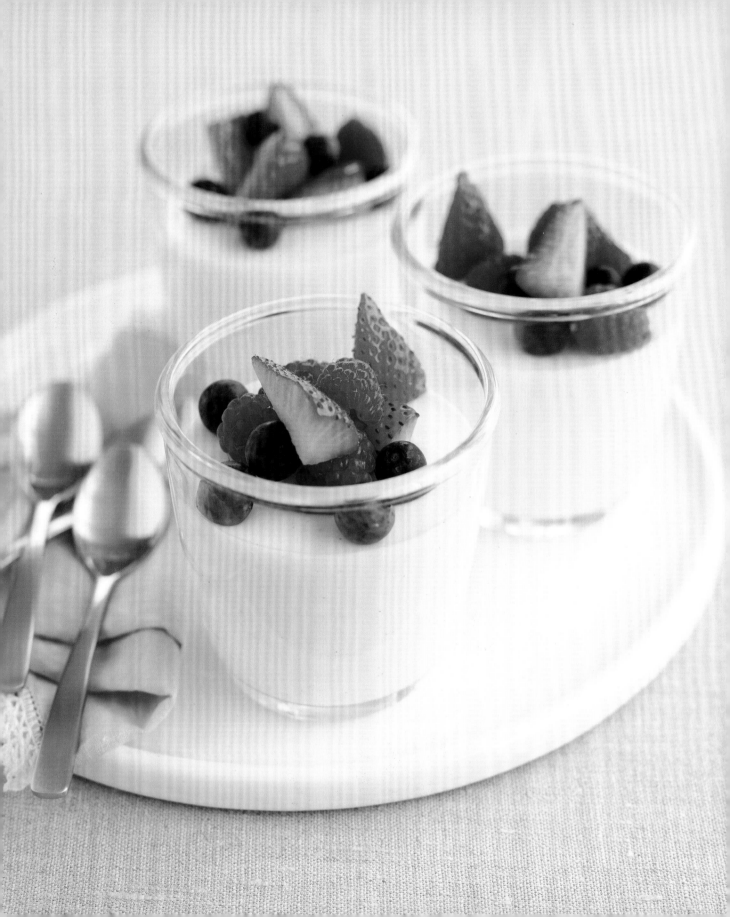

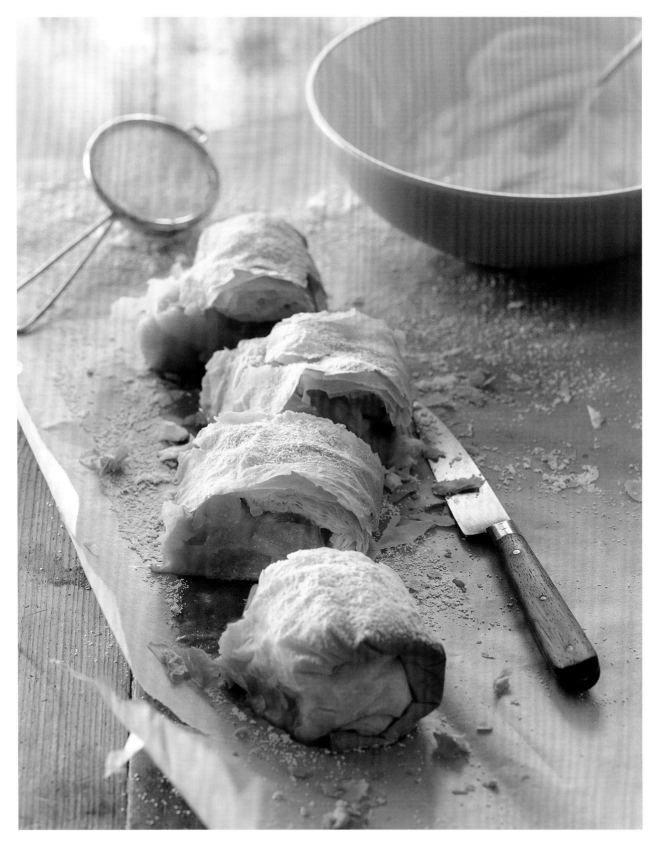

Apricot strudel

SERVES 4   **PREP** 15 mins   **COOK** 25 mins

1 × 400 g tin apricot pie fruit
  or apricot halves in juice,
  well drained
25 g slivered almonds
4 sheets filo pastry
olive oil spray
icing sugar, for dusting

Crisp pastry and a warm fruit filling make this dessert feel like a real indulgence, but the good news is you can enjoy it guilt-free.

1   Preheat the oven to 200°C and line a baking tray with baking paper.

2   Roughly chop the apricots and combine with the almonds in a bowl.

3   Lay one sheet of pastry on a clean work surface and spray lightly with olive oil. Place the remaining sheets on top, spraying each with olive oil as you go. With the longest edge closest to you, spoon the apricot mixture into a log shape across the centre of the pastry (you should have about a quarter of the width of the pastry on each side of the fruit log). Fold the edge closest to you over the fruit, then bring in the sides and roll up firmly.

4   Place the strudel, seam-side down, on the prepared baking tray and spray lightly with olive oil. Bake for 20–25 minutes or until golden. Dust lightly with icing sugar and serve with reduced-fat vanilla yoghurt or a dairy dessert from your daily dairy allowance, if liked.

TIP   For a different filling, replace the apricots with tinned apple pie fruit or cherries, or a combination of the two.

Eve's pudding

SERVES 4   PREP 10 mins   COOK 40 mins

500 g tinned apple pie fruit, drained
500 g fresh or tinned berries

SPONGE TOPPING
2 eggs
¹⁄₃ cup (75 g) powdered sweetener
2 tablespoons plain flour
2 tablespoons self-raising flour
2 tablespoons cornflour
icing sugar, for dusting

This is a lighter version of a traditional British pudding made with apples and a sponge cake topping.

1 Preheat the oven to 180°C.

2 Place the fruit in an 18 cm round baking dish.

3 To make the sponge topping, place the eggs and sweetener in a medium bowl and beat until thick and creamy. Sift the flours together in a separate bowl, then fold into the egg mixture.

4 Spoon the sponge mix over the fruit and bake for 30–40 minutes or until golden and firm. Dust lightly with icing sugar and serve with reduced-fat yoghurt or dairy dessert from your daily dairy allowance, if liked.

TIP Replace this filling with your choice of frozen or tinned fruit, such as pear, mango, plum or berries, thawed or drained as applicable, or use 1 kg tinned apple pie fruit for the traditional version. If using berries, cook them first as they drop a lot of liquid while cooking. A combination of well-drained, cooked berries and apples would be a better choice. Fresh stewed fruit can also be used in place of tinned or frozen fruit.

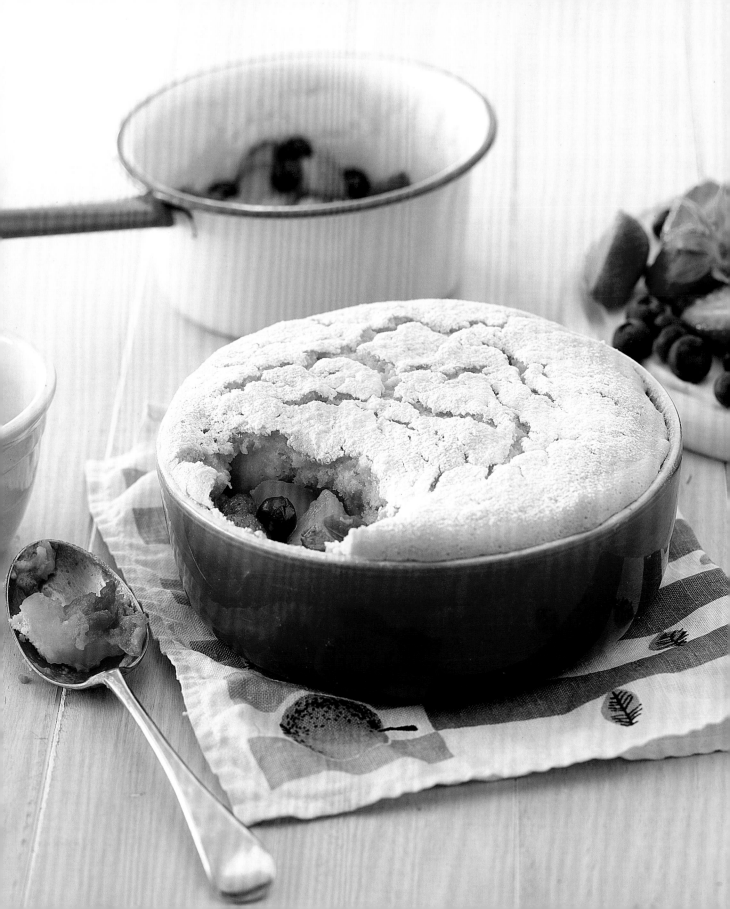

Summer pudding

SERVES 4 **PREP** 10 mins **COOK** 8 mins

600 g mixed fresh or frozen berries
¼ cup (55 g) powdered sweetener
140 g trimmed, unsliced
   day-old bread
400 g reduced-fat Greek-style yoghurt

Frozen berries are a great alternative to fresh: they are very cost-effective and no less delicious. Be sure to get an unsliced loaf of bread, so you can slice it very thinly yourself.

1 Place the berries and 2 tablespoons water in a small saucepan, then cover and bring to simmering point. Cook over low–medium heat for 5 minutes or until the berries have softened and released their juices. Stir in the sugar or sweetener, then leave to cool to room temperature.

2 Using a sharp serrated knife, cut the bread into very thin slices – the thinner you can make them, the better. Place half the bread over the base of a 22 cm × 16 cm baking dish, breaking off pieces of bread to fit and cover the base. Spoon over half the berry mixture, spreading to cover the bread. Place the remaining bread in a single layer over the top, then spoon over the remaining berry mixture.

3 Cover the dish with plastic wrap, then refrigerate for 1 hour or until chilled. Spread the yoghurt over the top, then serve.

TIP Day-old bread works best for this recipe.

Baked custard

SERVES 4   PREP 5 mins   **COOK** 40 mins

400 ml reduced-fat milk
1 teaspoon Equal
1 teaspoon vanilla essence
4 eggs
2 teaspoons ground cinnamon

1   Preheat oven 150°C.

2   Heat milk, Equal and vanilla essence in a saucepan over medium heat. Do not let mixture boil. Allow to cool slightly.

3   In a bowl, whisk eggs with half the cinnamon. Slowly add milk mixture to eggs, whisking constantly. Pour into a 1.5-litre capacity ovenproof dish. Place dish in a deep baking dish and pour enough warm water into the dish to come halfway up sides of custard dish.

4   Carefully transfer to oven and bake for 35 minutes, or until just set. Sprinkle with remaining cinnamon and serve.

Baked apples with cinnamon and ricotta

SERVES 4   PREP 10 mins   **COOK** 20 mins

2 large green apples
¹/₃ cup (30 g) rolled oats
¼ cup (40 g) mixed dried fruit
½ teaspoon ground cinnamon
½ cup (120 g) reduced-fat ricotta
2 tablespoons maple syrup
400 g reduced-fat vanilla yoghurt

1   Preheat oven to 200°C.

2   Peel, core and halve apples and place, cut-side up, on a baking tray lined with baking paper. In a bowl, mix oats, dried fruit, cinnamon and ricotta. Spoon mixture into the core of each apple half, making a small mound. Drizzle with maple syrup and bake for 20 minutes. Serve warm with vanilla yoghurt.

Coconut-sago pudding with mango

SERVES 4   PREP 10 mins + 1 hour soaking time   COOK 15 mins

¹/₃ cup (65 g) sago
¹/₃ cup (75 g) powdered sweetener
1 cup (250 ml) reduced-fat coconut-flavoured evaporated milk
1 mango, peeled and stone removed, flesh cut into 1 cm pieces

This is the perfect antidote to a steamy summer's day, and a great way to enjoy mango when it's at its seasonal best.

1   Soak the sago in cold water to cover for 1 hour, then drain well. Combine the drained sago and 2 cups (500 ml) water in a saucepan and slowly bring to simmering point. Cook the mixture, stirring often, over low–medium heat for 15 minutes or until the sago is translucent.

2   Stir in the sweetener and evaporated milk, then remove from the heat and leave to cool slightly. Serve warm or at room temperature with the mango.

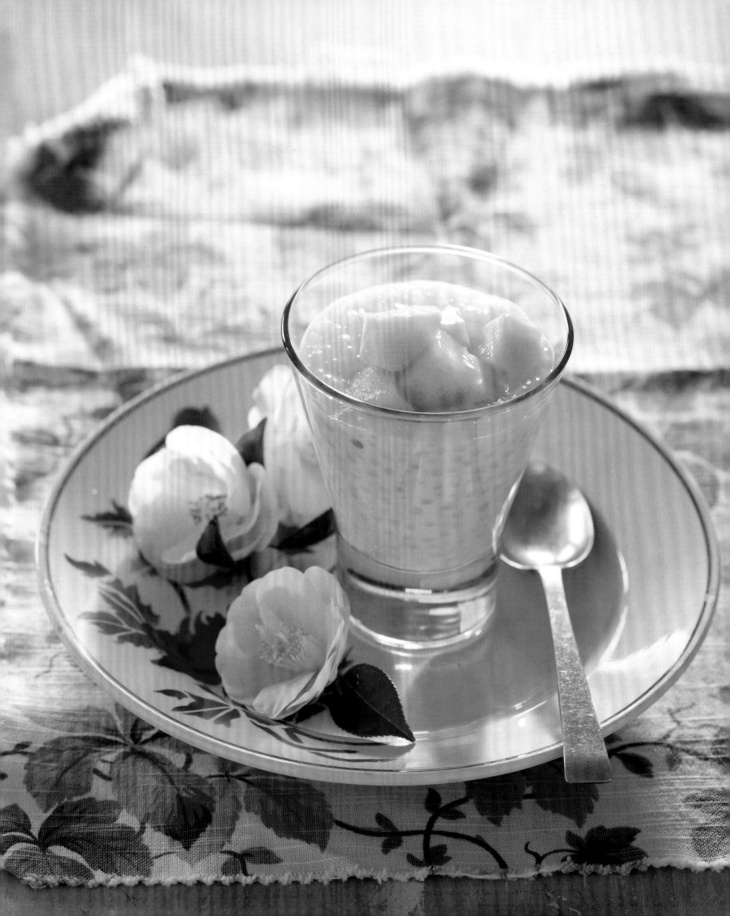

Berry cheesecake

SERVES 8   PREP 10 mins + cooling time   COOK 35 mins

olive oil spray
400 g reduced-fat ricotta
1 tablespoon plain flour
¼ cup (55 g) sugar or
    powdered sweetener
2 eggs
finely grated zest of 1 lime
1 teaspoon vanilla extract
150 g berries, lightly crushed and
    very well drained if frozen, plus
    extra berries to garnish (optional)
icing sugar, for dusting (optional)

Cheesecake is an old-time favourite, but almost always a big 'no-no' when you're watching your nutritional intake. But thanks to this clever recipe, you can have your cheesecake and eat it too, while staying within the guidelines of your daily food allowance.

1   Preheat the oven to 160°C. Spray an 18 cm springform tin with olive oil and line the base with baking paper.

2   Combine all the ingredients, except the berries, in a food processor and process until smooth. Spoon half the mixture into the prepared tin, then sprinkle the berries over the top and lightly swirl through. Finish with the remaining ricotta mixture and smooth the top of the cake.

3   Bake for 30–35 minutes or until just set. Turn the oven off and allow the cake to cool in the oven for 1 hour. Remove and cool completely before serving. If you're not eating the cake as soon as it has cooled, refrigerate until ready to serve. Garnish with extra berries and lightly dust with icing sugar if you like.

TIP You can use fresh or frozen berries for this cake. The best fresh berries to use are raspberries, blueberries or blackberries. Packets of frozen mixed berries from the supermarket are also a good option. If you choose to use frozen berries, make sure you give them time to thaw before incorporating them into the mix, and drain them well.

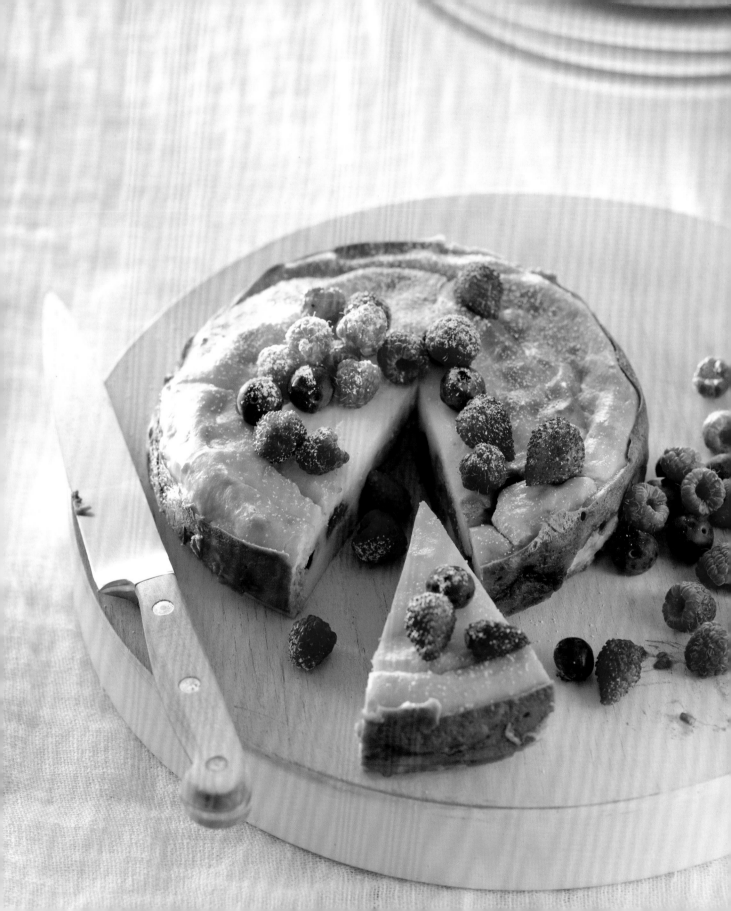

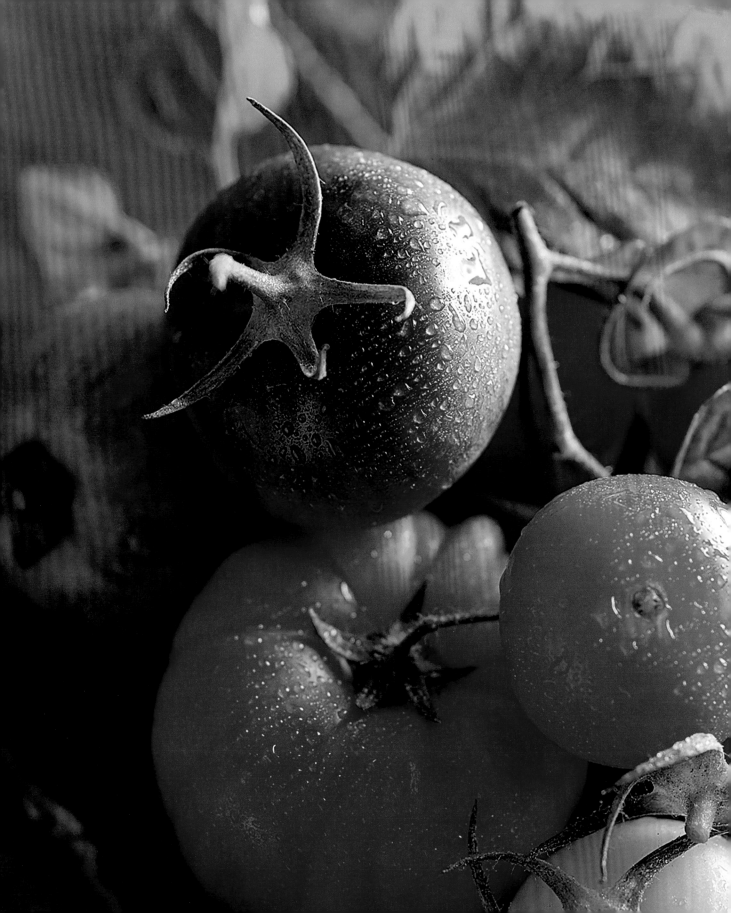

index

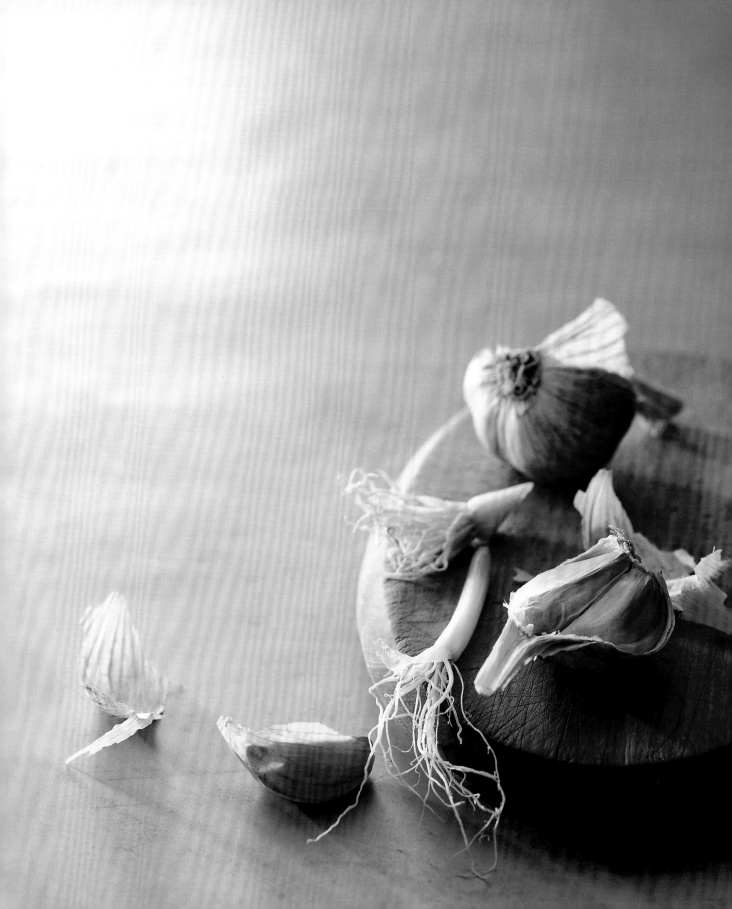

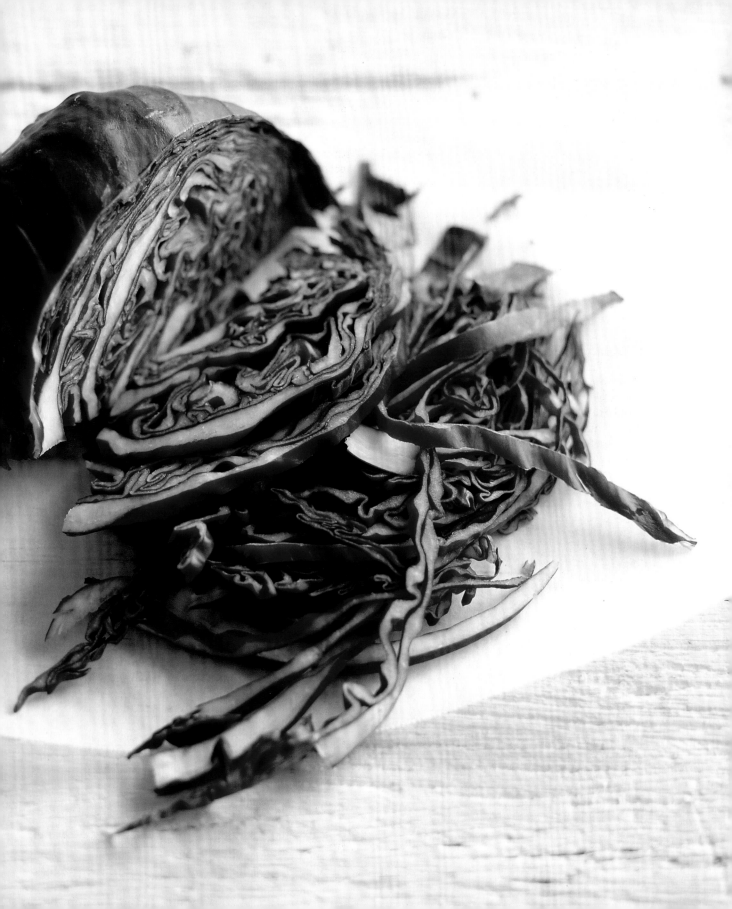

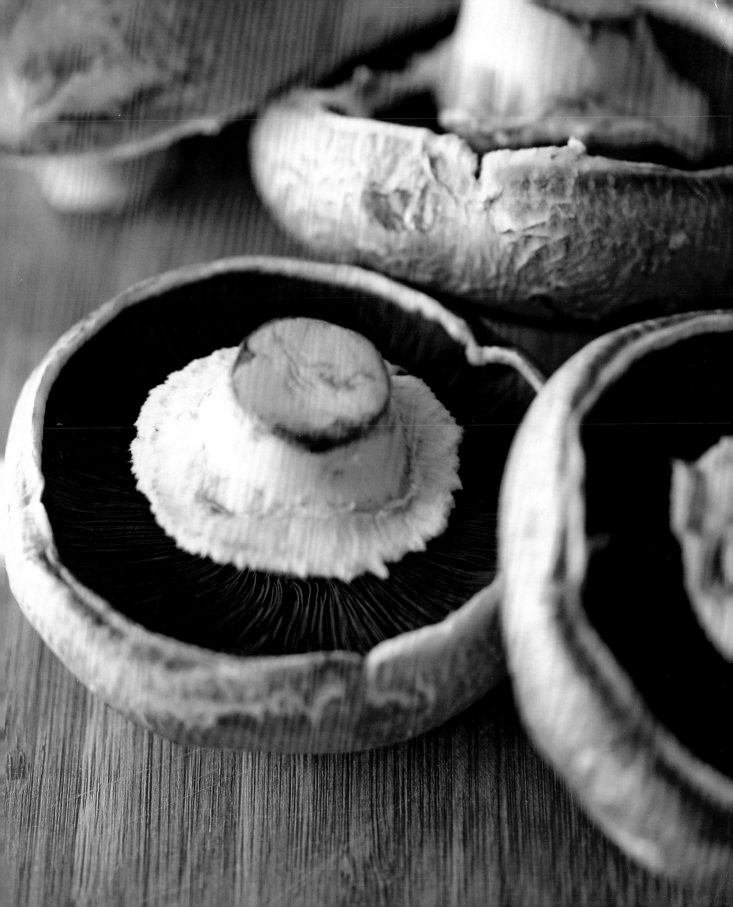

Penguin

UK | USA | Canada | Ireland | Australia
India | New Zealand | South Africa | China

Penguin Books is part of the Penguin Random House group
of companies whose addresses can be found at
global.penguinrandomhouse.com.

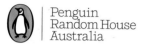
Penguin
Random House
Australia

First published by Penguin Group (Australia), 2015

10 9 8 7 6 5 4 3 2 1

Design by Hannah Schubert © Penguin Group (Australia)
Typeset in Myriad Pro 10/13.5pt by Post Pre-press Group,
Brisbane, Queensland
Colour separation by Splitting Image Colour Studio,
Clayton, Victoria
Printed and bound in China by C & C Offset Printing Co Ltd

National Library of Australia
Cataloguing-in-Publication data:

Noakes, Manny 1953- author.
The CSIRO total wellbeing diet: complete recipe collection/
Professor Manny Noakes.
9780670078530 (pbk)
Includes index.
Reducing diets--Recipes.
Weight loss.
Nutrition.
Other Creators/Contributors: CSIRO.

613.25

penguin.com.au

Photography credits:

Pages 6, 10, 39, 63, 73, 81, 91, 92, 100, 106, 109, 111, 119, 129,
133, 143, 145, 155, 160, 163, 175, 182, 179, 181, 207, 215, 231,
237, 246, 253, 257, 261, 265, 275, 276, 315, 281, 293, 312, 325,
326, 328, 335, 336, 343, 353, 359, 363, 371, 373, 377, 391, 393,
405, 407, 409, 410, 413, 419, 437, 451, 454, 451, 463, 501, 542,
544, 555, 561, 562, 577, 581, 588, 591, 595, 597, 598, 605, 617,
front cover middle, right and back cover – top left, top right,
bottom right © Alan Benson

Pages ii, iv, vi, 5, 9, 26, 29, 31, 32, 36, 57, 68, 81, 98, 103, 112, 117,
120, 123, 124, 133, 140, 143, 151, 160, 171, 182, 189, 191, 201,
205, 207, 216, 221, 223, 234, 237, 254, 267, 281, 283, 285, 289,
293, 299, 301, 304, 307, 312, 323, 333, 341, 347, 362, 365, 381,
396, 443, 457, 464, 473, 477, 480, 483, 489, 489, 499, 501, 505,
511, 517, 521, 522, 527, 538, 547, 548, 553, 573, 581, 595, 610,
front cover left and back cover – top middle, bottom left and
bottom middle © Chris Chen

Pages 20, 23, 40, 53, 82, 101, 135, 136, 146, 159, 167, 168, 194,
202, 209, 210, 222, 238, 241, 249, 270, 294, 309, 320, 356, 367,
388, 399, 402, 422, 427, 434, 440, 449, 454, 459, 469, 494, 508,
535, 567, 574 © Petrina Tinslay

Page 17, 35, 45, 47, 58, 65, 71, 77, 84, 87, 88, 97, 153, 156, 176,
187, 197, 227, 245, 262, 317, 338, 348, 351, 374, 382, 385, 417,
431, 445, 491, 514, 559, 568, 583, 587 © Ian Wallace

Page 164 © Shutterstock